Inequalities in health
The evidence

Edited by David Gordon, Mary Shaw, Daniel Dorling
and George Dav*

**The evidence presen____ ___ __ ___ independent inquiry into
Inequalities in Health, chaired by Sir Donald Acheson**

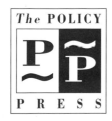

The POLICY
P~P
PRESS

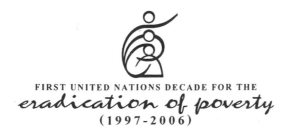

FIRST UNITED NATIONS DECADE FOR THE
eradication of poverty
(1997-2006)

First published in Great Britain in 1999 by

The Policy Press
University of Bristol
34 Tyndall's Park Road
Bristol BS8 1PY
UK

Tel   +44 (0)117 954 6800
Fax   +44 (0)117 973 7308
E-mail tpp@bristol.ac.uk
http://www.bristol.ac.uk/Publications/TPP

ISBN 1 86134 174 1

Studies in poverty, inequality and social exclusion
Series Editor: David Gordon

Poverty, inequality and social exclusion remain the most fundamental problems that humanity faces in the 21st century. This exciting new series, published in association with the Townsend Centre for International Poverty Research at the University of Bristol, aims to make cutting-edge poverty related research more widely available.

The series will:
• investigate the causes of poverty and inequality;
• enable a greater understanding of the ways in which poverty is measured using analysis of the costs and consequences of poverty for individuals, groups, families, communities and societies;
• examine theoretical and conceptual issues of definition and perceptions of poverty, inequality and social exclusion;
• encourage the production and adoption of practical policies and solutions to alleviate world poverty.

David Gordon is Head of the Centre for the Study of Social Exclusion and Social Justice, School for Policy Studies, **Mary Shaw** is a Research Fellow at the School of Geographical Sciences, **Daniel Dorling** is a Lecturer in Geography at the School of Geographical Sciences and **George Davey Smith** is Head of Epidemiology, Department of Social Medicine, all based at the University of Bristol.

Cover design by Qube Design Associates, Bristol
Photograph supplied by kind permission of www.johnbirdsall.co.uk
Printed in Great Britain by Hobbs the Printers Ltd, Southampton

Contents

Acknowledgements

We would like to thank Sir Donald Acheson, Margaret Whitehead, Hilary Graham, Ray Earwicker, Catherine Law and Yoav Ben Shlomo for their help and advice.

We would like to thank Liz Humphries and Helen Anderson for their assistance.

We would also like to thank Dawn Pudney and David Worth for their Herculean efforts in producing this book.

Introduction

This book consists of the 19 input papers that were submitted as evidence to the Independent Inquiry into Inequalities in Health, chaired by Sir Donald Acheson. It also includes a chapter by Professor Peter Townsend that discusses the crucially important issue of the cost of reducing inequalities in health (see pp xiv-xxi).

The report of the Independent Inquiry into Inequalities in Health, which was published in November 1998, is potentially one of the most significant public health reports written in the 20th century. Unfortunately, the Independent Inquiry was only able to publish a summary of the evidence that it based its 39 recommendations upon. This book makes available to both professionals and the general public the bulk of the evidence considered by the Inquiry. It is therefore an essential complement to the main report of the Independent Inquiry into Inequalities in Health, which can be obtained either through The Stationery Office or at http://www.official-documents.co.uk/document/doh/ih/.

The Independent Inquiry was commissioned by the Labour government in July 1997, just two months after their landslide General Election victory, and was carried out over a 12-month period. The task of the Inquiry was to review the evidence on inequalities in health in England and to identify areas for policy development likely to reduce these inequalities. The Inquiry's terms of reference were:

- To moderate a Department of Health review of the latest available information on inequalities in health, using data from the Office for National Statistics, the Department of Health and

elsewhere. The data review would summarise the evidence of inequalities of health and expectation of life in England and identify trends.
- In the light of that evidence, to conduct – within the broad framework of the government's overall financial strategy – an independent review to identify priority areas for future policy development, which scientific and expert evidence indicate are likely to offer opportunities for the government to develop beneficial, cost-effective and affordable interventions to reduce health inequalities.
- The review was to be reported to the Secretary of State for Health and this report was to be published. Its conclusions, based on evidence, would contribute to the development of a new strategy for health.

The purpose of the Independent Inquiry was essentially the same as that of the Black Committee on Inequalities in Health that had been commissioned by the previous Labour government at the end of the 1970s (DHSS, 1980; Townsend and Davidson, 1988). The Black Committee's Report was not published until 1980 and was met with hostility by the then Conservative government led by Margaret Thatcher. There was no official press release or conference for the report, only 260 copies were produced and government Ministers dismissed the Report's recommendations as unrealistic and too expensive to implement. Despite this hostility, the Black Report was hugely influential, both in Britain and internationally (Davey-Smith et al, 1990).

The Black Committee argued that there was overwhelming evidence that poverty and inequality in material well-being underlie inequalities in health:

While the Health care service can play a significant part in reducing inequalities in health, measures to reduce differences in material standards of living at work, in the home and in everyday social and community life are of even greater importance.

Their key policy recommendation to reduce inequalities in health was:

Above all, we consider that the abolition of child poverty should be adopted as a national goal for the 1980s. (DHSS, 1980)

After reviewing the huge mass of evidence that has been published since the Black Report, the Independent inquiry into Inequalities in Health came to very similar conclusions. The three key recommendations repeatedly emphasised in the independent Inquiry's report are:

There are three areas which we regard as crucial:

- all policies likely to have an impact on health should be evaluated in terms of their impact on health inequalities;
- a high priority should be given to the health of families with children;
- further steps should be taken to reduce income inequalities and improve the living standards of poor households. (DoH, 1998)

In total, the Independent Inquiry into Inequalities in Health made 39 policy recommendations which are listed at the end of this chapter. The publication of the input papers in this book will allow readers to consider how and to what extent the recommendations of the commissioned experts were taken on board in the advice that was presented to government.

One of the criticisms that has been made of the Independent Inquiry's report was that their 39 policy recommendations were not costed (Davey Smith et al, 1998). This means that it is impossible to weigh up the costs, benefits and opportunity costs of implementation or inaction. It is thus also impossible to judge the extent to which the recommendations are 'cost-effective'. The issue of costing is addressed in an additional chapter we have commissioned for this book (see pp xiv-xxi), written by Peter Townsend, one of the authors of the original Black Report.

The government's response

The report of the Independent Inquiry into Inequalities in Health was met with a much more welcoming response by the government than that given to the Black Committee's Report. The Minister of Health, Frank Dobson, stated that:

The whole Government, led from the top by the Prime Minister, is committed to the greatest ever reduction in health inequalities. (Dobson and DoH, 1998)

In July 1999, eight months after the publication from the Independent Inquiry into Inequalities in Health, the government responded with a White paper on Public Health (*Saving lives: Our healthier nation*, DoH, 1999a) and an action report on *Reducing health inequalities* (DoH, 1999b). Somewhat surprisingly, the White Paper was made widely available via The Stationery Office shops around the country but the action report was only available from the Department of Health which guaranteed it a much more restricted circulation. (It is available at http://www.doh.gov.uk/ohn/inequalities.htm.)

The action report represents a comprehensive response to the 39 recommendations made by the Independent Inquiry into Inequalities in Health. The government has taken the Acheson Report seriously and responded in some detail. The action report details plans to cut the number of people sleeping rough by two thirds by 2002 and to halve the rate of conception among under-18s in England by 2010. Officials are discussing with the food industry the possibility of reducing salt levels in processed food and the Social Exclusion Unit is examining ways of improving shopping access in deprived areas. A week's course of nicotine replacement therapy will be provided free to the poorest smokers. Government-funded researchers are investigating why fewer poor mothers breast feed and infant feeding advisers have been appointed to increase the prevalence of breast feeding. Resource packs will be provided to schools to increase awareness of healthy eating under the healthy schools initiative, school breakfast clubs are to be encouraged and research is to be conducted to establish practical ways of encouraging children to eat fruit and vegetables. National nutritional standards for school meals will be re-established at some point in the future (DoH, 1999a, 199b; Burke, 1999).

However, while these are all laudable plans, they are very unlikely to have a major impact on health inequalities at a national level.

The White Paper on Public Health (DoH, 1999a) set clear and unambiguous targets for improving "the health of the population as a whole". Targets to be achieved by the year 2010 included reducing the death rate in people aged under 75 years from coronary heart disease by at least two fifths; from cancers by a fifth; from accidents by a tenth; and from mental illness by a fifth. The total number of deaths from these causes is to be reduced by 300,000 over the next 10 years. A budget of £96m has been allocated to these programmes through a public health development fund over the next three years.

However, none of this £96m has been allocated to reducing health inequalities, nor did the White Paper set any national targets for reducing health inequalities. Instead of national targets with clear and unambiguous goals on inequalities in health, the White Paper requires health authorities to set their own local targets. These local targets for reducing the health divide are to be met from the health authorities' existing funds. Despite the fact that the White Paper claims that its goals are "consistent with the World Health Organisations (Europe)'s new programme for the 21st century *Health 21*", to which the United Kingdom is a signatory, the government was clearly unwilling to include Target 2 of the *Health 21* strategy in the White Paper which states: "By the year 2020, the health gap between socio-economic groups within countries should be reduced by at least one quarter in all member states, by substantially improving the level of health of disadvantaged groups" (WHO Europe, 1999). This is not even a particularly ambitious target on reducing health inequalities but it is clearly a more ambitious plan than the government is currently prepared to commit itself to.

Child poverty

Despite this initially somewhat disappointing response to the recommendations made by the Independent Inquiry into Inequalities in Health, the new Labour government has firmly committed itself to implementing their key recommendation of ending child poverty.

In his Beveridge Lecture on 18th March 1999, Tony Blair committed the government to "lifting 700,000 children out of poverty by the end of the Parliament" and "to end child poverty for ever" over the next 20 years (Blair, 1999; Walker, 1999). He argued that "We have made children our top priority because as the Chancellor memorably said in his Budget 'they are 20% of the population but they are 100% of the future'".

Although it is not yet clear how the government intends to meet this commitment to end child poverty 'for ever', if it does succeed, then the scientific evidence presented in this book shows that it will also have a major long-term impact on reducing inequalities in health. The report of the Independent Inquiry into Inequalities in Health may then be regarded as one of the most important scientific reports of the 20th century and the input papers published in this book will have been hugely influential. However, if the new Labour government does not succeed then these reports may be consigned to just a footnote in history. Only time will tell which is to be their ultimate fate.

Finally, we hope that by making these input papers on inequalities in health available to the interested reader we will further fuel debate on health inequalities, and most crucially, help drive their reduction.

List of Recommendations made by the Independent Inquiry into Inequalities in Health

General recommendations

1   We **recommend** that as part of health impact assessment, all policies likely to have a direct or indirect effect on health should be evaluated in terms of their impact on health inequalities, and should be formulated in such a way that by favouring the less well off they will, wherever possible, reduce such inequalities.

1.1   We recommend establishing mechanisms to monitor inequalities in health and to evaluate the effectiveness of measures taken to reduce them.

1.2   We recommend a review of data needs to

improve the capacity to monitor inequalities in health and their determinants at a national and local level.

2   We **recommend** a high priority is given to policies aimed at improving health and reducing health inequalities in women of childbearing age, expectant mothers and young children.

Poverty, income, tax and benefits

3   We **recommend** policies which will further reduce income inequalities, and improve the living standards of households in receipt of social security benefits. Specifically:

3.1   We recommend further reductions in poverty in women of childbearing age, expectant mothers, young children and older people should be made by increasing benefits in cash or in kind to them.

3.2   We recommend uprating of benefits and pensions according to principles which protect and, where possible, improve the standard of living of those who depend on them and which narrow the gap between their standard of living and average living standards.

3.3   We recommend measures to increase the uptake of benefits in entitled groups.

Education

4   We **recommend** the provision of additional resources for schools serving children from less well off groups to enhance their educational achievement. The Revenue Support Grant formula and other funding mechanisms should be more strongly weighted to reflect need and socio-economic disadvantage.

5   We **recommend** the further development of high quality pre-school education so that it meets, in particular, the needs of disadvantaged families. We also recommend that the benefits of pre-school education to disadvantaged families are evaluated and, if necessary, additional resources are made available to support further development.

6   We **recommend** the further development of 'health-promoting schools', initially focused on, but not limited to, disadvantaged communities.

7   We **recommend** further measures to improve the nutrition provided at school, including: the promotion of school food policies; the development of budgeting and cooking skills; the preservation of free school meals entitlement; the provision of free school fruit; and the restriction of less healthy food.

Employment

8   We **recommend** policies which improve the opportunities for work and which ameliorate the health consequences of unemployment. Specifically:

8.1   We recommend further steps to increase employment opportunities.

8.2   We recommend further investment in high quality training for young and long-term unemployed people.

9   We **recommend** policies to improve the quality of jobs, and reduce psychosocial work hazards. Specifically:

9.1   We recommend employers, unions and relevant agencies take further measures to improve health through good management practices which lead to an increased level of control, variety and appropriate use of skills in the workforce.

9.2   We recommend assessing the impact of employment policies on health and inequalities in health (see also Recommendation 1).

Housing and environment

10   We **recommend** policies which improve the availability of social housing for the less well off within a framework of environmental improvement, planning and design which takes into account social networks, and access to goods and services.

11   We **recommend** policies which improve housing provision and access to healthcare for both officially and unofficially homeless people.

12   We **recommend** policies which aim to improve the quality of housing. Specifically:

12.1   We recommend policies to improve insulation and heating systems in new and existing buildings in order to reduce further the prevalence of fuel poverty.

12.2 We recommend amending housing and licensing conditions and housing regulations on space and amenity to reduce accidents in the home, including measures to promote the installation of smoke detectors in existing homes.

13 We **recommend** the development of policies to reduce the fear of crime and violence, and to create a safe environment for people to live in.

Mobility, transport and pollution

14 We **recommend** the further development of a high quality public transport system which is integrated with other forms of transport and is affordable to the user.

15 We **recommend** further measures to encourage walking and cycling as forms of transport and to ensure the safe separation of pedestrians and cyclists from motor vehicles.

16 We **recommend** further steps to reduce the usage of motor cars to cut the mortality and morbidity associated with motor vehicle emissions.

17 We **recommend** further measures to reduce traffic speed, by environmental design and modification of roads, lower speed limits in built up areas, and stricter enforcement of speed limits.

18 We **recommend** concessionary fares should be available to pensioners and disadvantaged groups throughout the country, and that local schemes should emulate high quality schemes, such as those of London and the West Midlands.

Nutrition and the Common Agricultural Policy

19 We **recommend** a comprehensive review of the Common Agricultural Policy (CAP)'s impact on health and inequalities in health.

19.1 We recommend strengthening the CAP Surplus Food Scheme to improve the nutritional position of the less well off.

20 We **recommend** policies which will increase the availability and accessibility of foodstuffs to supply an adequate and affordable diet. Specifically:

20.1 We recommend the further development of policies which will ensure adequate retail provision of food to those who are disadvantaged.

20.2 We recommend policies which reduce the sodium content of processed foods, particularly bread and cereals, and which do not incur additional cost to the consumer.

Mothers, children and families

21 We **recommend** policies which reduce poverty in families with children by promoting the material support of parents; by removing barriers to work for parents who wish to combine work with parenting; and by enabling those who wish to devote full-time to parenting to do so. Specifically:

21.1 We recommend an integrated policy for the provision of affordable, high quality day care and pre-school education with extra resources for disadvantaged communities (see also Recommendation 5).

22 We **recommend** policies which improve the health and nutrition of women of childbearing age and their children with priority given to the elimination of food poverty and the prevention and reduction of obesity. Specifically:

22.1 We recommend policies which increase the prevalence of breastfeeding.

22.2 We recommend the fluoridation of the water supply.

22.3 We recommend the further development of programmes to help women to give up smoking before or during pregnancy, and which are focused on the less well off.

23 We **recommend** policies that promote the social and emotional support for parents and children. Specifically:

23.1 We recommend the further development of the role and capacity of health visitors to provide social and emotional support to expectant parents, and parents with young children.

23.2 We recommend local authorities identify and address the physical and psychological health needs of looked-after children.

Young people and adults of working age

24 We **recommend** measures to prevent suicide among young people, especially among young men and seriously mentally ill people.

25 We **recommend** policies which promote sexual health in young people and reduce unwanted teenage pregnancy, including access to appropriate contraceptive services.

26 We **recommend** policies which promote the adoption of healthier life-styles, particularly in respect of factors which show a strong social gradient in prevalence or consequences. Specifically:

26.1 We recommend policies which promote moderate intensity exercise including: further provision of cycling and walking routes to school, and other environmental modifications aimed at the safe separation of pedestrians and cyclists from motor vehicles; and safer opportunities for leisure.

26.2 We recommend policies to reduce tobacco smoking including: restricting smoking in public places; abolishing tobacco advertising and promotion; and community, mass media and educational initiatives.

26.3 We recommend increases in the real price of tobacco to discourage young people from becoming habitual smokers and to encourage adult smokers to quit. These increases should be introduced in tandem with policies to improve the living standards of low-income households and polices to help smokers in these households become and remain ex-smokers.

26.4 We recommend making nicotine replacement therapy available on prescription.

26.5 We recommend policies which reduce alcohol-related ill-health, accidents and violence, including measures which at least maintain the real cost of alcohol.

Older people

27 We **recommend** policies which will promote the material well-being of older people.

28 We **recommend** the quality of homes in which older people live be improved.

29 We **recommend** policies which will promote the maintenance of mobility, independence, and social contacts.

30 We **recommend** the further development of health and social services for older people, so that these services are accessible and distributed according to need.

Ethnicity

31 We **recommend** that the needs of minority ethnic groups are specifically considered in the development and implementation of policies aimed at reducing socio-economic inequalities.

32 We **recommend** the further development of services which are sensitive to the needs of minority ethnic people and which promote greater awareness of their health risks.

33 We **recommend** the needs of minority ethnic groups are specifically considered in needs assessment, resource allocation, healthcare planning and provision.

Gender

34 We **recommend** policies which reduce the excess mortality from accidents and suicide in young men (see also Recommendation 24).

35 We **recommend** policies which reduce psychosocial ill-health in young women in disadvantaged circumstances, particularly those caring for young children.

36 We **recommend** policies which reduce disability and ameliorate its consequences in older women, particularly those living alone.

The National Health Service

37 We **recommend** that providing equitable access to effective care in relation to need should be a governing principle of all policies in the NHS. Priority should be given to the achievement of equity in the planning, implementation and delivery of services at every level of the NHS. Specifically:

37.1 We recommend extending the focus of clinical governance to give equal prominence to equity of access to effective healthcare.

37.2 We recommend extending the remit of the National Institute for Clinical Excellence to include equity of access to effective healthcare.

37.3 We recommend developing the National Service Frameworks to address inequities in access to effective primary care.

37.4 We recommend that performance management in relation to the national performance management framework is focused on achieving more equitable access, provision and targeting of effective services in relation to need in both primary and hospital sectors.

37.5 We recommend that the Department of Health and NHS Executive set out their responsibilities for furthering the principle of equity of access to effective health and social care, and that health authorities, working with Primary Care Groups and providers on local clinical governance, agree priorities and objectives for reducing inequities in access to effective care. These should form part of the Health Improvement Programme.

38 We **recommend** giving priority to the achievement of a more equitable allocation of NHS resources. This will require adjustments to the ways in which resources are allocated and the speed with which resource allocation targets are met. Specifically:

38.1 We recommend reviewing the 'pace of change' policy to enable health authorities that are furthest from their capitation targets to move more quickly to their actual target.

38.2 We recommend extending the principle of needs-based weighting to non-cash limited General Medical Services (GMS) resources. The size and effectiveness of deprivation payments in meeting the needs and improving the health outcomes among the most disadvantaged populations, including ethnic minorities, should be assessed.

38.3 We recommend reviewing the size and effectiveness of the Hospital and Community Health Service (HCHS) formula and deprivation payments in influencing the healthcare outcomes of the most disadvantaged populations, and to consider alternative methods of focusing resources for health promotion and public healthcare to reduce health inequalities.

38.4 We recommend establishing a review of the relationship of private practice to the NHS with particular reference to access to effective treatments, resource allocation and availability of staff.

39 We **recommend** Directors of Public Health, working on behalf of health and local authorities, produce an equity profile for the population they serve, and undertake a triennial audit of progress towards achieving objectives to reduce inequalities in health.

39.1 We recommend there should be a duty of partnership between the NHS Executive and regional government to ensure that effective local partnerships are established between health, local authorities and other agencies and that joint programmes to address health inequalities are in place and monitored.

References

Blair, T. (1999) Beveridge Lecture at Toynbee Hall London on 18 March, London: Cabinet Office.

Burke, K. (1999) 'Doctors fear that inequalities are slipping down the agenda', *British Medical Journal*, vol 319, p 144.

Davey Smith, G., Bartley, M. and Blane, D. (1990) 'The Black Report on socioeconomic inequalities in health 10 years on', *British Medical Journal*, vol 310, pp 373-7.

Davey Smith, G., Morris, J.N. and Shaw, M. (1998) 'The independent inquiry into inequalities in health', *British Medical Journal*, vol 317, pp 1465-6.

DHSS (Department of Health and Social Security) (1980) *Inequalities in health: Report of a working group*, London: DHSS (Black Report).

DoH (Department of Health) (1998) *Independent Inquiry into Inequalities in Health*, London: The Stationery Office (also http://www.official-documents.co.uk/document/doh/ih/).

DoH (1999a) *Saving lives: Our healthier nation*, Cmd 4386, London: The Stationery Office (also http://www.offical-documents.co.uk/documents/cm43/4368/4368.htm).

DoH (1999b) *Reducing health inequalities: An action report*, London: DoH (also http://www.doh.gov.uk/ohn/inequalities.htm).

Dobson, F. and DoH (1998) 'Government committed to greatest ever reduction in health inequalities' says Dobson, Acheson Report into Inequalities in Health welcomed, DoH Press Release 98/0547, 26 November.

Townsend, P. and Davidson, N. (1988) *Inequalities in health: The Black Report* (2nd edn), London: Penguin Books.

Walker, R. (ed) (1999) *Ending child poverty: Popular welfare for the 21st century*, Bristol: The Policy Press.

WHO (World Health Organisation) Europe (1999) *Health 21 – Health for all in the 21st century*, Copenhagen: WHO Regional Office for Europe.

A structural plan needed to reduce inequalities of health

Peter Townsend

The Black Report of 1977-80 (Black Report, 1980; and Townsend and Davidson, 1982) showed that inequalities in health had been widening since the 1950s, that this trend was principally related to inequalities of material deprivation, and that a programme across departments of higher benefits and better distribution of income, as well as action on housing and services, was required. The Report was rejected by the Conservative government at the time of its publication, especially on grounds of cost, and yet it continued to exert influence on research and the structural action necessary to achieve better population health. For example, a report for the Health Education Council in 1987 listed hundreds more papers with new research evidence (Whitehead, 1987; and see Townsend et al, 1992).

After winning the election of May 1997 the Labour government set up a scientific advisory group under the chairmanship of Sir Donald Acheson to review further evidence, and this reported in December 1998 (Acheson Report, 1998).

The central thrust of the recommendations reflected those put forward in the Black Report. This is significant and should be explained. The Report demonstrated the heightened problem created by dramatically widening living standards since the late 1970s. There were 39 principal recommendations. The all-important one is No 3, which specifies the need for policies to "reduce income inequalities and improve the living standards of households in receipt of social security benefits" (Acheson Report, 1998, p 36). Benefits in cash or in kind had to be increased to reduce "poverty in women of childbearing age, expectant mothers, young children and older people." That also applied to pensioners. No 3 is the core recommendation because there are nine supporting recommendations (nos 8, 13, 20, 21, 22, 27, 31, 35, 36) that are explicitly linked to it to reinforce the call for integrated action on unemployment, ethnicity, elderly people and disability, as well as generally on families with children, to bring about increases in levels of benefit and real living standards. Moreover, another 10 of the Acheson recommendations (nos 5, 7, 11, 12, 16, 17, 18, 19, 28, 30) are concerned with meeting material needs in schools, housing, the environment, transport, and in relation to diet.

The Report is extensive. Some commentators fastened onto particular recommendations which, though important, are not central. Because there seemed to be some danger of the central thrust being missed, the original members of the 1977-80 Black Committee issued a report in March 1999 calling for a government plan to phase in better benefits for health (Black et al, 1999).

In July 1999 the government issued an action plan on inequalities of health (DoH, 1999a). Unfortunately this was published along with a White Paper (DoH, 1999b, Cm 4386) putting forward a series of measures "focussed on the main killers – cancer, coronary heart disease and stroke, accidents and mental illness" and giving most importance to healthcare and preventive healthcare policies. As a result, the action report on inequalities, and especially the cursory treatment of income distribution and the absence of comment on benefit levels, was not widely reported. Both reports were issued by the Department of Health.

The White Paper *Saving lives: Our healthier nation* makes almost no mention of the growing inequality of income and of measures to boost the inadequate incomes of the poor, other than a reference to the minimum wage and to the Working Families Tax Credit and the Childcare Tax Credit (DoH, 1999b, Cm 4386, p 45). The government's initiatives on cancer, heart disease, accidents and mental illness are welcome, as is its acceptance that "while the roots of health inequality run deep, we refuse to accept such inequality as inevitable" (p 44). But the key message about the substantial structural action required to turn round the growing divisions in society, especially by addressing the inadequacy of many current social security benefits, is not raised or discussed in that report.

The 1999 action report on inequalities of health

Does the action report on 'reducing health inequalities' from the DoH take up this missing theme? It describes progress in addressing all 39 recommendations. On the key recommendation, No 3, attention is called to the government's commitment to tackle worklessness, including the New Deals for employment, tax and benefit reforms to "make sure that work pays, reform of the employer's contribution to help remove barriers to employment, and policies to improve skills through education and training." The report continues, "But we recognise the need to provide security for those who cannot work" (DoH, 1999a, p 6). There is no discussion of the exact meaning of security, or of minimally adequate standards of income for families with children, lone parents, disabled people and pensioners. The measures are listed in the box below.

Families with children

- An increase of £4.70 a week from October 1999 in the child premium in the income related benefits (IRBs) for children under 11.

- Additional increases from April 2000 in the family and child premiums in the IRBs to match increases in Child Benefit.

Disabled people

- *Extra help for young people disabled early in life:* reform of Severe Disablement Allowance (SDA) to give people who are disabled and claim benefit before the age of 20 access to a higher rate of benefit than they would get from SDA and Income Support. The age limit is extended to 25 for those in higher education and vocational training whose course began before they were 20.

- *Extra help for severely disabled people with the greatest care needs and the lowest incomes:* Disability Income Guarantee will provide extra help in IRBs for people who receive the highest rate care component of Disabled Living Allowance (DLA).

Pensioners

- A new Minimum Income Guarantee (at least £75 a week for single pensioners; £116.60 for a couple). This will make the poorest pensioners at least £160 a year better off in real terms from April 1999.

- The Minimum Income Guarantee will be uprated relative to earnings in April 2000 so that single pensioners will be an estimated £250 a year better off than in April 1998.

- A fivefold increase in the winter fuel payment and a new, more generous, Home Efficiency Scheme.

There is no doubt of the government giving greater priority than the preceding governments of the 1980s and 1990s to inequalities in health. Equally there is no doubt that a range of measures, external to healthcare policy and not only internal to such policy are now in play. This is welcome. But serious questions remain: (i) the scale of action so far, (ii) effective management of the distribution of earnings and of disposable income, (iii) adequacy of income and of living standards generally of many millions of people with no prospect of having paid employment, and (iv) urgent documentation of structural trends, as well as the effects of major policies, from year to year.

How must this be demonstrated in the best summary form, so that pressure from those concerned about health can be placed on those responsible in government? The first step is to deal with scale and range of possible policies by referring back to the original Black Report. What were its priorities – derived from its attempt to illustrate what policies followed from its demonstration of growing inequalities of health?

Some of the recommendations made at the time, either on pragmatic grounds or derived from the principles of equity, later underpinned in the 1998 Acheson Report, gained credibility from the continuing stream of research evidence. The four members of the Black Research Working Group said then: "We have tried to confine ourselves to matters which are practicable now, in political, economic and administrative terms, and which will, nonetheless, properly maintained, exert a long-term structural effect.... We have continued to feel it right to give priority to young children and mothers, disabled people and measures concerned with prevention.... Above all the *abolition of child poverty should be adopted as a national goal...*" (Black Report, 1980, p 195; author's emphasis).

Following the new evidence reviewed by Sir Donald Acheson and his colleagues, it would be possible to reach a scientific and popular consensus about the necessary combination of measures required in the first stages of tackling the problem. Reproduced below in Table 1 are the principal recommendations made in the Black Report, with estimates of cost made at the time by the previous government, updated by the Department of Health to 1998. While recognising that exact current costs would depend on changed sources of potential revenue as well as changes in the population affected, this may be a useful basis on which agreement about the package of measures required to implement the Acheson Report might be reached.

Table 1: Annual cost of meeting the principal recommendations of the Black Report on Inequalities of Health, as estimated in 1982 and in 1996 prices

No	Recommendation	£m (1982 prices) (1)	£m (1996 prices) (2)
10	Free milk for under-5s	300	700
12	Expansion of day care for under-5s	550*	1,250
23	Special programmes in 10 areas with highest mortality	65	150
24	Child Benefit increased to 5.5% of average gross male earnings	950+	2,200
25	Age-related Child Benefit	1,275‡	2,900
26	Maternity grant increased to £100	60	140
27	Infant care allowance	440§	1,000
28	Free school meals for all children (net extra cost)	640μ	1,460
29	Comprehensive disablement allowance	1,175¶	2,700
	Total annual cost	5,455	12,500
	Total cost (as % GDP)	2.2	1.7
	Total cost (as % social security)	13	11.7

Notes: *An initial capital cost of possibly £300-£400m would also be required.

+ Cost of raising Child Benefit to £7.57 per week.

‡ Assuming average increase of £3 per week for children aged 5-15.

§ The cost of a £5.85 per week benefit if half the 2.9 million women at home looking after children had a child under 5.

μ Assuming 70% take-up.

¶ As estimated by the Disability Alliance in 1981.

Source: (1) *Hansard* 16 December 1982, cols 242-3, reply by Kenneth Clarke MP to Gwynneth Dunwoody MP. (2) Reply by Tessa Jowell, Minister of State for Public Health, to a Parliamentary Question from Jean Corston MP, 25 November 1998

Although the cost of implementing the recommendations was not as high as it was made out to be in the Secretary of State's (Patrick Jenkins) 'Foreword' to the 1980 Report, nevertheless, then as now, affordability is a key issue. History shows that governments can introduce radical changes but that when they occur they are ordinarily built on precedents and are divided into a succession of steps. To be influential, scientific advice has to be pitched in a practicable and manageable as well as desirable form. What matters first in the year 2000 is for the government to change the direction of trends making for increased poverty and inequality. This depends on mobilising popular support for a number of principal measures, and introducing new institutions at the same time as strengthening existing ones. There exists overwhelming evidence of support, in a series of representative and reliable opinion polls, for the kind of measures listed in Table 1 (Jowell, 1991-98).

In 1980 there were in theory many alternative options available to help meet the UK's divisive problem. The Black Research Working Group recommended a combination of measures, most of which could be introduced on the basis of existing legislation, which could be shown to have a great deal of public support, and which would make a substantial and measureable initial difference to meet what was then, and is even more so now, a huge national and social problem.

At the time objections were raised about cost. Policy recommendations should routinely be costed. This was done in the case of the Black Report. As Table 1 shows, in relation to national measures of Gross Domestic Product, or even the current cost of social security, the extra resources envisaged were not unachievable. In today's terms, as the table shows, significant advances could be made with under 2% of GDP, or about a tenth of the current expenditure on social security – even if further steps need to be considered after five or ten years. The total amount is of an order illustrated by the Chancellor's decisions in 1997-98 to introduce the windfall tax (which should generate £5bn between 1997 and 2002), and to change tax allowances and National Insurance Contributions. Another indicator is the surplus of £2.5bn of contributions over payments in the National Insurance Fund in 1997-98, rising to £7bn a year in the following two years.

Policies causing divergences in standard of living

The task ahead in the early years of the new millennium is daunting but must be accepted. One problem, which has not been examined by successive governments in the last two decades, is the effect of specific past and present *policies* on trends in the inequalities of living standards and hence health. The nearest attempt to doing this was in a report for the Joseph Rowntree Foundation (Hills, 1995; and see also Hills, 1998). The biggest influences on structural trends need to be identified and explained. In Britain these policy influences must include (i) the abolition of the link between social security benefits and earnings; (ii) the restraints on the value of Child Benefit; (iii) the abolition of lone parent allowances and of the earnings-related addition to Incapacity Benefit, which allowed people disabled before pensionable age to draw early on their entitlement to the State Earnings Related Pension Scheme; and (iv) the substitution of means-tested benefits for universal social insurance and for non-contributory benefits for particular population categories like pensioners and disabled people.

What would be required to restore the UK to the much reduced range of inequality experienced 20 years ago? If the Conservative government had not re-cast and reduced social security benefits it can be estimated that the poorest 20% of the population would today have about £5bn, or 20%, more in aggregate disposable income, that the ratio between richest and poorest 20% would be reduced from about 9:1 or 10:1 to 5:1, and that poverty by European standards would have been reduced by more than a third. Instead, the UK experienced the most severe growth of social inequality and of poverty, especially child poverty, of any European country.

In the 1998 budget statement the Chancellor announced a welcome increase in the rate of Child Benefit, together with improvements in Income Support rates for children. However, the increase applies only to the eldest or only child in the family and, since the real value had fallen in previous years, primarily represents a catching-up exercise. If the Chancellor also decides to tax the Benefit, as has been suggested but for which there is little rational support (Clarke and McCrae, 1998; Dilnot, 1998;

Bradshaw, 1998; Bradshaw and Barnes, 1999: forthcoming), that may lead to the benefit being withdrawn altogether from higher earning households at a later stage, and being converted into a means-tested benefit. In 1999 the government will also replace Family Credit with Working Families Tax Credit, which is designed to increase the level of benefit as well as the numbers entitled to it. This is also a means-tested scheme, intended to raise the numbers of low-earning families receiving such a tax credit by 400,000. On the basis of written answers to Parliamentary questions (for example, *Hansard*, 28 July 1998, cols 188-90), and investigations on the minimum necessary family income, some experts have concluded after protracted research that the new credit "will not provide Low Cost Allowance level incomes to two-parent families" (Parker, 1998, p 88). On all the available evidence, means-tested benefits are poor in coverage, costly to administer, do not encourage savings, and are generally inadequate in meeting need as well as unpopular.

The scale of poverty

The problem of poverty is larger than is often represented. There are numerous independent reports (for example, Cohen et al, 1992; NCH, 1995, 1998; Kempson, 1996; Gordon and Pantazis, 1997; Bradshaw, 1998). Even narrowly drawn government statistics, for example, the annual Department of Social Security reports on *Households Below Average Income* (HBAI) (DSS, 1998) reveal a serious divergence of living standards in the 1980s and 1990s. Thus, as summarised in Table 2, the number of adults and children with incomes below the low income

standards set for 1979 has remained as high as, or even higher than, in 1979 itself. The latest HBAI report shows that there were 1.2 million children below half average 1979 household income after housing costs in 1979 but, despite a big increase in average national living standards and especially of the rich in the intervening 17 years, there were 1.3 million children below that same absolute 1979 standard in 1996-97 (DSS, 1998, p 229). If we look at the 'relative' situation in both 1979 and 1996-97 then the number of children in households with below half the average household income grew sharply from 1.2 million to 3.9 million.

The denial of even half average household living standards to so many of the nation's children is bound to stultify health and access to education, and gravely diminish the stock of national skill. The problem of two nations has been returning with a vengeance, from which escape must be found.

On latest data the problem is still growing. The latest national survey data from the Office for National Statistics shows that the poorest 20% of households (nearly 12 million people), who depend for 80% of their income on benefits, had an average disposable weekly income of only £86 a week (at 1997-98 prices) in the financial year 1994-95 and, three years later, £87. The richest 20% of households had an average of £707 in 1994-95 and advanced to £753 in 1997-98. The richest 20% had 8.2 times the income of the poorest 20% in 1994-95 and 8.6 times their income in 1997-98 (ONS, 1998, Table 8.3). At the end of the 1990s the widening of disposable income on the part of major sections of the population is still continuing.

Table 2: Number in population living below the government's two 1979 standards of low income, and below half contemporary average household income in real terms, excluding self-employed (millions)

Standard	1979	1993-94	1994-95	1995-96
Below 1979 median income of lowest decile	2.8	3.0	2.9	3.0
Below half 1979 average household income	4.5 (children 1.2m)	4.35	4.25	4.4 (children 1.3m)
Below half contemporary average household income	4.5 (children 1.2m)	11.6	12.1	12.2 (children 3.9m)

Note: The data are adjusted according to the retail prices index for the years in question. The corresponding totals, including the self-employed, are not given for these years, although they were given in earlier HBAI reports. These tended to show that the number of self-employed with incomes smaller than the two measures of low income had increased much faster than the number of employed.

Source: DSS (*Households Below Average Income* 1996, 1997, 1998, pp 226 and 229; 234 and 237; and 227, 229 and 231 respectively)

The part played by successive policies in redirecting income trends has not been picked up and examined in reports on the public health, almost as if there were no connection between government measures and dramatic changes in the structure of society. The links between the two have to be shown. Sir Donald's Report begins this task, pointing out that while average household income has grown by 40% in real terms during the last two decades, it has grown much faster among the richest in the population. "For the poorest tenth average income increased by only 10 per cent (before housing costs) or fell by 8 per cent (after them)" (Acheson Report, 1998, p 32). However, this statement is not precise and calls for clarification, and for an account of the exact contributions made to the trend in different years by particular changes in policy. Indeed, a tantalisingly brief paragraph on income distribution early in the report intended to set the socio-economic scene appears to contradict this statement. This describes increases in "median real household disposable income *before* housing costs" (author's emphasis), showing that "the bottom decile point rose by 62 per cent from £74 per week to £119 per week" (Acheson Report, 1998, p 16). But the reader finds that this covers the period 1961 to 1994 when, as the Report later admits, there was, in the 1960s and 1970s, a movement towards greater equality, followed in later years by a 'reversal' of this trend.

These two periods of recent British history have to be distinguished. What might be sponsored by government is a computerised simulation of the national distribution of income, whereby the effect on trends of different specific recent and prospective policies can be adequately described and the appropriate conclusions drawn.

Adequacy of benefit

A second problem neglected by successive governments is the adequacy of benefit. Internationally and scientifically the definition of a poverty line is becoming increasingly highlighted. A breakthrough occurred in 1995 with the agreement to issue a Declaration and Programme of Action after the World Summit on Social Development called by the UN, signed by the heads of state of 117 countries (UN, 1995). In this Declaration individual nation-states committed themselves to the preparation of

national plans to eradicate poverty, applying two standard measures of 'absolute' and 'overall' poverty. In Britain a national opinion poll carried out in late 1997 by MORI (Townsend et al, 1997) found that 20% of the population perceived themselves as living in 'absolute' poverty. People in the sample survey went on to give estimates of income need which, when aligned with the composition of households, showed that they considered that Income Support levels were generally from 25% to 50% too low. Expert statistical and scientific work on household income needs, some of it very recent, broadly confirms this scale of shortfall (for example, Parker, 1998). The combination of scientific investigation and democratically representative opinion provides forceful evidence of the severity of this national crisis.

The Acheson Group argue for policies which "increase the income of the poorest" and show how important it will be to raise benefit levels, restore the earnings link to National Insurance and other universal benefits and introduce more progressive taxation (Acheson Report, 1998, pp 32-6). The government's action report of July 1999 (DoH, 1999a) is intended to address this central recommendation but does not succeed. It remains unexamined. The plea to equalise incomes and raise different social security benefits for millions of poor people still needs to be turned into exact operational elements of a bold integrated national plan.

Social exclusion and poverty

How might an effective anti-poverty programme be related to the government's declared strategy to reduce social exclusion? In its third report to the Prime Minister in September 1998 (Cm 4045) the Social Exclusion Unit proposes a broad programme for "tackling poor neighbourhoods". A New Deal for Communities will begin in 17 districts, with more areas able to bid in later years. There will be funds to develop and implement local community-based plans covering everything from jobs and crime to health and housing. Ten Whitehall departments will be involved. Their assignments include getting more people into work, better management of neighbourhoods and housing, reducing anti-social behaviour, extending schools and youth facilities, improving access to shops, financial services and information technology and making the government work better.

The strategy is imaginative and undoubtedly obliges different departments and specialists to work together. However, some observers believe that, with pilot work going on in 17 districts, the strategy is tilted too far towards the long-term and that urgent action needs to be taken to remedy some of the worst problems concerned with poverty. There is a structural problem of the first magnitude – addressed above – which needs to be dealt with immediately. The work of the Downing Street Unit is distinct from that concerned with poverty. In its approach the Unit is interdepartmental, pump-priming and experimental, and clearly preoccupied with anti-social behaviour as well as with access to services and to jobs and other opportunities.

There is one paragraph in the command paper about social security. "Problems with the benefit system are being addressed by welfare reform, the Working Families Tax Credit, and the minimum wage.... The relationship between housing policy and housing benefit is being reviewed." Most revealingly, poor pensioners are to be helped by "boosting income support levels to provide a guaranteed minimum income", getting more pensioners to apply, and paying an annual sum towards winter fuel bills (Social Exclusion Unit, 1998, p 52). Alternative, and more promising, strategies to reduce poverty have not yet been discussed.

Conclusion

The three crucial reports dealing with inequalities of health in the UK have been described. The Black and Acheson Reports argued in favour of raising the benefit levels of poor groups, especially families with children. The Department of Health's action report on reducing health inequalities begins to address the problem, but gives insufficient signs of the scale of change required to bring about significant change. With support from authoritative recent reviews of income and of health, including those formally sponsored by many of the principal organisations acting on behalf of medicine – the Royal Colleges of General Practitioners, Nursing, and Physicians, the Faculty of Public Health Medicine, Action in International Medicine and the *British Medical Journal*

(for example, Wilkinson, 1994; Davey-Smith et al, 1997, 1998a, 1998b, 1999; Hills, 1998) the harmful effects on the distribution of income of particular policies – such as the abandonment of the link between earnings and benefits, cuts or reductions of benefits for some vulnerable groups and the flagging level of Child Benefit – have to be identified as obstacles to the reduction in inequalities of health.

What are the necessary recommendations for the government to consider? First, future proposed policies affecting income should be accompanied invariably with estimates of their effects on the structural distribution of incomes, and second, priority should be given by the government to the determination annually of what are 'adequate' levels of benefit.

Badly needed is, third, the preparation of a government report giving the minimum income and benefit needs for differently constituted families as the basis for developing a phased programme to raise benefits of impoverished groups with little likelihood of getting back into paid employment. That is the top priority. This would represent the necessary step towards implementing the recommendations of both the Black and Acheson Committees – making substantial real improvements in Child Benefit, Lone Parent Benefit, Incapacity and Disabled Living Allowance Benefits and the basic state retirement pension.

References

Acheson Report (1998) *Independent Inquiry into Inequalities in Health*, Report of the Scientific Advisory Group, Chairman, Sir Donald Acheson, London: The Stationery Office.

Black Report (1980) *Inequalities of health*, Report of a Research Working Group, Chairman, Sir Douglas Black, London: DHSS.

Black, D., Morris, J.N., Smith, C. and Townsend, P. (1999) 'Better benefits for health: plan to implement the central recommendation of the Acheson Report', *British Medical Journal*, vol 318, pp 724-7.

Bradshaw, J. (1998) 'The prevalence of child poverty in the UK: a comparative analysis', Children and Social Exclusion Conference, University of Hull.

Bradshaw, J. and Barnes, H. (1999: forthcoming) 'Relating inputs to outcomes: child poverty and family transfers in comparative perspective', in H. Emanuel (ed) *Issues in social security*, Aldershot: Ashgate.

Clarke, T. and McCrae, J. (1998) *Taxing Child Benefit*, Commentary 74, London: Institute for Fiscal Studies, December.

Cohen R., Coxall J., Craig G. and Sadiq-Sangster A.S. (1992) *Hardship in Britain: Being poor in the 1990s*, London, Child Poverty Action Group.

Davey Smith, G., Dorling, D., Gordon, D. and Shaw, M. (1998a) *The widening health gap – What are the solutions?*, Bristol: Townsend Centre for International Poverty Research, University of Bristol.

Davey Smith, G., Dorling, D., Gordon, D. and Shaw, M. (1999) 'The widening health gap: what are the solutions?', *Critical Public Health*, vol 9, no 2, pp 151-70.

Davey Smith, G., Morris, J.N. and Shaw, M. (1998b) 'The Independent Inquiry into Inequalities in Health', *British Medical Journal*, vol 317, pp 1465-6.

Davey Smith, G., Hart, C., Blane, D., Gillis, C. and Hawthorne, V. (1997) 'Lifetime socioeconomic position and mortality: prospective observational study', *British Medical Journal*, vol 314, pp 547-52.

Dilnot, A. (1998) Evidence to Social Security Committee, 16 December.

DoH (Department of Health) (1999a) *Reducing health inequalities: An action report*, London: DoH.

DoH (1999b) *Saving lives: Our healthier nation*, Cm 4386, London: The Stationery Office.

DSS (Department of Social Security) (1998) *Households Below Average Income*, London: The Stationery Office.

Gordon, D. and Pantazis, C. (eds) (1997) *Breadline Britain in the 1990s*, Aldershot: Ashgate.

Haines, A. and Smith, R. (1997) 'Working together to reduce poverty's damage: doctors fought nuclear weapons, now they can fight poverty', *British Medical Journal*, vol 3124, pp 529-30.

Hills, J. (1995) *Income and wealth, Vol 2*, York: Joseph Rowntree Foundation.

Hills J. (1998) *Income and wealth: The latest evidence*, York, Joseph Rowntree Foundation.

Jowell, R. (ed) (1991-98) *British Social Attitudes, 8th to 15th Reports*, London: CPSR.

Kempson, E. (1996) *Life on a low income*, York, Joseph Rowntree Foundation.

NCH Action for Children (1995) *Factfile '95*, Rochester: NCH Action for Children.

NCH Action for Children (1998) *Factfile '99*, Rochester: NCH Action for Children.

ONS (Office for National Statistics) (1998) *Family spending, Report of the Family Expenditure Survey*, London: The Stationery Office.

Parker, H. (ed) (1998) *Low cost but acceptable: A minimum income standard for the UK: Families with young children*, Bristol: The Policy Press.

Social Exclusion Unit (1998) *Bringing Britain together: A national strategy for neighbourhood renewal*, Cm 4045, London: The Stationery Office.

Townsend, P. and Davidson, N. (1982) *Inequalities in health: The Black Report*, Harmondsworth: Penguin Books.

Townsend, P., Davidson, N. and Whitehead, M. (1988, and 3rd edn, 1992) *Inequalities in health: The Black Report and the health divide*, Harmondsworth: Penguin Books.

Townsend, P., Gordon, D., Bradshaw, J. and Gosschalk, B. (1997) *Absolute and overall poverty in the UK in 1997: What the population themselves say: Bristol Poverty Line Survey*, Report of the Second MORI Survey, Bristol: Bristol Statistical Monitoring Unit.

UN (United Nations) (1995) *The Copenhagen Declaration and Programme of Action*, World Summit for Social Development 6-12 March, New York, NY: United Nations Department of Publications.

Whitehead, M. (1987) *The health divide: Inequalities in health in the 1980s*, London: Health Education Council.

Wilkinson, R.G. (1994) *Unfair shares: The effects of widening income differences on the welfare of the young*, Ilford: Barnardo's.

Notes on contributors

Peter Aggleton is a Professor in Education and Director of the Thomas Coram Research Unit at the Institute of Education, University of London.

Sara Arber is Professor of Sociology and Head of Department at University of Surrey, Guildford. She has written extensively on inequalities in women's health and later life. Her books include co-author of *Gender and later life* (Sage, 1991), *Connecting gender and ageing* (Open University Press, 1995) and *The myth of generational conflict* (Routledge, 1999: forthcoming).

Michaela Benzeval is a Senior Lecturer at the Department of Epidemiology and Public Health, University of London.

Richard Best is Director of the Joseph Rowntree Foundation.

David Blane is Reader in Medical Sociology at Imperial College of Science, Technology and Medicine and a member of the International Centre for Health and Society.

George Davey Smith is Professor of Clinical Epidemiology, Department of Social Medicine, University of Bristol.

Adrian Davis is a transport consultant specialising in the health impacts of road transport. Adrian is author of the 1997 British Medical Association report *Transport and health*. He has particular research interests in children's independent mobility, and intersectoral collaboration for health. He is currently a part-time Research Fellow with the Transport Studies Group at the University of Westminster.

Anna Donald is a Honorary Lecturer at the Department of Epidemiology and Public Health, University College, London.

Daniel Dorling is a Lecturer in Geography at the School of Geographical Sciences, University of Bristol.

Michael Farrell is Senior Lecturer and Consultant Psychiatrist at the National Addiction Centre and Institute of Psychiatry, London. He works part time in the Policy Division of Public Health at the Department of Health and is a member of the Expert Committee on Drug Dependence, World Health Organisation. He is Assistant Editor for *Addiction*.

Eva Garmarnikow is a Lecturer in Human Rights and Education in the Policy Studies Group at the Institute of Education, University of London.

Sir David Goldberg was until recently Director of Research and Development at the Institute of Psychiatry, King's College, London. He has conducted research into common mental disorders in the community, and his interests include medical education, rehabilitation for patients with schizophrenia and health economics.

David Gordon is Head of the Centre for the Study of Social Exclusion and Social Justice, School for Policy Studies, University of Bristol.

Melvyn Hillsdon is a Lecturer in the Health Promotion Research Unit based at the London School of Hygiene and Tropical Medicine.

Bobbie Jacobson is Director of Public Health at the East London and The City Health Authority.

Martin Jarvis is a Principal Scientist with the Imperial Cancer Research Fund's Health Behaviour Unit, and Professor of Health Psychology at the Department of Epidemiology and Public Health, University College, London. He has been researching tobacco issues for over 20years, with special interests in the role of nicotine, social and family influences on smoking, smoking cessation methods and passive smoking. He is a member of the Department of Health's Scientific Committee on Tobacco and Health, and a board member of ASH.

Kay-Tee Khaw is Professor of Clinical Gerontology at the University of Cambridge School of Clinical Medicine and Fellow of Gonville and Caius College, Cambridge. Her research interests are the maintenance of health in later life and the causes and prevention of chronic diseases such as cardiovascular disease, cancer and osteoporosis with a particular focus on nutrition and other environmental factors.

Catherine Law is a Senior Research Fellow and Honorary Consultant in Public Health Medicine at the MRC Environmental Epidemiology Unit (University of Southampton).

Barbara MacGibbon was a consultant to the MRC Institute for Environment and Health. Previous experience has included a post as Senior Lecturer/Honorary Consultant in Haematology at St Thomas' Hospital and Medical School, Head of the Division of Toxicology and Environmental Protection at the Department of Health and Social Security and Medical Assistant Director at the National Radiological Protection Board. She chaired the Energy Panel of the Commission on Health and Environment, which reported in 1992.

Sally Macintyre is Director of the Social and Public Health Sciences Unit, Medical Research Council, University of Glasgow.

James Y. Nazroo is Senior Lecturer in Sociology in the Department of Epidemiology and Public Health at University College London. His work has particularly focused on ethnic inequalities in health and ethnic differences in health beliefs and behaviours. He has also carried out a range of work on gender issues.

Michael Nelson is Senior Lecturer in Nutrition in the Department of Nutrition and Dietetics at King's College London. His main interests are nutritional epidemiology, food poverty and the nutrition of children.

Mary Shaw is a Research Fellow at the School of Geographical Sciences, University of Bristol.

Aubrey Sheiham is Professor of Dental Public Health in the Department of Epidemiology and Public Health, University College London Medical School.

Stephen Sutton is currently Senior Scientist and Reader in Social/Health Psychology in the Health Behaviour Unit, University College London, and Visiting Professor of Psychology in the Department of Psychosocial Sciences, University of Bergen, Norway. His research involves the application of social-psychological models of risk perception and health behaviour to smoking uptake and cessation and to participation in screening and genetic testing programmes.

Margaret Thorogood is an epidemiologist and Reader in Public Health and Preventative Medicine in the Health Promotion Research Unit at the London School of Hygiene and Tropical Medicine. Her research interests include cost-effective interventions for the prevention of coronary heart disease, pharmacoepidemiology, especially the safety of oral contraceptives, and the health effects of a vegetarian diet.

Peter Tyrer was a Research Officer at the Institute of Education, University of London and is now a Research Officer at Lancaster University.

Jane Wardle is Professor of Clinical Psychology and Director of the ICRF Health Behaviour Unit, Department of Epidemiology and Public Health, University College London Medical School.

Richard G. Watt is Senior Lecturer in Dental Public Health in the Department of Epidemiology and Public Health, University College London Medical School.

Patrick West is a Medical Sociologist at the Medical Research Council's Social and Public Health Sciences Unit in Glasgow. He leads the Youth Programme in the Unit and his interests include young people's health (particularly mental health), health behaviours (particularly smoking), life-styles and youth culture, school influences, family life and health inequalities. These issues are being investigated through the West of Scotland Twenty-07 study and, more recently, the 11 to 16 study.

Geoff Whitty is the Karl Mannheim Professor of Sociology of Education and Director of the Health and Education Research Unit at the Institute of Education, University of London.

Richard Wilkinson is Professorial Research Fellow at the Trafford Centre for Medical Research, University of Sussex, and Visiting Professor at the International Centre for Health and Society at University College London. For many years his research has been focused on the social and economic determinants of health inequalities and poopulation health in developed countries. He is specially interested in the tendency for more egalitarian societies to be healthier than less egalitarian ones, and in the psychosocial pathways linking health to material circumstances.

Preface

Sir Donald Acheson

In July 1997, I was asked by the Secretary of State for Health for England to review health inequalities and identify priority areas for policy development to help reduce them. I was supported in this work by the Scientific Advisory Group* and Secretariat who constituted the Inquiry team. In developing our report *The Independent Inquiry into Inequalities in Health*, the team was assisted by the contribution of many experts and practitioners in the field both from within and outside the UK.

The first stage of the Inquiry was provided by experts who agreed to provide us with summaries of the scientific and expert evidence on specific topics, and to identify possible policy recommendations to address some of the key issues. I am very grateful to colleagues who undertook this task, often at short notice and in competition with their other work pressures. These resulting 'input papers' which are reproduced in this book provided one of the foundations on which our final report was based.

These 'input papers' were part of a wider process which helped us meet the terms of reference we had been set by the Secretary of State. A considerable amount of written expert evidence was submitted separately to the Inquiry – over 300 items in all – and there were a number of oral presentations and briefings to the Scientific Group and to the Secretariat. We assessed all this information in reaching our conclusions, and are grateful to many colleagues for giving so generously of their time and expertise.

I believe that this volume will provide an important introduction to the input papers considered by the Inquiry. I welcome its publication as a contribution to the debate on tackling inequalities in health, which remains a challenge for science and for government.

Sir Donald Acheson
Chairman of the Independent Inquiry
into Inequalities in Health

* The members of the Scientific Advisory Group were Professor David Barker FRS, Director of the MRC Environmental Epidemiology Unit, University of Southampton; Dr Jacky Chambers, Director of Public Health, Birmingham Health Authority; Professor Hilary Graham, Director of ESRC's Health Variation Programme, Lancaster University; Professor Michael Marmot, Professor of Epidemiology, University College London and Director of the International Centre for Health and Society; Dr Margaret Whitehead, Visiting Fellow, King's Fund, London.

Mother, fetus, infant, child and family: socio-economic inequalities

Catherine Law

Executive summary

General

Policies to reduce socio-economic inequalities in child health should promote the health of women of childbearing age, and support parents in bringing up their children. Policies should also recognise that part of the inequalities in adult health are set in utero and in the first few years of life. They should recognise that reductions in these inequalities may take at least one generation.

Policy recommendations

[Unless stated otherwise the benefits are to people in lower social classes.]

1 **Policy** **Affordable day care should be available for all children.**

  Policy **Pre-school education should be provided for all children over the age of three years. Where appropriate this should be combined with day care provision.**

  Benefits • Improved short- and long-term educational achievement and increased social skills.

  • Decreased accidental injuries.

  • Decrease in family poverty.

  • Increased educational achievement.

Evidence Experiments in day care/pre-school education have shown desirable educational and social skills outcomes in the short, medium and long term. Affordable day care would allow return to work in some instances, thus relieving family poverty and dependence on benefits.

2 **Policy** **Transport policies should encourage walking, cycling and the use of public transport.**

  Policy **Roads should be modified in ways which reduce traffic volume and speed.**

  Benefits • Decreased child pedestrian injury.

  • Increased exercise in childhood, and decreased levels of obesity.

  • Decreased air pollution.

  • Improved access to facilities and services.

  Evidence Child pedestrian injuries are associated with increased traffic volume and speed. Evaluated interventions in this country and elsewhere have shown that environmental modification reduces such injuries.

3 **Policy** **Appropriate programmes to help women give up smoking before or during pregnancy should be available.**

Benefits   • Increase in birthweight in the babies of mothers who were formerly smokers (with decreases in early mortality).
   • Decreased smoking-related morbidity in mothers.
   • Decreased Sudden Infant Death Syndrome (SIDS).

Evidence   Maternal smoking is clearly established as a risk factor for lower birthweight, and SIDS. Effective methods for helping women to quit smoking during pregnancy have been identified.

Summary of inequalities in health in mothers, infants and children

This section summarises information on mortality, morbidity and health-related behaviours by socio-economic status. For morbidity and health-related behaviours much information exists, particularly in ad hoc surveys and in the research literature. However, it is not always available nationally (or in nationally representative samples) or by social class. The data in this section are mainly those which are collected nationally. For the purposes of this paper childhood is deemed to end on the child's 11th birthday (although the statistics quoted are not always published in compatible age groups).

Mortality

Stillbirth, perinatal and infant mortality rates show long-standing differences between social classes. The differences in stillbirth rates have remained fairly constant over the past 20 years, during which there have been marked falls in absolute rates. By contrast, infant and perinatal mortality rates have shown some narrowing in the ratio of the rates for social classes IV/V to I/II, although the gradients are still marked, especially for postneonatal deaths. Cause-specific infant mortality rates suggest some widening of the ratio for SIDS, albeit based on small numbers.

Despite declines in overall mortality rates for children from 1 to 15 years over the past 10 years, the social class differences in mortality have widened, from an excess of 61% to one of 68% of classes IV/V over classes I/II (Figure 1) (F. Drever, personal

communication to the Independent Inquiry into Inequalities in Health, 1997). The widening has occurred in mortality rates for 10-15 years, although ratios in younger age groups are also pronounced. The differential is particularly pronounced for death rates from injury and poisoning (the commonest cause of death), which has increased from a threefold difference of classes IV/V over classes I/II to a fivefold difference (Roberts and Power, 1996).

Figure 1: Age-specific mortality rates, children (England and Wales, selected years)

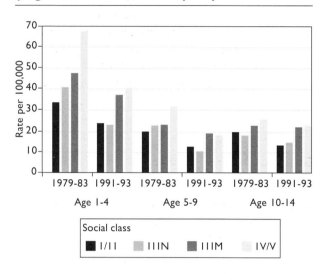

Morbidity

Mean birthweight is lower for babies whose fathers are in manual social classes. This trend has been fairly constant since 1982. Mean birthweight is even lower for babies whose birth is registered solely by the mother (ONS, 1997a).

Children in manual classes are more likely to suffer from chronic sickness (reported by an adult of their household as part of the General Household Survey) than children in non-manual classes, although this difference may be decreasing (ONS, 1997b). Children living in council housing are more likely to consult their GP, particularly for serious conditions, than those living in owner-occupied housing (McCormick et al, 1995).

Health-related behaviour

Mothers with husbands/partners in manual classes are more likely to smoke during pregnancy than those in non-manual classes. This difference has increased over the last 10 years, despite a small fall in overall rates of maternal smoking (Foster et al, 1997). Babies of fathers from social class I are more likely to be breastfed than those in social class V, but this difference has decreased over the last 10 years. Continued breastfeeding is much less common in lower social classes (Foster et al, 1997). The diet of children from a manual background has less emphasis on fruit and whole grain cereals (MAFF, 1997). The rates of obesity in children are increasing, but there are not marked differences between social classes (Duran-Tauleria et al, 1995), and no evidence that any differences are increasing (Chinn and Rona, 1994). The rates of obesity and level of body mass index in children are strongly predicted by those of their parents (Duran-Tauleria et al, 1995). Adult body mass index is inversely related to social class, especially in women (Prescott-Clarke and Primatesta, 1997).

Socio-economic status

Families with children (both couples and single parents) are over-represented at the bottom end of the income distribution. They form 4.5 million out of 7.9 million (57%) of the poorest group, with less than 40% of average household income, but comprise over 45% of the population (Benzeval and Webb, 1995). This trend is increasing (Spencer, 1996; Graham and Blackburn, 1998). The number of families accepted as homeless by local authorities rose steeply from 1980 to 1992, since when there has been some decrease. There are similar time trends for the number of families in local authority temporary accommodation. These trends may be partly explained by demographic changes (the 'baby boomers'), as well as changes in the provision of housing by local authorities (Best, 1995).

Introduction to evidence

The inequalities in direct measures of maternal and child health have been illustrated above. There are, in addition, arguments for policy investment in early life as a means of reducing inequalities in health in adult life. These will be summarised briefly (with references to reviews or summaries of the areas).

a) *Neurological and cognitive development* (see Ball, 1994 and Perry et al, 1995)
    Neuronal connections are developed in utero and the first years of life. They develop partly in response to external signals, and are therefore potentially modifiable. The extent to which neurological development is modifiable (for the better) is not known, although so-called 'natural' experiments have demonstrated profound effects in cases of inhumane treatment, for instance, children in war-time orphanages (Spitz and Wolf, 1946).

b) *Psychological health* (see Kraemer and Roberts, 1996)
    The capacity of children to be successful and healthy adults is strongly determined by early experiences with caregivers, when patterns of attachment are laid down. These are not irreversible, but are harder to alter later on. Furthermore, those who have good attachments to their parents have a greater chance of forming good attachments with their own children. Children and young people with insecure attachments are more at risk of delinquency and bullying, accidental injury, abuse by strangers, eating disorders, depression, chronic non-specific ill-health, and addictions, particularly at times of change or loss.

c) *Adult cardiovascular disease* (see Barker, 1994)
    Reduced growth in fetal life is associated with increased rates of death from cardiovascular disease, and higher levels of its major risk factors, hypertension, raised levels of cholesterol and fibrinogen, and impaired glucose tolerance. These associations cannot be explained by potential confounders operating in adult life. Fetal growth shows differences between social classes.

There are, no doubt, other examples of the association of early life with later health. What is missing from most, if not all, is an understanding of how differing human experiences, unfolding over time, initiate and sustain processes which lead to differing levels of health among different socio-economic groups. Hertzman and Wiens have proposed two models to describe (and perhaps explain) these associations (Hertzman and Wiens, 1996). The first is the latency model in which an 'exposure' results in an outcome which is distant in time, without any intervening exposure. This model embraces experiments in animals which have demonstrated 'critical periods' in development when the organism is specially receptive to exposure. Exposure during such a critical period permanently alters structure and/or function, a phenomenon also referred to as programming (Barker, 1994). The second is the pathways model which describes a temporal sequence of circumstances throughout the life-course of individuals. In this model differentials in health are a reflection of the enduring and (perhaps) cumulative effects of damaging physical and social environments (Hertzman and Wiens, 1996; Kuh and Ben-Shlomo, 1997). At their most simplistic, the policy corollary of the latency model is a one-shot social investment strategy for childbearing women and young children, and that of the pathways model is a cradle-to-grave social contract. However, these models are not necessarily contradictory. An early life event which causes a latent effect can also be the first step along a lifelong pathway which might have implications for health (Hertzman and Wiens, 1996). Policy approaches should also be complementary. However, the implication from both models, and from research that tends to one or the other (Barker, 1994; Kuh and Ben-Shlomo, 1997) is that reductions in inequalities in health may take more than one generation to achieve.

In the sections that follow, the evidence which supports a number of policy options is reviewed. In principle, interventions which have multiple benefits and more immediate outcomes (as opposed to only long-term outcomes) have been chosen. Health has been viewed widely, and thus some interventions aimed principally at correlates or determinants of health (such as employment, educational achievement and criminal behaviour) have been included.

Improving the physique of mothers and their children

Mothers: the offspring of women who are thin, having either a low body mass index (weight/length^2) or thin skinfolds, are at increased risk of developing non-insulin dependent diabetes and raised blood pressure (Godfrey et al, 1994; Ravelli et

al, 1998; Clark et al, 1998). The offspring of women who are overweight are at increased risk of coronary heart disease (Forsen et al, 1997). This effect is stronger among women with short stature. Short, overweight women are more common among low socio-economic groups.

Babies: reduced birthweight is associated with increased mortality and morbidity in the first year of life (The Scottish Low Birthweight Study Group, 1992; Vik et al, 1996), and throughout childhood (Mutch et al, 1992; Hack et al, 1993; Middle et al, 1996). People who had low birthweight, or who are thin or stunted at birth, are at increased risk of cardiovascular disease and the disorders related to it (Barker, 1994). Reduced fetal growth is more common in deprived areas of Britain (Law et al, 1993). Birthweight is mainly determined by the weight and height of the mother, which reflects her growth in childhood. The generally agreed 'healthy diet' in pregnancy may have long-term benefits in reducing the babies' later risk of cardiovascular disease (Campbell et al, 1996; Ravelli et al, 1998). Mothers on state benefits may not be able to afford a healthy diet (Dallison and Lobstein, 1995); and in the United States guaranteeing a minimum income to pregnant women has been shown to increase birthweight (Kehrer and Wolin, 1979).

Maternal smoking is associated not only with reduced birthweight, but also with an increased risk of SIDS (Blair et al, 1996), adverse effects on the mother's health, and the health of those with whom she shares her home (Chollat-Traquet, 1992; Royal College of Physicians, 1992; Faculty of Public Health Medicine Committee on Health Promotion, 1995). Recent work also suggests that educational achievement at 23 years is decreased in the offspring of mothers who smoke, over and above the effect expected by reduction of birthweight and other socio-economic factors (Fogelman and Manor, 1988). A systematic review of randomised controlled trials found that behavioural self-help approaches to smoking cessation were more effective than advice and feedback in reducing smoking in pregnancy (Arblaster et al, 1997). Given the differences in cessation rates by social class (Jarvis, 1997), more information may be needed to target interventions appropriately. Smoking in pregnancy is also likely to be susceptible to other approaches to reduction of smoking (addressed in Chapter 16).

Children: obesity is entrained during childhood and adolescence (Bourchard and Bray, 1996). The effects of obesity on the development of coronary heart disease, non-insulin dependent diabetes and hypertension are more severe in people who had low birthweight (Hales et al, 1991; Frankel et al, 1996; Leon et al, 1996; Lithell et al, 1996).

Summary

In general, policies should promote the avoidance of excessive thinness or overweight and a healthy diet for women of childbearing age. They should promote avoidance of excessive weight gain in children. Appropriate programmes to help women give up smoking before or during pregnancy should be available.

Parental support

The majority of those living in poverty wish to, and do, protect and promote the health of their children under the most unpromising conditions (Barnardo's, submission to the Independent Inquiry into Inequalities in Health Inquiry, 1997; Roberts, 1997). This section reviews the evidence that personal support to parents (especially mothers) will enhance their capacity to do so. Education as a means of preparation for parenthood is dealt with in Chapter 10.

The potency of even short periods of personal support is demonstrated by a review of the effects of continuous professional or social intrapartum support. In a number of settings women who received support from a trained person had shorter labours, less analgesia and operative delivery, and their babies had improved APGAR scores (Hodnett, 1998a). However, most studies have used longer periods of social support, aimed at reducing stress and enhancing self-esteem and confidence during pregnancy and the early part of parenthood. The effect of home visiting during pregnancy alone on birthweight and other pregnancy outcomes is inconsistent (Oakley, 1992; Roberts, 1997; Hodnett, 1998b). Some studies, while not showing an effect on physical health, have found social and behavioural effects. For instance, a review of controlled trials of social support in pregnancy concluded that women receiving support were less likely than controls to

feel unhappy, nervous and worried during pregnancy, and were more likely to be breastfeeding after birth (Elbourne et al, 1989).

Home visiting in the first two years of life has been associated with beneficial effects during childhood. A systematic review found that programmes of home visits by professional or specially trained lay care givers tended to be associated with decreased rates of childhood injury (Hodnett and Roberts, 1998). They may also reduce rates of child abuse, incomplete immunisations, hospital admission, and morbidity in infancy (eg severe nappy rash), although the evidence is not conclusive for these outcomes. Specifically differential surveillance between intervention and control arms may bias estimates of the outcomes, especially child abuse. The applicability of these studies to the UK is unknown. However, in the UK at least two studies have shown that a short training course for health visitors in the detection and management (mostly through counselling) of postnatal depression was associated with more rapid remission of symptoms (Barnardo's, submission to the Independent Inquiry into Inequalities in Health Inquiry, 1997), fewer problems in the relationship between the mother and the child at four months and fewer child behaviour problems at 18 months (Seeley et al, 1996). Although postnatal depression does not show a marked gradient with socio-economic status, the long-term effect of maternal depression on cognitive and emotional behaviour of the offspring is more marked in the presence of socio-economic disadvantage (Murray, 1997).

In the UK several experiments in home-based strategies to help parents be more self-confident and skilful in their child's development have been initiated. These have used specially trained health visitors or 'community mothers', training teams of volunteers (Barker et al, 1994; Whitehead, 1995). Early results indicate that those in the intervention arms feel more positive and have higher self-esteem during early motherhood, and the children have more complete immunisations, and less early weaning onto cow's milk. Longer-term outcomes are awaited (Barnardo's, submission to the Independent Inquiry into Inequalities in Health Inquiry, 1997; Whitehead, 1995). A systematic review of parent-training programmes in improving the behaviour of children between three and 10 years concluded that group-based programmes were the most effective. However, there is insufficient evidence to show which aspects of such programmes are important (Barlow, 1997).

Few studies have yet included long-term outcomes. However, in a 15-year follow-up of an American randomised controlled trial, those who had received home visits during pregnancy and the first two years were less likely to have been identified as perpetrators of child abuse. Among those who were socio-economically disadvantaged at the time of the intervention, those in the intervention arm had fewer subsequent births, increased birth interval, received Income Support for a shorter period, had fewer behavioural impairments associated with the use of alcohol and other drugs, and had fewer arrests (Ramey et al, 1990). A seven-year follow-up in the UK has found improved health in children and mothers who had midwife-provided social support in pregnancy (Oakley et al, 1996).

A number of general issues arise in the best way of providing parental support. The best evaluated studies are the randomised controlled trials. However, these tend to be conducted in particular settings, especially those of the health services. It is not clear whether the beneficial effects observed are the consequence of a particular type of support or would be seen with the provision of any support, even if of very different content (eg childcare). In addition, the quality of support offered in an experimental setting may not be reproducible in service. Thus the nature of support, who should offer it, when, and for how long is still under debate. Secondly, the applicability to the UK of the results of studies conducted outside this country is uncertain. Thirdly, the effect on some outcomes have only been tested in single trials, and have to be regarded with caution. Fourthly, the identification of those most likely to benefit from support needs to be refined. The trials have mostly been conducted among high risk populations. Lastly, the best way of translating research findings based on parental empowerment into service provision which does not patronise or stigmatise users needs to be addressed (Whitehead, 1995).

Summary

The evidence points to the importance of supporting parents (both mothers and fathers) in bringing up their children. However, the best ways of support, and its cost-effectiveness, are unknown. Further research, especially randomised trials, is needed before a specific policy can be recommended.

Pre-school education and day care

Out of home day care and pre-school education are two services which overlap in providing learning and care for those below current statutory school age. Currently the provision of these services varies by area. Often the services are only available for those who can pay the full or subsidised fees (Ball, 1994). A 1990 survey carried out by the Department of Health found that over 40% of mothers of three- and four-year-olds not attending day nursery would like them to do so (Meltzer, 1994). Provision of early out of home day care and education might reduce inequalities in health because:

1. The intervention is applied when the individual is sensitive to it (the critical period).
2. The intervention will be applied at a point in the life-course which can then influence the next (eg school 'readiness', primary schooling) step of the life-course.
3. Some parents, particularly single parents, find themselves in a benefit dependent poverty trap, and might seek work if affordable day care were available. It is thus a potential way to alleviate family poverty (Duncan and Giles, 1996).
4. It would increase choice to those currently denied it.

Assessment of the most rigorous evaluations is found in a systematic review of randomised controlled trials of non-parental out of home day care before the age of five years (Zoritch and Roberts, 1998). This assessed eight trials, all conducted in the USA. In total, 2,203 children were randomised to receive day care or to be in a control group. In four studies the intervention started when the children were infants. Length of follow-up ranged from six months to 27 years. Most of the studies targeted families of lower socio-economic status. Nearly all studies included an element of home visiting and targeted parental training. The formal educational component varied, although all were concerned with the attainment of cognitive concepts. The review was not able to determine the effects of different parts of the programmes.

Although all studies showed that IQ was increased by participation in day care, this effect did not persist much after the end of the intervention. However, measures of educational performance tended to be persistently higher in the intervention groups. Furthermore, there were no adverse effects of day care on behaviour. Other advantages included better maternal educational, employment and financial achievement in the intervention groups shown in some, but not all of the studies. In one of the studies, the Perry Project (later called Highscope), follow-up to 27 years of age showed that the intervention group were more likely to have desirable social outcomes such as high school graduation, employment, fewer arrests, better earnings, less single parenthood and more home ownership.

Few outcomes measured health directly, although enhanced cognitive development and educational achievement are associated with beneficial effects on the life-course (eg employment), which are themselves associated with health. Although not measured in the trials cited, day care might reduce childhood injuries, by providing a safe environment.

In a more general review, Sylva draws a number of conclusions from the sometimes conflicting results between trials and observational studies, and between countries. Firstly, she concludes that weaknesses in design and evaluation have led to some of the apparently contradictory findings. Secondly, pre-school education/day care may be especially effective in improving the abilities of the most disadvantaged, although this will not necessarily bring them up to the level of their more advantaged peers (as in the US federally funded 'Headstart' programme). Thirdly, the content and quality of the programmes are crucial: indeed, she concludes that low quality provision is associated with adverse outcome. Training of the carers is an important issue in quality. Lastly, she quotes studies which show that investment in pre-school provision is associated with financial gain to society in the long term (Sylva, 1994).

Issues that remain are:

1. The applicability of the evidence to the UK.
2. The nature of the interventions. Many of those

tested included multiple components. The impact of a different package of components, or of the individual components is unknown.
3. The quality of the interventions in the trials is likely to be high. Is this achievable in practice?
4. The optimal age for day care. Consensus about advantages for those over three years is greater than that for younger children, especially infants, although there is no evidence for an optimal age (Sylva, 1994; Zoritch and Roberts, 1998).

Summary

Overall, the evidence appears to be sufficient to recommend a policy of affordable day care combined with pre-school education. The issues above would need to be resolved.

Creation of safe environments and the prevention of injury from child pedestrian accidents

Fatal and non-fatal injuries from child pedestrian accidents has been declining in absolute terms, despite an increase in traffic volume. Some of this reduction may be related to lower pedestrian exposure, with an increasing tendency for children to be transported by car. Children from disadvantaged families are less likely to have access to a car. As a result they cross more roads and are exposed to greater injury risk (Roberts et al, 1996). The social class gradient for deaths from pedestrian injures is steep, and increasing. Furthermore, fatalities represent the tip of the iceberg, with ten times as many children being injured as killed.

Policies which might reduce childhood pedestrian injuries fall into two categories: broad land use and transport policies, and environmental modification of the roads. These have been fully reviewed by Towner et al (1996) whose findings are summarised below.

Broad land use and transport policies: policies which encourage walking, cycling and the use of public rather than private transport might reduce pedestrian injuries, particularly by decreasing traffic volume. If traffic volume were less, the number of 'escort' journeys made by parents for their children might also decrease, further reducing volume. This would have the additional effect of increasing physical exercise in children and decreasing air pollution. Improving public transport should also improve access to services or facilities by children experiencing disadvantage. Changes to the layout of residential districts (for instance, removal of on-street parking) may also lead to fewer pedestrian accidents. The potential for such policies to cause change is suggested by the greater rates of decline in childhood pedestrian fatalities in other European countries.

Environmental modification of the roads: a variety of approaches have been tried to reduce traffic volume and speed. In general, these have been associated with a decrease in accidents, including pedestrian injuries. The size of the decrease has varied by place. Local participation in the schemes may be necessary for success. Studies suggest that the interventions may result in cost savings.

Summary

Transport policy which encourages walking, cycling and the use of public transport should reduce child pedestrian injuries and have other benefits. Environmental modification of the roads should also reduce such injuries.

Acknowledgements

I am grateful to many colleagues for their advice. In particular I should like to thank Jim Appleyard, Frances Drever, David Hall, Lynn Murray, Roberto Rona, Chris Power, Helen Roberts, Ian Roberts, and Sarah Stewart-Brown. The opinions expressed in this paper are my own.

References

Arblaster, L., Entwistle, V., Fullerton, D., Glanville, J., Forster, M., Lambert, M., Sheldon, T., Sowden, A. and Watt, I. (1997) *A review of the effectiveness of health promotion interventions aimed at reducing inequalities in health*, York: NHS Centre for Reviews and Dissemination.

Ball, C. (1994) *Start right: The importance of early learning*, London: Royal Society of Arts.

Barker, D. (1994) *Mothers, babies, and disease in later life*, London: British Medical Journal Books.

Barker, W., Anderson, R. and Chalmers, C. (1994) *Child protection: The impact of the child development programme (evaluation document 14)*, Bristol: Early Child Development Unit, University of Bristol.

Barlow, J. (1997) *Systematic review of the effectiveness of parent-training programmes in improving behaviour problems in children aged 3-10 years*, Oxford: Health Services Research Unit, University of Oxford.

Benzeval, M. and Webb, S. (1995) 'Family poverty and poor health', in M. Benzeval, K. Judge and M. Whitehead (eds) *Tackling inequalities in health: An agenda for action*, London: King's Fund, pp 69-81.

Best, R. (1995) 'The housing dimension', in M. Benzeval, K. Judge and M. Whitehead (eds) *Tackling inequalities in health: An agenda for action*, London: King's Fund, pp 53-68.

Blair, P., Fleming, P., Bensley, D., Smith, I., Bacon, C., Taylor, T., Berry, J., Golding, J., Tripp, J., LESDI Coordinators and Researchers (1996) 'Smoking and the sudden infant death syndrome: results from 1993-5 case-control study for Confidential Enquiry into Stillbirths and Deaths in Infancy', *British Medical Journal*, vol 313, pp 195-8.

Bourchard, C. and Bray, G. (1996) *Regulation of body weight*, Chichester: John Wiley.

Campbell, D., Hall, M., Barker, D., Cross, J., Shiell, A. and Godfrey, K. (1996) 'Diet in pregnancy and the offspring's blood pressure 40 years later', *British Journal of Obstetrics Gynaecology*, vol 103, pp 273-80.

Chinn, S. and Rona, R. (1994) 'Trends in weight-for-height and triceps skinfold thickness for English and Scottish children, 1972-1982 and 1982-1990', *Paediatric and Perinatal Epidemiology*, vol 8, pp 90-106.

Chollat-Traquet, C. (1992) *Women and tobacco*, Geneva: World Health Organisation.

Clark, P., Allen, C., Law, C., Shiell, A., Godfrey, K. and Barker, D. (1998) 'Weight gain in pregnancy, triceps skinfold thickness and blood pressure in the offspring', *Obstetrics and Gynaecology*, vol 91, pp 103-7.

Dallison, J. and Lobstein, T. (1995) *Poor expectations: Poverty and undernourishment in pregnancy*, London: NCH Action for Children and The Maternity Alliance.

Duncan, A. and Giles, C. (1996) 'Should we subsidise pre-school child-care, and if so, how?', *Fiscal Studies*, vol 17, pp 39-61.

Duran-Tauleria, E., Rona, R. and Chinn, S. (1995) 'Factors associated with weight for height and skinfold thickness in British children', *Journal of Epidemiology and Community Health*, vol 49, pp 466-73.

Elbourne, D., Oakley, A. and Chalmers, I. (1989) 'Social and psychological support during pregnancy', in I. Chalmers, M. Enkin and M. Keirse (eds) *Effective care in pregnancy and childbirth, vol 1*, Oxford: Oxford University Press, pp 221-36.

Faculty of Public Health Medicine Committee on Health Promotion (1995) *Women and smoking: Health promotion report no 39*, London: Royal College of Physicians, Faculty of Public Health Medicine.

Fogelman, K. and Manor, O. (1988) 'Smoking in pregnancy and development into early adulthood', *British Medical Journal*, vol 297, pp 1233-6.

Forsen, T., Eriksson, J., Tuomilehto, J., Teramo, K., Osmond, C. and Barker, D. (1997) 'Mother's weight in pregnancy and coronary heart disease in a cohort of Finnish men: follow up study', *British Medical Journal*, vol 315, pp 837-40.

Foster, K., Lader, D. and Cheesbrough, S. (1997) *Infant feeding 1995*, London: The Stationery Office.

Frankel, S., Elwood, P., Sweetnam, P., Yarnell, J. and Davey Smith, G. (1996) 'Birthweight, body-mass index in middle age, and incident coronary heart disease', *Lancet*, vol 348, pp 1478-80.

Godfrey, K., Forrester, T., Barker, D., Jackson, A., Landman, J., Hall, J., Cox, V. and Osmond, C. (1994) 'Maternal nutritional status in pregnancy and blood pressure in childhood', *British Journal of Obstetrics Gynaecology*, vol 101, pp 398-403.

Graham, H. and Blackburn, C. (1998) 'The socio-economic patterning of health and smoking behaviour among mothers with young children on income support', *Sociology of Health and Illness*, vol 20, pp 215-40.

Hack, M., Weissman, B., Breslau, N., Klein, N., Borawski-Clark, E. and Fanaroff, A. (1993) 'Health of very low birthweight children during their first eight years', *Journal of Pediatrics*, vol 122, pp 887-92.

Hales, C., Barker, D., Clark, P., Cox, L., Fall, C., Osmond, C. and Winter, P. (1991) 'Fetal and infant growth and impaired glucose tolerance at age 64', *British Medical Journal*, vol 303, pp 1019-22.

Hertzman, C. and Wiens, M. (1996) 'Child development and long-term outcomes: a population health perspective and summary of successful interventions', *Social Science and Medicine*, vol 43, pp 1083-95.

Hodnett, E. (1998a) 'Support from caregivers during childbirth', in The Cochrane Database of Systematic Reviews (ed) *The Cochrane Library, Issue 2, 1998*, Oxford: Update Software (updated quarterly).

Hodnett, E. (1998b) 'Support from caregivers during at-risk pregnancy', in The Cochrane Database of Systematic Reviews (ed) *The Cochrane Library, Issue 2, 1998*, Oxford: Update Software (updated quarterly).

Hodnett, E. and Roberts, I. (1998) 'Home-based social support for socially disadvantaged mothers', in The Cochrane Database of Systematic Reviews (ed) *The Cochrane Library, Issue 2, 1998*, Oxford: Update Software (updated quarterly).

Jarvis, M. (1997) 'Patterns and predictors of smoking cessation in the general population', in C. Bolliger and K. Fagerstrom (eds) *Progress in respiratory research: The tobacco epidemic*, Basel: S Karger AG.

Kehrer, B. and Wolin, V. (1979) 'Impact of income maintenance on low birthweight, evidence from the Gary experiment', *Journal of Human Resources*, vol 14, pp 434-62.

Kraemer, S. and Roberts, J. (1996) *The politics of attachment: Towards a secure society*, London and New York, NY: Free Association Books.

Kuh, D. and Ben-Shlomo, Y. (eds) (1997) *A life course approach to chronic disease epidemiology*, Oxford: Oxford University Press.

Law, C., Barker, D., Richardson, W., Shiell, A., Grime, L., Armandsmith, N. and Cruddas, A. (1993) 'Thinness at birth in a northern industrial town', *Journal of Epidemiology and Community Health*, vol 47, pp 255-9.

Leon, D., Koupilova, I., Lithell, H., Berglund, L., Mohsen, R., Vagero, D., Lithell, V.-B. and McKeigue, P. (1996) 'Failure to realise growth potential in utero and adult obesity in relation to blood pressure in 50 year old Swedish men', *British Medical Journal*, vol 312, pp 401-6.

Lithell, H., McKeigue, P., Berglund, L., Mohsen, R., Lithell, U. and Leon, D. (1996) 'Relation of size at birth to non-insulin dependent diabetes and insulin concentrations in men aged 50-60 years', *British Medical Journal*, vol 312, pp 406-10.

McCormick, A., Fleming, D. and Charlton, J. (1995) *Morbidity statistics from general practice fourth national study 1991-92*, London: The Stationery Office.

MAFF (Ministry of Agriculture Fisheries and Food) (1997) *National food survey*, London: HMSO.

Meltzer, H. (1994) *Day care services for children: A survey carried out on behalf of the Department of Health in 1990*, London: HMSO.

Middle, C., Johnson, A., Alderdice, F., Petty, T. and Macfarlane, A. (1996) 'Birthweight and health and development at the age of 7 years', *Childcare, Health and Development*, vol 22, pp 55-71.

Murray, L. (1997) 'Postpartum depression and child development', *Psychological Medicine*, vol 27, pp 253-60.

Mutch, L., Ashurst, H. and Macfarlane, A. (1992) 'Birth weight and hospital admission before the age of 2 years', *Archives of Disease in Childhood*, vol 67, pp 900-4.

Oakley, A. (1992) *Social support and motherhood*, Oxford: Blackwell.

Oakley, A., Hickey, O., Rajan, L. and Hickey, A. (1996) 'Social support in pregnancy: does it have long term effects?', *Journal of Reproductive Infant Psychology*, vol 14, pp 7-22.

ONS (Office for National Statistics) (1997a) *Series DH3 mortality statistics: Perinatal and infant: Social and biological factors*, London: The Stationery Office.

ONS (1997b) *Living in Britain: Results from the General Household Survey 1995*, London: The Stationery Office.

Perry, B., Pollard, R., Blakley, T., Baker, W. and Vigilante, D. (1995) 'Childhood trauma, the neurobiology of adaptation, and 'use-dependent' development of the brain: how 'states' become 'traits', *Infant Mental Health Journal*, vol 16, pp 271-91.

Prescott-Clarke, P. and Primatesta, P. (1997) *Health Survey for England 1995*, London: The Stationery Office.

Ramey, C., Bryant, D., Campbell, F., Sparling, J. and Wasik, B. (1990) 'Early intervention for high-risk children: The Carolina Early Intervention Programme', in C. Ramey (ed) *Early childhood programs*, Binghampton, NY: The Haworth Press, pp 33-57.

Ravelli, A., van der Meulen, J., Michels, R., Osmond, C., Barker, D., Hales, N. and Bleker, O. (1998) 'Glucose tolerance in adults after prenatal exposure to the Dutch famine', *Lancet*, vol 351, pp 173-7.

Roberts, H. (1997) 'Children, inequalities, and health', *British Medical Journal*, vol 314, pp 1122-5.

Roberts, I. and Power, C. (1996) 'Does the decline in child injury death rates vary by social class?', *British Medical Journal*, vol 313, pp 784-6.

Roberts, I., Norton, R. and Taua, B. (1996) 'Socioeconomic and ethnic differences in child pedestrian injury: the importance of exposure to risk', *Journal of Epidemiology and Community Health*, vol 50, pp 162-5.

Royal College of Physicians (1992) *A report of a working party on smoking in the young*, London: Royal College of Physicians.

Seeley, S., Murray, L. and Cooper, P. (1996) 'The outcome for mothers and babies of health visitor intervention', *Health Visitor*, vol 69, pp 135-8.

Spencer, N. (1996) *Poverty and child health*, Oxford: Radcliffe Medical Press.

Spitz, R. and Wolf, K. (1946) 'Anaclitic depression: an inquiry into the genesis of psychiatric conditions in early childhood', *Psychoanalytic Study of the Child*, vol 2, pp 313-42.

Sylva, K. (1994) 'The impact of early learning on children's later development', in C. Ball (ed) *Start right: The importance of early learning*, London: Royal Society of Arts, pp 84-96.

The Scottish Low Birthweight Study Group (1992) 'The Scottish Low Birthweight Study 1: survival, growth, neuromotor and sensory impairment', *Archives of Disease in Childhood*, vol 67, pp 675-81.

Towner, E., Dowswell, T., Simpson, G. and Jarvis, S. (1996) *Health promotion in childhood and young adolescence for the prevention of unintentional injuries*, London: Health Education Authority.

Vik, T., Vatten, L., Markestad, T., Ahlsten, G., Jacobsen, G. and Bakketeig, L. (1996) 'Morbidity during the first year of life in small for gestational age infants', *Archives of Disease in Childhood*, vol 75, pp F33-F37.

Whitehead, M. (1995) 'Tackling inequalities: a review of policy initiatives', in M. Benzeval, K. Judge and M. Whitehead (eds) *Tackling inequalities in health: An agenda for action*, London: The King's Fund, pp 22-52.

Zoritch, B. and Roberts, I. (1998) 'The health and welfare effects of day care for pre-school children: a systematic review of randomised controlled trials', in The Cochrane Database of Systematic Reviews (ed) *The Cochrane Library, Issue 2, 1998*, Oxford: Update Software (updated quarterly).

2

Youth

Patrick West

Introduction

Definition of youth

It is notoriously difficult to define 'youth' with any precision principally because its meaning, and therefore its boundaries, have changed over time. In general terms, it refers to a period in the life-course between childhood and adulthood during which dependence on parents is replaced by the independence of adulthood. Its key defining features in contemporary society are that it encompasses the years of secondary (and tertiary) education, it is a period of intense involvement with peers, and it is infused by one or more youth cultures which shape identity and behaviour for young people (Jones and Wallace, 1992; Furlong and Cartmell, 1997; Wyn and White, 1997). While it is somewhat easier to define the beginning of this period as entry into secondary school (the word 'transition' is commonly used to describe this), it is almost impossible to define an end point (West, 1997). This is because over the last decade or so the youth–adult transition has become both extended and fragmented with the consequence that young people are now dependent on parents for longer periods of time (both for finance and housing needs) and experience the transition in a much less consistent way (eg getting a job, leaving home and forming a stable relationship are less integrated than before) (Morrow and Richards, 1996; Furlong and Cartmell, 1997). One view is that the endpoint of youth is definable only when young people achieve the full citizenship rights of adulthood (Jones and Wallace, 1992) which in the present context would be age 25 (the age at which the full adult benefit rate is paid). Another is

that this is too finite and fails to recognise the diverse ways adult status is achieved, for example, by becoming a parent (West, 1997). Either way, it is a problem but in general terms most authorities would agree that it spans the years 12-25, an age range corresponding to the World Health Organisation definition.

In thinking about the factors which influence health, however, it is not sensible to consider the period of youth in an undifferentiated way. In particular, it is important to distinguish the stage of 'early' youth from 'later' youth. The former principally refers to the period of secondary schooling (though it might extend to further and higher education), at which time the constellation of influences stemming from the school, the peer group and youth culture are at their maximum. Any influences arising from these sources which cut across social class therefore have the potential for reducing health inequalities at that time (West, 1997). 'Later' youth, by contrast, though containing many of the same features (eg youth culture), refers to the post-school years and as such involves exposure to a range of new environments and risks associated with the work situation, unemployment or homelessness. The distinction allows us to think about different influences arising during these two periods and it clearly makes a nonsense of health statistics which refer to the age group 12-25. A much more useful distinction is between young people aged 12-15/16 and those aged 17-25, though it is acknowledged that this is imperfect. The distinction between 'early' and 'later' youth informs the interpretation of health variations described below.

Health, health behaviours and other risks

An important question arises as to what are the best indicators of health in youth. There are two distinct perspectives here. The first is that youth is a time of maximum healthiness (mortality is rare) and that in consequence attention should be directed towards indicators of underlying health potential (eg height) or indicators of risk for future morbidity (eg health behaviours). The second questions the assumption of 'youthful healthiness' (Bennett, 1985) and points to the high prevalence of health problems in youth, most notably symptoms of one kind or another (West, 1997), accidents and injuries (Woodroffe et al, 1993) and mental health problems (Rutter and Smith, 1995). Each of these approaches tends to be associated with a different emphasis on the issue of class variation in health in youth, the first stressing the existence of (or potential for) health inequalities (Davey Smith et al, 1994), the second stressing the relative lack of health inequalities in youth (Glendinning et al, 1992; West, 1997). Both perspectives are valid and the approach taken here is to incorporate a range of indicators referring to current health, health potential and health risk.

There is, however, a third perspective on the issue which derives in large part from a life-course perspective. This is that it is not only important to direct attention to health and health behaviours in youth but also to consider other processes which may not impact directly on health at that time but which nevertheless have implications for health, and health inequalities, later in life. Recent research has highlighted the 'adolescent' period as of considerable importance for health inequalities, particularly in relation to the consequences of low educational attainment and 'conduct disorder' for future health and class position (Power et al, 1991, 1997). Another interpretation of this relationship suggests that young people who are disengaged from school, and who are involved in deviant and risky life-styles, are more likely to experience both reduced life-chances (eg unemployment) and later health problems. This perspective offers a different, and longer-term, view of the relevance of youth for health inequalities, and points up particular strategies for tackling the problem.

The measurement of inequality

The conventional measure of inequality in youth (as in childhood) is social class of background as measured by parental occupation. This remains the most usual measure, but it may not adequately reflect newer forms of inequality, and there is some evidence that the poorest health occurs in those people who cannot be classified into a social class (eg young people in lone-parent families) (Judge and Benzeval, 1993). An additional problem of classification occurs in youth because own occupation is known to be an unreliable indicator of achieved adult class position up to age 25. In addition to measures of class of background, it is useful to identify the labour market position young people occupy in later youth, distinguishing, for example, between those in tertiary education, work or those who are unemployed. The particular health problems associated with unemployment will be referred to, as will other particularly vulnerable groups such as homeless youth.

Description of health (in)equalities in youth

Six dimensions of health are considered: mortality, chronic illness/disability, general health, symptoms, non-fatal accidents and mental health, together with physical measures (height, body mass index [BMI], respiratory function and blood pressure), distinguishing where possible the patterns for early and later youth.

- *Mortality:* despite the view that mortality is not a good indicator of health in youth (Blane et al, 1994), successive Decennial Supplements attest to class differences in mortality in both early and later youth. In the most recent (1991-93), in the age group 10-14 mortality rates increased from 15/100,000 in social class I to 41/100,000 in class V for males, and from 13/100,000 to 17/100,000 for females (see Table 1). These differences, particularly for females, are less marked than that observed in later youth (age 20-24), where rates for males rise from 98/100.000 in class I to 368/100,000 in class V (see Table 2). Throughout youth, and especially in early youth, class gradients in mortality are predominantly attributable to accidents/injuries, with particularly high rates among young people in social class V (Roberts and Power, 1996), a pattern also applying to suicide (Hawton et al, 1993). Mortality due to other causes shows much less class variation; in the ONS Longitudinal Survey, for example, there are no health inequalities found for 'medical mortality' in the age group 10-14 (Blane et al, 1994). This relative lack of class differentiation in mortality from causes other than accidents has led some commentators to characterise the period of early youth as one of 'relative equality' (West, 1988, 1997), a view challenged by others (Judge and Benzeval, 1993; Dennehy et al, 1997) who see this as an artefact of the social class measure used.

Table 1: Childhood mortality rates, rate per 100,000 (England and Wales, 1991-93) aged 10-14

	Boys	Girls
Social class		
I – Professional	15	13
II – Managerial and Technical	14	12
IIIN – Skilled (non-manual)	17	12
IIIM – Skilled (manual)	25	18
IV – Partly skilled	26	15
V – Unskilled	41	17

Source: After Drever and Whitehead (1997, Table 7.6, p 92)

Table 2: Age-specific mortality rates, by social class, men aged 20-24, all causes (England and Wales, 1991-93)

Social class	Age 20-24
I – Professional	98
II – Managerial and Technical	139
IIIN – Skilled (non-manual)	158
IIIM – Skilled (manual)	219
IV – Partly skilled	195
V – Unskilled	368
England and Wales	246

Source: After Drever and Whitehead (1997, Table 8.3, p 98)

- *Chronic illness/disability:* using the conventional General Household Survey measure of chronic illness/disability, a number of studies report little or no variation in rates of long-standing, or limiting long-standing, illness by social class in either early or later youth (Power et al, 1997; West, 1997). However, with more severe chronic illness, there is evidence of health inequalities.

Using the 1991 Census question (limiting long-term illness, health problem or handicap), rates of 'severe' chronic illness are higher in the lower social classes in most single year groups in the age range 10-19, and highest of all in the 'no social class' category (see Table 3). This finding complements those of other more focused studies, where class gradients have been found for some conditions, particularly respiratory problems (but not asthma) and hearing impairment.

Table 3: Long-term limiting illness (%) by social class (HoH) in youth (10-19), males and females (Census 1991 2% sample)

	I	II	IIIN	IIIM	IV	V	No s/c§	Total
Males								
10	2.6	2.0	2.5	2.2	3.4	2.5	4.7	2.4
11	2.2	2.1	2.9	3.0	1.8	3.9	4.2	2.5
12	2.6	2.7	3.0	2.6	3.3	4.2	6.3	2.9
13	1.7	2.4	3.2	2.3	2.6	5.2	5.4	2.6
14	2.3	1.7	2.6	2.0	2.7	5.7+	6.4	2.3
15	0.8	2.5	0.9	2.9	3.2	2.4	4.1	2.4
16	2.8	2.2	2.2	2.7	2.6	4.6	4.0	2.6
17	2.6	1.5	3.1	3.2	3.0	5.5‡	6.8	2.7
18	3.3	1.9	2.6	2.6	2.8	1.9	8.3	2.5
19	1.9	2.2	3.0	3.5	3.5	3.2*	7.8	3.6
Females								
10	0.9	1.1	1.7	1.9	2.3	1.8+	2.8	1.6
11	1.0	1.1	1.5	1.8	3.6	1.4‡	4.6	1.8
12	0.5	2.1	1.7	2.8	2.0	5.2+	4.5	2.4
13	1.3	1.3	2.6	2.1	3.0	1.5*	4.5	1.5
14	1.1	1.8	2.3	1.8	3.0	3.3*	5.2	2.1
15	1.4	1.6	1.6	1.5	3.3	3.9+	3.4	1.9
16	1.7	1.7	2.0	2.1	3.3	2.0	4.8	2.1
17	2.8	1.8	2.8	2.1	3.3	4.4*	7.7	2.4
18	1.7	1.6	3.0	3.1	3.9	3.5‡	6.5	2.7
19	2.0	2.7	2.4	2.8	2.6	4.0	9.2	2.7

Notes: *$p < 0.05$
+ $p < 0.01$
‡ $p < 0.001$ (χ^2 trend with 1 *df*)
§ No social class (s/c) consists of all individuals without information on HoH occupation together with inadequately described occupations and Armed Forces.
Source: Reprinted form West (1997, Table 2, p 842), with permission from Elsevier Science. Original source: Samples of Anonymised Records from the 1991 Census, 2% Individual Sample, Crown Copyright

- *General (self-rated) health:* the findings for another commonly used General Household Survey measure, self-rated health, are mixed. Some studies have found little or no relationship with social class in early youth (Glendinning et al, 1997) while others have (Currie et al, 1997). By later youth, however, more evidence of class differentiation is found (Power et al, 1991; West, 1997), especially in relation to unemployed 18-year-olds (West and Sweeting, 1996).

- *Symptoms:* very little information exists on the class patterning of symptoms in either early or later youth. What little there is suggests remarkably little differentiation. Among 18-year-olds in the West of Scotland, dysmenorrhoea was the only symptom related to class of background (see Table 4). In the same group, malaise symptoms (but not physical symptoms) were higher among the unemployed (West and Sweeting, 1996). In an unpublished study of rural youth, somatic and affective symptoms showed no significant relationship with social class but 14- and 16-year-olds who were 'unclassifiable' exhibited higher symptoms (see Table 5)

- *Non-fatal accidents/injuries:* despite the evidence of health inequalities in fatal accidents, the association between social class and non-fatal accidents is much less clear-cut. Several studies find no relationship with social class in either early (Williams et al, 1997) or later youth (Bijur et al, 1991), although hospital admissions for accidents (possibly more severe) are higher among lower class youth (Bijur et al, 1991). In one study of head injuries in Scotland, a relatively slight relationship with area of deprivation among 10- to 14-year-olds translated to a very strong one among 15- to 19-year-olds (Figure 1). Not surprisingly, the circumstances in which accidents occur and their type vary by social class and area, with implications for injury prevention strategies.

- *Mental health:* findings vary between different dimensions and diagnostic categories. With respect to measures of *general well-being* (eg General Health Questionnaire [GHQ]), there is little or no evidence of class variation in early youth though by later youth, particularly in consequence of the greater experience of unemployment among lower class youth, a pattern of health inequalities is emerging (West, 1997). For *emotional disorders* (eg depression), there is also not much evidence of class variation in youth though rates may be elevated among those in situations of extreme poverty (Wallace et al, 1998). Among unemployed youth (Fombonne, 1996), and especially those who are homeless (Wrate and McLaughlin, 1997), rates of depression are significantly elevated. *Conduct disorders*, by contrast, are class differentiated throughout youth, are associated with poorer school performance, smoking and drug use, and teenage pregnancy (Maughan and Lindelow, 1997).

Table 4: Symptoms reported at age 18 (previous month) by social class of background, males and females (Twenty-07 Study)

		NM	IIIM	IV-V	Total
Physical					
Colds/flu	M	45.0	44.2	47.6	45.2
	F	49.2	50.3	56.9	51.3
Sinus/catarrh	M	37.0	39.0	35.4	37.4
	F	36.5	36.3	27.5	34.5
Wheezy chest	M	10.1	15.5	13.4	12.7
	F	9.6	11.7	12.7	11.1
Persistent cough	M	12.2	7.1	6.1	9.2
	F	8.1	13.5	13.7	11.3
Stiff, painful joints	M	25.4	29.0	29.3	27.5
	F	23.4	19.9	15.7	20.4
Back trouble	M	16.4	13.0	15.9	15.1
	F	15.2	14.6	17.6	15.5
Ear trouble	M	7.9	7.7	7.3	7.7
	F	8.1	12.9	9.8	10.2
Eye trouble	M	10.6	18.1	11.0	13.4
	F	13.2	17.0	18.6	15.7
Allergies	M	5.8	9.1	4.9	6.8
	F	12.7	8.2	4.9	9.4*
Palpitations/	M	3.7	5.2	6.1	4.7
breathlessness	F	7.1	6.4	7.8	7.0
Skin problems	M	17.5	13.6	12.2	15.1
	F	19.8	15.8	15.7	17.4
Kidney/bladder	M	–	–	–	0.0
problems	F	3.6	4.1	1.0	3.2
Mixed					
Headaches/migraine	M	29.6	20.6	30.5	26.5
	F	47.7	44.4	42.2	45.3
Sickness/diarrhoea	M	14.8	11.6	14.6	13.6
	F	19.3	30.4	23.5	24.3
Fainting/dizzines	M	3.7	5.8	6.1	4.9
	F	11.7	10.5	10.8	11.1
Constipation	M	1.1	0.0	2.4	0.9
	F	9.1	12.9	11.8	11.1
Indigestion	M	14.3	13.5	14.6	14.1
	F	17.3	25.7	22.5	21.5
Malaise					
Sleep difficulties	M	20.1	23.9	17.1	20.9
	F	27.9	17.5	21.6	22.8
Always tired	M	23.3	24.0	24.4	23.8
	F	36.5	31.0	31.4	33.4
Concentration	M	15.3	10.3	12.2	12.9
difficulties	F	19.8	8.2	12.7*	14.0
Worrying	M	9.5	9.0	4.9	8.5
	F	16.8	21.6	16.7	18.5
Nerves	M	9.0	6.5	2.4	6.8
	F	12.7	11.7	10.8	11.9
Eating difficulties	M	3.7	7.1	0.0	4.2
	F	8.1	11.1	8.8	9.4
Female					
Dysmenorrhoea		31.6	39.4	48.5+	38.1
Premenstrual tension		26.5	17.1	14.9*	20.6
Vaginal discharge		11.2	15.3	18.6	14.3

Notes: *p < 0.05

+ p < 0.01 (χ^2 trend with 1 *df*).

Source: Reprinted from West (1997, Table 3, p 847), with permission from Elsevier Science

Table 5: Self-reported symptoms (checklist) over last four weeks by social class of HoH among 14- and 16-year-olds in Northern Ireland (1997)

Symptoms (out of 12)	14-year-olds				16-year-olds			
	I/II	IIIN&IIIM	IV/V	Unclass'd	I/II	IIIN&IIIM	IV/V	Unclass'd
Mean score	4.8	4.8	4.9	5.3	4.8	5.0	4.7	6.0
Bases (n =)	292	316	138	49	344	354	147	59

A: Somatic symptoms (ie headache, aching limbs, cold, stomach ache) in last four weeks

Somatic symptoms	14-year-olds				16-year-olds			
	I/II (%)	IIIN&IIIM (%)	IV/V (%)	Unclass'd (%)	I/II (%)	IIIN&IIIM (%)	IV/V (%)	Unclass'd (%)
None or one	36	30	31	25	33	31	28	30
Two	24	26	29	24	32	28	29	26
Three or more	40	44	40	51	35	41	43	44
Bases (n=100%)	292	316	138	49	344	354	147	59

B: Affective symptoms (ie anxious, depressed, bad-tempered, lonely) in last four weeks

Affective symptoms	14-year-olds				16-year-olds			
	I/II (%)	IIIN&IIIM (%)	IV/V (%)	Unclass'd (%)	I/II (%)	IIIN&IIIM (%)	IV/V (%)	Unclass'd (%)
None or one	56	57	61	48	46	50	50	47
Two	19	17	19	20	25	22	20	16
Three or more	25	26	20	32	29	28	30	37
Bases (n=100%)	292	316	138	49	344	354	147	59

Source: Glendinning and Hendry (nd), funded by the Scottish Office, Department of Health, Grant No K/OPR/2/2 D281, in association with the Department of Sociology, University of Aberdeen

• *Physical measures:* as at all stages of the life-course, in youth *height* is directly related to social class. *Obesity*, which is not class differentiated in early youth, is by later youth. *Respiratory function* in males, but not females, is class differentiated at age 15 (Table 6) while *blood pressure* shows no relationship with social class throughout youth (Sweeting et al, 1998).

Figure 1: The age-specific incidence of head injury events per 1,000 male population by deprivation category (Scotland 1990-92)

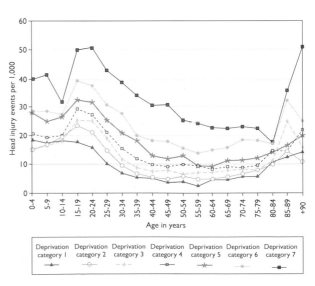

Source: Smith (1995, Figure 4.3.8)

Table 6: Physical measures by social class and sex

Health measure		NM	IIIM	IV-V	Total	Overall	Trend
Anthropometric							
Height (cm)	M	172.7	170.6	170.8	171.6	$p < 0.01$	$p < 0.01$
	F	162.9	160.5	161.6	161.7	$p < 0.001$	$p < 0.05$
Weight (kg)	M	61.6	58.6	58.6	59.9	$p < 0.01$	$p < 0.01$
	F	56.0	54.1	56.0	55.3	ns	ns
BMI (weight/height²)	M	21.0	20.6	20.8	20.8	ns	ns
	F	21.5	21.9	22.2	21.8	ns	ns
Waist/hip ratio	M	0.91	0.91	0.91	0.91	ns	ns
	F	0.82	0.82	0.82	0.82	ns	ns
Cardiovascular function							
Systolic blood	M	115.8	113.7	112.9	114.4	ns	$p < 0.05$
pressure (mm Hg)	F	108.8	108.4	110.3	108.9	ns	ns
Diastolic blood	M	66.9	65.4	64.8	65.9	ns	ns
pressure (mm Hg)	F	67.0	66.2	66.1	66.5	ns	ns
Pulse rate (beats/min)	M	71.4	69.9	70.0	70.6	ns	ns
	F	72.8	74.3	76.5	74.2	$p < 0.01$	$p < 0.01$
Respiratory function							
FEV_1 (litres)	M	3.6	3.4	3.3	3.5	$p < 0.01$	$p < 0.01$
	F	2.9	2.8	2.9	2.9	ns	ns
Standardised FEV_1 *	M	0.06	0.04	−0.06	0.00	ns	$p < 0.05$
	F	−0.03	0.01	0.03	0.00	ns	ns

Note: * Deviation from mean FEV_1, standardised for height for each sex.
Source: Reprinted from West et al (1990, Table 5, p 669), with permission from Elsevier Science

Summary

There are six main conclusions to be drawn from this overview. (i) There is no consistent pattern of association between health measures and class of background in youth. (ii) The measures most clearly related to class are mortality (principally mortality from accidents), severe chronic illness/disability, 'conduct disorder' and height. (iii) With respect to mortality and chronic illness, social class V together with the 'unclassifiable' group are distinguished as being in particularly poor health (an underclass?). (iv) The measures least related to class are symptoms, non-fatal accidents, general well-being and emotional disorders, and blood pressure. (v) Health inequalities increase between early and later youth for mortality and begin to emerge at the later period for some types of non-fatal accidents, obesity and poorer psychological well-being/emotional health. (vi) Unemployment is strongly related to poorer mental health and, though affecting fewer young people, homelessness is related to very much poorer physical and mental health. Overall, youth (particularly early youth) may be characterised as a period of relative equality in health; where inequalities exist they are generally shallower than at other stages of the life-course; where they are absent they have either yet to develop or they may have diminished relative to childhood by processes of equalisation associated with the school, peer group or youth culture (West, 1997).

Description of health behaviour (in)equalities in youth

Six health behaviours are considered: smoking, drinking, illicit drug use, diet, exercise and sexual behaviour.

- *Smoking:* evidence about the relationship between social class and smoking is equivocal, with some studies finding higher rates among lower class youth (Fogleman, 1983; Green et al, 1991), others finding no relationship (Currie et al, 1993; Glendinning et al, 1997) and still others finding higher rates among middle-class youth (Robertson et al, 1994). It is possible that class differences in smoking in youth have narrowed over time though a very recent study of rural youth (14- and 16-year-olds) in Scotland has found clear evidence of a class gradient (Glendinning, personal communication). In later youth, higher rates of smoking-are associated with unemployment (Montgomery, 1996) and homelessness (Wrate and McLauglin, 1997).
- *Drinking:* most studies have found drinking to be either unrelated to class of background (Plant et al, 1985) or more common among middle-class youth (Green et al, 1991; Currie et al, 1993) though the experience of drunkenness has been reported as higher among young people in areas of highest deprivation (Carey et al, 1996; Wallace

et al, 1998). In later youth, drinking remains largely undifferentiated by class with some groups (eg students) having particularly high levels of consumption.

- *Illicit drug use:* there has been a dramatic increase in the proportion of young people using drugs in recent years, principally for recreational purposes and associated with rave culture (cannabis, LSD and Ecstasy being the main ones). Possibly because their use is so widespread, most of the evidence suggests that there is little relationship to class of background (Barnard, 1996; Forsyth et al, 1997). In one study of 12- to 15- and 16- to 19-year-olds in Glasgow, experience of drugs was highest in the second most affluent and most deprived areas (L. Carey, personal communication). In later youth, being unemployed (Steptoe and Butler, 1996) and being homeless (Wrate and McLaughlin, 1997) are each associated with higher rates of drug use. It is possible that the consequences of drug use are more severe for lower-class than higher-class youth.

- *Diet:* of all the health behaviours, diet shows the most consistent relationship with social class. Several studies have shown that young people from lower-class backgrounds consume more fatty foods, snack foods and less fruit and vegetables (Anderson et al, 1994; Currie et al, 1994; Sweeting et al, 1994). An additional problem is associated with unemployment (Sweeting et al, 1994) and homelessness (Wrate and McLaughlin, 1997).

- *Exercise:* much less research has been conducted on this issue but what there is suggests that vigorous physical exercise is directly related to social class in early youth (Currie et al, 1993), a pattern which magnifies after school-leaving, particularly among females (Steptoe and Butler, 1996).

- *Sexual behaviour:* a wide range of heterosexual behaviours and outcomes are associated with social class in youth. Young people from lower classes are more likely to have intercourse at an earlier age (West et al, 1993; Johnson et al, 1994), lower contraceptive use (Johnson et al, 1994), higher rates of STDs (Faculty of Public Health Medicine, 1995) and higher teenage pregnancy rates (NHS Centre for Reviews and Dissemination, 1997). While teenage pregnancy should not be regarded as an inevitably negative outcome, there is evidence that young mothers experience poorer mental health (West and Sweeting, 1996).

Summary

There are five main conclusions to be drawn. (i) The relationship between social class and health behaviours is inconsistent, both between the behaviours themselves and between studies. (ii) There is some evidence that recent social changes (particularly in youth culture) may have narrowed the class gap in smoking and drug use. (iii) The clearest evidence of inequalities in health behaviours occurs for diet and exercise, with some aspects of sexual behaviour also being class-associated. (iv) Unemployment, and homelessness, involve additional risks for poor diet, smoking and drug use. (v) Some of these behaviours are associated, particularly smoking, drug use and sexual behaviour, and constitute components of life-styles that carry additional risk to health.

Other indirect risks

In addition to the effects of social class on health and health behaviours, there are a number of more indirect ways that class impacts on health. Class is related to educational achievement and attitude to school. Young people who underachieve and/or are disengaged from school are more likely to engage in life-styles involving smoking, drug use and early sexual behaviour (West and Sweeting, 1996). They are also more likely to become unemployed with the additional health risks involved. Low expectations are an additional factor affecting both health and life chances. Longer term, through a process of accumulating disadvantage and exposure to risk, they are much more likely to end up in low-status occupations, or no occupation at all, and constitute a major group contributing to the health inequalities seen in early adulthood (Power et al, 1991, 1997).

Interventions

Many of the anti-poverty strategies and interventions of relevance to the population as a whole have applicability to youth. There are, however, several areas which relate specifically to their situation.

- *Youth unemployment:* research has consistently documented the negative effect of unemployment for mental health. Although the experience of unemployment now affects young people from varied backgrounds it is much more likely among those (particularly class V) and is a major cause of health inequalities. High levels of youth unemployment also affect the expectations of young people with deleterious consequences both for their health and life-styles. Among 11-year-olds in the West of Scotland, one in five expected to be unemployed (Sweeting and West, 1996). Policies to reduce youth unemployment therefore have the highest priority and have the potential to make a major contribution to reducing health inequalities in later youth and in changing expectations in early youth. Welfare to Work must involve good training and real jobs if it is to succeed.

- *Disengaged youth:* evidence of the link between low educational achievement, 'conduct disorder', and later health inequalities highlights the problem of disengaged youth. Consideration of ways of re-engaging them has high priority. This would almost certainly involve a radical change in the meaning of 'school' for these young people, including a different use of school buildings (eg after school or holiday provision of clubs), greater emphasis on sports, a different curriculum and even different staff. An alternative view is that the school is an inappropriate place for disengaged youth and that their training needs are best met elsewhere and at an earlier age.

- *School meals:* the strongest relationship between class and health behaviours is with diet. Consideration must be given to ways in which the school can provide nutritious meals which effectively compete with the food industry and youth culture. The reintroduction of free school milk for all young people might be well received.

- *Health education:* one explanation for the 'education' effect on health behaviours is that it reflects different levels of knowledge about health risk, one component of which is health education. Reviews of school-based programmes conclude, however, that they are largely

ineffective (Michell, 1994). A similar assessment has been made of the community-based 'Smokebusters' club (Teijlingen and Friend, 1993). Most, though, are teacher- (or other adult-) led, information-based and conventional in content. There is scope for the development of much more innovative approaches, both in and out of school, involving input from youth workers, health promotion officers and peer leaders. While such programmes are relevant to all young people, they can be targeted at specific schools.

- *Health promoting school:* the health promoting school takes an holistic approach and seeks to promote health within the school context by reference to both the formal and hidden curriculum, the provision of healthfull resources (eg healthy meals) and the development of positive relationships between members of the community. A major emphasis is on the development of self-esteem and a positive view of the future. The health promoting school movement is gathering momentum, has many advocates, but has yet to be thoroughly evaluated. Evidence in support of the potential of the health promoting school comes from several studies showing wide variation in health behaviours between schools with similar intake (Swan et al, 1991). In Finland, school league tables of health behaviours like smoking are made public.

- *Health promoting youth culture:* it is well known that young people are strongly influenced by advertising and role models. More emphasis could be given to youth specific adverts and to the involvement of sports and rock stars in promoting healthy life-styles. Leisure venues could also be utilised more effectively with an emphasis on harm reduction. Youth cafes and youth pubs, in which young people have space with a minimum of adult supervision, are an interesting development.

- *Services for young people:* in general, young people are not well served, particularly in relation to mental health and GP services. Greater awareness of their needs, a youth-friendly approach and the involvement of young people in planning and running services are all warranted. The role of youth workers, as health coordinators, in areas of deprivation is worth exploring.

Acknowledgements

In preparation for this paper, the author circulated a short questionnaire to a number of researchers and health professionals relating to evidence about health inequalities in youth and interventions to reduce them. He would like to thank the following individuals for responding and/or providing additional information and in some cases new data: Marina Barnard, Joanne Barton, Neville Belton, Andy Biggart, Robin Bunton, Lynette Carey, Candace Currie, George Davey Smith, Danny Dorling, Andy Furlong, Anthony Glendinning, Hiliary Graham, Gillian Grant, Stephen Jarvis, Trevor Lakey, Mike Lean, Barbara Maughan, Neil McKeganey, Stephen Pavis, Chris Power, Debi Roker, David Stone, Helen Sweeting, Liz Towner, Edwin van Teijlingen, Lawrence Weaver and Daniel Wight. Data from the SARS were provided by the Census Microdata Unit, University of Manchester, with support from the ESRC, JISC and DENI. Thanks go to Tracey Schofield for preparing data for Table 3 used here. Patrick West is supported financially by the Medical Research Council of Great Britain.

References

Anderson, A., Macintyre, S. and West, P. (1994) 'Dietary patterns among adolescents in the West of Scotland', *British Journal of Nutrition*, vol 71, pp 111-22.

Barnard, M. (1996) *An analytical review of recent surveys of drug misuse among young people in the United Kingdom*, Glasgow: Centre for Drug Misuse Research, University of Glasgow.

Bennett, D.L. (1985) 'Young people and their health needs: a global perspective', *Seminars in Adolescent Medicine*, vol 1, no 1, pp 1-14.

Bijur, P.E., Kurzon, M., Hamelsky, V. and Power, C. (1991) 'Parent-adolescent conflict and adolescent injuries', *Developmental and Behavioural Paediatrics*, vol 12, no 2, pp 92-8.

Blane, D., Bartley, M., Davey Smith, G., Filakti, H., Bethune, A. and Harding, S. (1994) 'Social patterning of medical mortality in youth and early adulthood', *Social Science & Medicine*, vol 39, pp 361-6.

Carey, L., Farrow, K. and Thornton, A. (1996) *Drugs and alcohol: A prevalence study of 12-15 year olds in Greater Glasgow*, Health Promotion Department, Greater Glasgow Health Board.

Currie, C.E., Todd, J. and Thomson, C. (1994) *Health behaviours of Scottish schoolchildren, Report 4: The cross national perspective: Scotland compared to other European countries and Canada*, Edinburgh: RUHBC.

Currie, C.E., Todd, J. and Wijckmans, K. (1993) *Health behaviours of Scottish schoolchildren Report 2: Family peer, school and socio-economic influences*, Edinburgh: RUHBC and HEBS.

Currie, C., Elton, R.A., Todd, J. and Platt, S. (1997) 'Indicators of socio-economic status for adolescents: the WHO Health Behaviour in School-aged Children Survey', *Health Education Research*, vol 12, no 3, pp 385-97.

Davey Smith, G., Blane, D. and Bartley, M. (1994) 'Explanations for socio-economic differentials in mortality', *European Journal of Public Health*, vol 4, pp 131-44.

Dennehy, A., Smith, L. and Harker, P. (1997) *Not to be ignored: Young people, poverty and health*, London: CPAG.

Drever, F. and Whitehead, M. (1997) *Health inequalities: Decennial supplement*, ONS Series DS, No 15, London: The Stationery Office.

Faculty of Public Health Medicine (1995) *Guidelines for health promotion No 42: Sex education for young people*, Royal College of Physicians of the UK, 4 St Andrews Place, London, NW1 4LB.

Fogleman, K. (ed) (1983) *Growing up in Great Britain*, London: Macmillan.

Fombonne, F. (1996) 'Depressive disorder: time trends and possible explanatory mechanisms', in M. Rutter and D.J. Smith (eds) *Psychosocial disorders in young people: Time trends and their causes*, Chichester: John Wiley, pp 544-615.

Forsyth, A., Barnard, M., Anderson, L. and McKeganey, N. (1997) *Levels of drug use in a sample of Scottish independent secondary school pupils*, Glasgow: Centre for Drug Misuse Research, University of Glasgow.

Furlong, A. and Cartmell, F (1997) *Young people and social change: Individualisation and risk in late modernity*, Buckingham: Open University Press.

Glendinning, A. and Hendry, L.B. (nd) *Health, lifestyles and health concerns of rural youth: 1996-98*, Aberdeen: Department of Sociology, University of Aberdeen.

Glendinning, A., Hendry, L. and Shucksmith, J. (1997) 'Lifestyle, health and social class in adolescence', *Social Science & Medicine*, vol 41, pp 235-48.

Glendinning, A., Love, J.G., Hendry, L.B. and Shucksmith, J. (1992) 'Adolescence and health inequalities: extensions to Macintyre and West', *Social Science & Medicine*, vol 35, pp 679-87.

Green, G., Macintyre, S., West, P. and Ecob, R. (1991) 'Like parent like child? Associations between drinking and smoking behaviour of parents and their children', *British Journal of Addiction*, vol 86, pp 745-58.

Hawton, K., Fagg, S. and Hawkins, M. (1993) 'Factors associated with suicide after parasuicide in young people', *British Medical Journal*, vol 306, pp 1641-4.

Johnson, A.M., Wadsworth, J., Wellings, K. and Field, J. (1994) *Sexual attitudes and lifestyles*, London: Blackwell Scientific.

Jones, G. and Wallace, C. (1992) *Youth, family and citizenship*, Buckingham: Open University Press.

Judge, K. and Benzeval, M. (1993) 'Health inequalities: new concerns about the children of single mothers', *British Medical Journal*, vol 306, pp 677-80.

Maughan, B. and Lindelow, M. (1997) 'Secular change in psychosocial risks: the case of teenage motherhood', *Psychological Medicine*, vol 27, pp 1129-44.

Michell, L. (1994) *Smoking prevention programmes for adolescents – A literature review*, Oxford: The National Adolescent and Student Health Unit.

Montgomery, S.M. (1996) *The relationship of unemployment with health and health behaviour among young men*, PhD Thesis, City University, London.

Morrow, V. and Richards, R. (1996) *Transitions to adulthood: A review of research*, York: Joseph Rowntree Foundation.

NHS Centre for Reviews and Dissemination (1997) 'Preventing and reducing the adverse effects of unintended teenage pregnancies', *Effective Health Care Bulletin*, vol 3, no 1.

Plant, M.A., Peck, D.F. and Sammel, F. (1985) *Alcohol, drugs and school leavers*, London: Tavistock.

Power, C., Manor, O. and Fox, J. (1991) *Health and class: The early years*, London: Chapman and Hall.

Power, C., Hertzman, C., Matthews, S. and Manor, O. (1997) 'Social differences in health: life-cycle effects between ages 23 and 33 in the 1958 British birth cohort', *American Journal of Public Health*, vol 87, no 9, pp 1499-503.

Roberts, I. and Power, C. (1996) 'Does the decline in child injury mortality vary by social class? A comparison of class specific mortality in 1981 and 1991', *British Medical Journal*, vol 313, 28 September, pp 784-6.

Robertson, W., Bedford, S., Gabb, A., Parfitt, D. and Field, N. (1994) 'Smoking prevalence in 15-16 year old pupils in Solihull, 1987-93: impact on health education practice', *Health Education Journal*, vol 53, pp 375-84.

Rutter, M. and Smith, D.J. (eds) (1995) *Psychosocial disorders in young people: Time trends and their causes*, Chichester: John Wiley.

Smith, G. (1995) *Head injury in Scotland: An epidemiological study of mortality and morbidity 1990-1992*, Thesis, Department of Public Health, University of Glasgow.

Steptoe, A. and Butler, N. (1996) 'Sports participation and emotional well-being in adolescents', *Lancet*, vol 347, pp 1789-92.

Swan, A.V., Murray, M. and Jarrett, P. (1991) *Smoking behaviour from pre-adolescence to young adulthood*, Aldershot: Avebury.

Sweeting, H. and West, P. (1996) *The health of 11 year olds in the West of Scotland: Results from the First Stage of the 11-16 Study: Teenage health*, Glasgow: MRC Medical Sociology Unit, Glasgow University.

Sweeting, H., Anderson, A. and West, P. (1994) 'Socio-demographic correlates of dietary habits in mid to late adolescence', *European Journal of Clinical Nutrition*, vol 48, pp 736-48.

Sweeting, H., Lever, A. and Macintyre, S. (1998) 'Correlates of blood pressure at age 18 in a cohort of Scottish adolescents', *Journal of Epidemiology & Community Health*, vol 52, pp 133-4.

Teijlingen, E.R. van and Friend, J.A.R. (1993) 'Smoking habits of Grampian School children and an evaluation of the Grampian Smoke Busters Campaign', *Health Education Research Theory & Practice*, vol 8, no 1, pp 97-108.

Wallace, S.A., Crown, J.M., Cox, A.D. and Berger, M. (1998) *Epidemiologically based needs assessment: Child and adolescent mental health*, Winchester: Wessex Institute of Public Health.

West, P. (1988) 'Inequalities? Social class differentials in health in British youth', *Social Science & Medicine*, vol 27, no 4, pp 291-6.

West, P. (1997) 'Health inequalities in the early years: is there equalisation in youth?', *Social Science & Medicine*, vol 44, no 6, pp 833-58.

West, P. and Sweeting, H. (1990) 'Young people's lifestyles; origins and consequences for health, health behaviour and transitions to adulthood', Paper presented at EHSMS Conference, Budapest.

West, P. and Sweeting, H. (1996) 'Nae job nae future: young people and health in a context of unemployment', *Health and Social Care in the Community*, vol 4, no 1, pp 50-62.

West, P., Wight, D. and Macintyre, S. (1993) 'Heterosexual behaviour of eighteen year olds in the Glasgow area', *Journal of Adolescence*, vol 16, no 4, pp 367-96.

West, P., Macintyre, S., Annandale, E. and Hunt, K. (1990) 'Social class and health in youth: findings from the West of Scotland Twenty-07 Study', *Social Science & Medicine*, vol 30, pp 665-73.

Williams, J.M., Currie, C.E., Wright, P., Elton. R.A. and Beattie, T.F. (1997) 'Socio-economic status and adolescent injuries', *Social Science & Medicine*, vol 44, no 12, pp 1881-91.

Woodroffe, C., Glickman, M., Barker, M. and Power, C. (1993) *Children, teenagers and health: The key data*, Buckingham: Open University Press.

Wrate, R.M. and McLaughlin, P. (1997) *Feeling bad: The troubled lives and health in young homeless people in Edinburgh*, Edinburgh: The Young People's Unit, Royal Edinburgh Hospital.

Wyn, J. and White, R. (1997) *Rethinking youth*, London: Sage Publications.

3

Adults of working age (16/18 to 65 years)

David Blane

Executive summary

General

Tackle motor vehicle traffic accidents and suicide for quick response reductions in health inequalities during the years of working life. For longer-term, but larger, reductions modernise welfare policies to prevent the accumulation of disadvantage and relaunch occupational health services to tackle new challenges. In addition, simple proposals concerning nicotine replacement, greengrocers in deprived areas and benefit shortfall should be subject to formal testing.

Policy recommendations

1 **Policy**   **Transfer responsibility for occupational road accidents to the Health and Safety Commission.**

 Benefits   • Would draw attention to a major occupational hazard which is at present largely unrecognised.

 • Would reduce motor vehicle traffic accidents by controlling those which effect manual workers in particular.

 Evidence   An estimated one third or more of road traffic accident (RTA) deaths and injuries are occupational and long distance drivers have comparable accident risks to coal miners.

 A 'Workplace Health and Safety' approach has been shown to reduce occupational road accidents.

2 **Policy**   **Invest in the training and employment of community psychiatric nurses.**

 Benefits   • Would reduce the suicide rate among disadvantaged social groups.

 Evidence   A Cochrane review of community mental health team management for those with severe mental illnesses and disordered personality suggests that such management reduces the incidence of violence and self-harm.

3 **Policy**   **Invest in high quality training for young and long-term unemployed (eg NVQ qualifications, cognitive-behavioural training and free childcare/nursery education).**

 Benefits   • Would prevent the accumulation of social, and consequently health, disadvantage among a highly vulnerable population.

 Evidence   Training to NVQ level will, to some extent, compensate for the loss of apprenticeships; a randomised controlled trial (RCT) suggests that cognitive-behavioural therapy may usefully repair the loss of self-esteem; historical and international experience shows that childcare is a crucial factor in parental behaviour.

4 Policy   Revitalise occupational health and safety.

Benefits • Would improve control of the presently prioritised physicochemical hazards, benefiting particularly manual workers.

• Would encourage control of the new hazards associated with the new patterns of work, which effect most employees and women workers in particular.

Evidence The combination of medical research (providing the knowledge base), legislation (providing the institutional framework) and workplace organisation (providing the local motive force) has in the past successfully reduced occupational accidents and diseases. It seems likely that a similar combination of medical research, legislation and workplace organisation will be required to meet the health challenge of new patterns of work.

5 Policy   Nicotine replacement on prescription.

Benefits • Might encourage smoking cessation, particularly among those exempt from prescription charges.

Evidence Successful smoking cessation is aided modestly by nicotine replacement. A large proportion of smokers attempt cessation at some time. Policy needs formal testing.

6 Policy   Waive rates for greengrocers in deprived areas.

Benefits • Might improve impoverished people's access to fresh fruit and vegetables.

Evidence Lack of locally available fresh fruit and vegetables may be one reason for their low consumption by people on low incomes. Policy needs formal testing. (It is assumed, despite sometimes conflicting evidence, that increased consumption will improve health.)

7 Policy   Reduce benefit shortfall through primary care intervention.

Benefits • Would, almost by definition, benefit only those on the lowest incomes. One of the few sources of substantial sums of money which have been budgeted for in the public finances, but not spent.

Evidence 'Reverse-J' cross-sectional relationship between income and health. Formal testing is required to establish causality and appropriateness of primary care as intervention site.

Evidence of socio-economic inequalities in health

The risk of an adult dying before the statutory retirement age is influenced by their social class position. This applies to both men and women, to each age group within adulthood and to the overwhelming majority of the most prevalent causes of death. Other aspects of health, such as the absence of disease and a healthy physiological state, show a broadly similar relationship with social class (Drever and Whitehead, 1997).

Inequality and deprivation are related but separate ideas which can be used to describe this phenomenon. The choice of concept has practical consequences because it affects the policy focus. When social class differences in health are seen as a form of inequality the whole social structure is brought into focus. This interpretation is supported by the way in which health differences are graded across the whole social hierarchy. The chances of premature death, for example (see Table 1), increase in a stepwise gradient from social class I (professionals) to social class V (unskilled), rather than being higher only among a disadvantaged minority. The concept of deprivation, in contrast, tends to focus attention on a disadvantaged or excluded minority. The mortality rates of social class V, which are markedly higher than those of other manual workers, and have improved least during the 20th century (Blane et al, 1997), could justify an additional emphasis on deprivation, as could evidence that mortality rates are rising among some age groups in the poorest areas of Britain (Phillimore et al, 1994; McLoone and Boddy, 1994).

Table 1: Age-specific mortality rates, by social class, men aged 20-64, all causes (England and Wales, 1991-93)

Social class	20-24	25-29	30-34	35-39	40-44	45-49	50-54	55-59	60-64
					(rate per 100,000)				
I – Professional	98	91	142	228	373	704	1,186	2,057	3,735
II – Managerial and Technical	139	146	197	279	380	722	1,230	2,148	3,992
IIIN – Skilled (non-manual)	158	181	319	448	600	1,125	1,773	2,975	5,414
IIIM – Skilled (manual)	219	221	279	429	619	1,141	1,989	3,521	6,736
IV – Partly skilled	195	260	325	485	681	1,244	2,020	3,491	6,227
V – Unskilled	368	489	660	950	1,334	2,047	3,430	5,534	9,341
England and Wales	246	250	307	425	579	1,035	1,745	2,966	5,181
Percentage classified	67	77	83	87	90	92	94	95	96

Source: Drever and Whitehead (1997, Table 8.3, p 98), by permission of the Office for National Statistics © Crown Copyright

Social class differences in premature death are widest in relative terms during early adulthood and become narrower as retirement age approaches. Class V has 4.5 times the mortality rate of class I in 30- to 34-year-old men, four times the mortality rate at ages 35 to 39 years and 2.5 times at ages 60 to 64 years (Table 1). This relative narrowing with age has theoretical and practical significance.

Its practical significance emerges when the causes of death are analysed using measures which take account of both the number of deaths and the age at which these deaths occur. Accidental and violent deaths tend to occur during the earlier years of working life, so they are responsible for the loss of approximately the same number of years of working life as ischaemic heart disease and malignant neoplasms (Table 2). In terms of years of potential life lost, accidents and violence also show a marked social class gradient (Blane et al, 1990). As accidents and violence could respond quickly to prevention, they should be an important target for interventions to reduce health inequalities, particularly among men where the absolute levels of risk from these causes are higher.

A life-course perspective is required to understand the other causes of death, apart from accidents and violence, which are preceded by chronic disease processes; most prevalently ischaemic heart disease, malignant neoplasms, respiratory diseases and stroke (Kuh and Ben-Shlomo, 1997; Marmot and Wadsworth, 1997). Physiological status and mortality risk at middle and older age are related to the amount of previous exposure to social disadvantages such as manual occupation, no educational qualifications and poor quality residence (Mare, 1990; Wunch et al, 1996; Davey Smith et al, 1997). In the West of Scotland Collaborative Study, for example, a wide range of measures of health are graded by the proportion of life spent in the manual social class group (Table 3).

Risk factor status and cause of death during adulthood may vary in their relationship to the life-course. Forms of behaviour which are risk factors for cardiovascular disease (cigarette smoking and recreational exercise) are related in the West of Scotland Collaborative Study to adult but not childhood social position. Most physiological risk factors, on the other hand (diastolic blood pressure, serum cholesterol concentration, lung function), are related to both childhood and adult social class, although more strongly to the latter (Blane et al, 1996). Plausibly, behaviour is influenced by the norms of current social position while physiological status reflects both past and especially present experience. Cause of death analyses in the same study show that adult stroke and stomach cancer mortality are particularly strongly associated with childhood social position: that adult coronary heart disease and respiratory disease mortality are associated with both childhood and adult social position, and that adult mortality due to accidents and violence and cancers other than stomach are predominantly associated with adult social position

Table 2: Annual age-adjusted rate of years of potential life lost per 1,000 population for principal causes of death in men aged 20-64 in England and Wales for 1970-72, 1979-80 and 1982-83, and 1991-93 (standardised to population of England and Wales, 1981)

Social class	1970-72	1979-80, 1982-83	1991-93
All causes of death			
I	48.7	36.5	28.0
II	51.9	42.2	31.6
IIIN	65.0	53.9	45.7
IIIM	66.0	58.0	50.5
IV	75.6	67.7	52.8
V	103.0	105.8	93.3
*Death from ischaemic heart disease**			
I	15.3	11.1	6.1
II	16.3	13.6	7.1
IIIN	21.2	17.9	10.6
IIIM	19.9	18.4	12.5
IV	20.5	19.7	12.8
V	22.8	26.7	20.4
Death from all malignant neoplasms+			
I	12.5	10.0	9.2
II	12.7	10.9	9.3
IIIN	14.8	13.0	12.2
IIIM	17.1	15.1	14.1
IV	17.9	16.2	13.6
V	20.7	21.6	19.3
Death from accident and violence‡			
I	8.5	7.1	5.5
II	9.1	8.1	6.4
IIIN	9.4	9.3	9.0
IIIM	10.7	11.2	11.9
IV	14.1	14.5	12.3
V	24.5	27.8	26.6

Notes: * ICD-9 codes 410-414.
+ ICD-9 codes 140-208.
‡ ICD-9 codes E800-E999.
Source: Blane and Drever (1998, p 255)

(Davey Smith et al, 1998). The stroke and stomach cancer findings are particularly significant because the large, unexplained fall in their mortality rates during the past 50 years may be an unintended consequence of 20th-century policy initiatives, stretching back to the 1904 Interdepartmental Committee, designed to improve the health and nutrition of children.

The life-course approach to adult disease does not give priority to any particular phase of life such as childhood, but stresses instead the way biological and social risk accumulate throughout life. There may, however, be critical transitions where social policy may prevent disease by preventing the further accumulation of risk. Critical transitions during the years of working life include entry to the labour market, leaving the parental home and establishing own residence, start of parenthood, job insecurity,

change or loss, onset of chronic illness and exit from labour market (Bartley et al, 1997). Social policies in relation to these events are relevant to health inequalities and need to be scrutinised from this point of view.

Explanations of health inequalities

The types of explanation of health inequalities identified by the Black Report (Black et al, 1980) have been clarified by subsequent research. The Office for National Statistics (ONS) (formerly Office of Population Censuses and Surveys [OPCS]) Longitudinal Study has helped to settle many of the issues. The design of the Longitudinal Study means that its estimates of the size of social class differences in mortality (Harding, 1995), and its demonstration that these socio-economic differentials are widening (Filakti and Fox, 1995), can no longer be dismissed as

Table 3: Health status according to cumulative social class and relative death rates (95% confidence intervals) by cumulative social class, adjusted for age and risk factors (values are-age adjusted means or proportions unless stated otherwise)

	All three non-manual	Two non-manual, one manual	Two manual, one non-manual	Total	All three manual	P value for trend
			Cumulative social class based on occupation			
Age at screening (years)*	47.5	47.7	48.6	48.6	48.2	<0.0001
Blood pressure (mm Hg)						
Systolic	131.1	132.2	134.1	136.1	134.1	<0.0001
Diastolic	82.4	83.1	84.1	84.7	83.9	<0.0001
Cholesterol (mmol/l)	6.3	6.1	5.8	5.7	5.9	<0.0001
Height (cm)	176.0	174.4	172.6	170.8	172.8	<0.0001
Body mass index	24.7	25.1	25.4	25.3	25.2	<0.0001
FEV_1 (%)	99.4	98.0	94.0	90.3	94.2	<0.0001
Percentage (No) of subjects						
With angina	4.4 (39)	5.4 (57)	6.5 (77)	7.5 (176)	6.3 (349)	0.0002
With electrocardiographic ischaemia	5.9 (55)	5.2 (57)	6.1 (74)	5.9 (143)	5.9 (329)	0.64
With bronchitis	0.6 (5)	0.5 (6)	2.9 (35)	3.4 (79)	2.2 (125)	<0.0001
Who had never smoked+	20.0 (194)	22.1 (254)	18.1 (209)	14.5 (330)	17.7 (987)	<0.0001
Who were current smokers+	45.4 (435)	46.8 (522)	55.4 (649)	63.5 (1,471)	55.3 (3,077)	<0.0001
Who were ex-smokers+	30.6 (289)	27.7 (306)	22.9 (270)	20.5 (482)	24.2 (1,347)	<0.0001
Average no of cigarettes smoked per day‡	19.6	18.3	19.2	18.9	19.0	0.58
Percentage (No) of subjects						
Who drove cars regularly	69.3 (669)	57.5 (646)	54.3 (632)	40.8 (938)	51.8 (2,885)	<0.0001
Living in area of residence of deprivation category 5-7	18.6 (173)	32.0 (354)	54.3 (638)	66.0 (1,539)	48.6 (2,704)	<0.0001
All causes						
Age	1	1.29 (1.08 to 1.56)	1.45 (1.21 to 1.73)		1.71 (1.46 to 2.01)	<0.0001
Age and risk factor§	1	1.30 (1.08 to 1.57)	1.33 (1.11 to 1.60)		1.57 (1.33 to 1.85)	<0.0001
Cardiovascular causes						
Age	1	1.51 (1.16 to 1.98)	1.90 (1.47 to 2.45)		1.94 (1.53 to 2.45)	<0.0001
Age and risk factor§	1	1.57 (1.20 to 2.05)	1.78 (1.37 to 2.31)		1.92 (1.51 to 2.45)	<0.0001
Cancer						
Age	1	1.04 (0.76 to 1.42)	1.06 (0.78 to 1.44)		1.44 (1.11 to 1.87)	0.001
Age and risk factor¶	1	1.04 (0.76 to 1.42)	1.01 (0.74 to 1.37)		1.34 (1.03 to 1.75)	0.009
Non-cardiovascular, non-cancer causes						
Age	1	1.31 (0.84 to 2.03)	1.16 (0.75 to 1.82)		1.75 (1.20 to 2.56)	0.002
Age and risk factor¶	1	1.30 (0.83 to 2.02)	1.02 (0.65 to 1.60)		1.42 (0.97 to 2.09)	0.09

Notes: *Not age adjusted.

+ Excluding 154 men who smoked a pipe or cigars and two men with missing data.

‡For current cigarette smokers only.

§ Adjusted for age, smoking, diastolic blood pressure, cholesterol concentration, body mass index, adjusted FEV_1, angina, bronchitis, electrocardiographic ischaemia.

¶ Adjusted for age, smoking, body mass index, adjusted FEV_1 and bronchitis.

Source: Davey Smith et al (1997)

possible artifacts of numerator-denominator bias. The Longitudinal Study has also largely settled the question of health selection by showing that it does not take place in the numbers and on the scale required to generate the observed inequalities (Goldblatt, 1989). Indeed the most recent evidence, based on the 1991 Census question concerning long-standing illness, suggests that health-related social mobility constrains or moderates the size of social class differences in health, rather than creating them or adding to their size (Bartley and Plewis, 1997). These new findings are potentially important because they could explain why health inequalities do not widen with increasing age (see above) as health-damage, due to, for example, lifelong cigarette smoking, accumulates.

Explanation of health inequalities must consequently be sought in terms of the types of explanation described by the Black Report as behavioural/ cultural and materialist. An early estimate of the contribution of the former type of explanation was provided by the Whitehall I Study's finding that differences in risk factors between the various grades of the Civil Service accounted for one third of the variation in the grades' relative risk of death from coronary heart disease (Marmot et al, 1984). This estimate of approximately one third of class differences in health being due to behavioural factors has proved resilient (Kunst, 1997). More recently, however, the issue of behaviour has been conceptualised usefully as comprising: (i) behaviour which is freely chosen or a personal preference; and (ii) behaviour which is conditioned by material circumstances (Mheen et al, 1998). In relation to nutrition, for example, this model would distinguish between (i) disliking fresh fruit; (ii) being unable to afford fresh fruit, or little or poor quality fresh fruit being available in local shops. A study which used this distinction found that 30-40% of health inequalities were due to behavioural factors and that, of this proportion, more than half was due to the influence of material circumstances on behaviour (Stronks, 1997).

Occupational factors contribute importantly to materialist explanations of inequalities during adult life. Large changes in the structure and organisation of work, however, mean that new concerns must be added to occupational health's traditional emphasis on the physicochemical hazards of manual work. A large proportion of paid employment now consists of white-collar work in offices. An impressive body of research has demonstrated in this setting that psychosocial factors are important determinants of health and particularly the risk of developing coronary heart disease (Siegrist, 1996; Marmot et al, 1997; Theorell et al, 1998). Labour market flexibility and segmentation into core and periphery mean that a large proportion of employees experience unemployment and job insecurity. Research is beginning to identify the health effects of these aspects of work (Bartley, 1994; Ferrie et al, 1995; Vahtera et al, 1997) and to situate them within a life-course perspective (Montgomery et al, 1996). The

female labour force participation rate is still rising; women currently make up some 40% of the workforce, approximately one half of female employees hold part-time contracts and women, whether in paid employment or not, continue to perform the great majority of domestic labour. The effects on the health of women of combining formal and domestic labour is emerging as an important but still under-researched area (Bartley et al, 1992; Weatherall et al, 1994).

Likely beneficial interventions to reduce inequalities in health

General points

- A policy response is demanded by widening health inequalities (Drever and Whitehead, 1997) and rising mortality rates among some of the most disadvantaged (Phillimore et al, 1994; McLoone and Boddy, 1994).
- Effective policies will need to improve health *and* differentially benefit manual workers and their families; policies which do not possess both characteristics may inadvertently widen health inequalities.
- An unprecedented level of research into health inequalities is currently under way and will be reporting over the next few years; the fruits of this investment by the Economic and Social Research Council, the Department of Health and the European Union, among others, needs to be fed into the policy process. Recognition of these opportunities should not be taken as an excuse to 'wait and see' (ie do nothing), but as requiring an ongoing policy mechanism which can absorb new information and use new resources as they become available.
- Policy proposals are more likely to be implemented if they relate to existing programmes (eg nursery education) and initiatives (eg Social Exclusion Unit).

Accidents and violence

Their marked social class gradient, their absolute importance in terms of years of potential life lost and their potential to respond rapidly to prevention make accidents and violence an intervention priority.

Motor vehicle traffic accidents and suicide are the two largest groups within this general category of causes of death.

Motor vehicle traffic accidents could be addressed by recognising:

- that the roads are the only setting in which the worlds of work and domesticity mingle in an unregulated manner;
- that a large but unrecorded proportion of motor vehicle traffic accidents involve trucks, vans and company cars and should be regarded as workplace accidents;
- that the accident risk of long distance driving is comparable with that of coal mining (RoSPA, 1997) and falls predominantly on manual workers (RoSPA, 1997);
- that pedestrians and cyclists are at greater risk than drivers from traffic accidents (RoSPA, 1996) and consequently are deterred from these healthy, cheap and sustainable forms of behaviour;
- that occupational road accidents should be separately registered and responsibility for preventing them should be brought within the powers of the Health and Safety Commission and Executive (including liability to the proposed new crime of corporate manslaughter);
- that a traffic policy which included the provision of safe and motor-free walking and cycling routes would prevent accidents and encourage low-cost exercise among all age groups, so addressing health problems such as obesity and osteoporosis.

Suicide could be addressed by recognising:

- that it is often preceded by major psychiatric illness, clinical depression or substance, particularly alcohol, misuse;
- that *Health of the nation* targeting has already given priority to this area;
- that the suicide rate is falling at older ages but rising among young people, arguably as a result of unemployment and scant prospects of satisfactory work;
- that employment policy is therefore relevant to suicide prevention (and, given workplace bans on cigarette smoking, also to smoking cessation);
- that community mental health teams may be able to prevent violence and self-harm (P. Tyrer, J. Coid, S. Simmonds, P. Joseph and S. Marriott, draft Cochrane review: Community mental

health team management for those with severe mental illnesses and disordered personality, personal communication) and that community psychiatric nurses are key personnel (Gournay and Brooking, 1995);

- funds to expand the training and employment of community psychiatric nurses should be a priority when new health service funding becomes available.

Life-course

Policy interventions need to:

- recognise that those most at risk of disadvantaged outcomes at any critical transition are likely to have experienced other disadvantages earlier in their lives (for example, those most at risk of unemployment during early adulthood are likely to have had a materially or emotionally deprived childhood – Montgomery et al, 1996);
- act as both safety nets, by preventing the accumulation of further disadvantage, and springboards, by maximising the chances that critical transitions will result in beneficial change (Bartley et al, 1997) (for example, enabling unemployed young adults to obtain a craft or technical training rather than unskilled work);
- modernise existing programmes to act as springboards, which may include addressing the physical and psychological sequelae of earlier disadvantage (in relation to the young and long-term unemployed for example, a springboard approach might include training to National Vocational Qualification level and a group training programme – Proudfoot et al, 1997).
- a springboard approach to the whole range of social welfare policies would be a most effective way to reduce health inequalities because it would, almost by definition, most benefit those at greatest risk of poor health.

Work

This is an area which should be considered for a major initiative. The old institutions of Workplace Inspectorate and Safety Representatives atrophied under the previous administration and labour market change has produced new challenges. A new knowledge base is needed to establish the health effects of a flexible labour market and workloads which combine domestic and formal labour and to test the most effective methods of preventing psychosocial job strain. The institutions of Inspectorate and Representatives need to be revitalised and expanded to implement this new knowledge, to take on new responsibility for the road safety of commercial vehicles and to police effectively the existing physicochemical priorities of musculoskeletal disorders, occupational lung disease, noise and dermatitis. Integrating these initiatives by establishing an occupational health service within the NHS should be considered.

Specific initiatives, for trial

Nicotine gum and patches on prescription: would it increase smoking cessation rates among people on low incomes? Would it quickly become self-financing so that prescription access can be limited to one week or one month? *Waive rates for greengrocers in deprived areas:* would easier local access to fresh fruit and vegetables increase the consumption of these foods by people on low incomes? *Welfare benefit advice in primary care:* annually £1.5bn-£3.0bn of budgeted and entitled benefit is unclaimed by those with least income (DSS, 1995). Would reducing this shortfall improve the health of the affected households? Would primary care be an appropriate place from which to address this problem and with what accuracy can households at risk of benefit shortfall be identified from a general practice patient list? What proportion of those not claiming their entitled benefit could be helped to do so by the Jarman computerised programme in their surgery waiting room plus the option of assistance from a welfare rights worker? (See Van Oorschot, 1995.) The York Review (NHS Centre for Reviews and Dissemination, 1998) identified this as a potentially valuable intervention which requires more rigorous investigation.

References

Bartley, M. (1994) 'Unemployment and ill health: understanding the relationship', *Journal of Epidemiology and Community Health*, vol 48, pp 333-7.

Bartley, M. and Plewis, I. (1997) 'Does health-selective mobility account for socioeconomic differences in health? Evidence from England and Wales, 1971 to 1991', *Journal of Health and Social Behaviour*, vol 38, pp 376-86.

Bartley, M., Blane, D. and Montgomery, S. (1997) 'Health and the life course: why safety nets matter', *British Medical Journal*, vol 314, pp 1194-6.

Bartley, M., Popay, J. and Plewis, I. (1992) 'Domestic conditions, paid employment and women's experience of ill-health', *Sociology of Health and Illness*, vol 14, pp 313-43.

Black, D., Morris, J.N., Townsend, P. and Smith, C. (1980) *Inequalities in health: Report of a research working group* (Black Report), London: DHSS.

Blane, D. and Drever, F. (1998) 'Inequality among men in standardised years of potential life lost, 1970-93', *British Medical Journal*, vol 317, p 255.

Blane, D., Bartley, M. and Davey Smith, G. (1997) 'Disease aetiology and materialist explanations of socioeconomic mortality differentials', *European Journal of Public Health*, vol 7, pp 385-91.

Blane, D., Davey Smith, G. and Bartley, M. (1990) 'Social class differences in years of potential life lost: size, trends and principal causes', *British Medical Journal*, vol 301, pp 429-32.

Blane, D., Hart, C., Davey Smith, G., Gillis, C., Hole, D. and Hawthorne, V. (1996) 'Association of cardiovascular disease risk factors with socioeconomic position during childhood and during adulthood', *British Medical Journal*, vol 313, pp 1434-8.

Davey Smith, G., Hart, C., Blane, D. and Hole, D. (1998) 'Adverse socioeconomic conditions in childhood and cause-specific adult mortality: prospective observational study', *British Medical Journal*, vol 316, pp 1631-5.

Davey Smith, G., Hart, C., Blane, D., Gillis, C. and Hawthorne, V. (1997) 'Lifetime socioeconomic position and mortality: prospective observational study', *British Medical Journal*, vol 314, pp 547-52.

Drever, F. and Whitehead, M. (eds) (1997) *Health inequalities*, ONS Series DS No 15, London: The Stationery Office.

DSS (Department of Social Security) (1995) *New official estimates of income-related benefit take-up*, December.

Ferrie, J., Shipley, M., Marmot, M., Stansfeld, S. and Davey Smith, G. (1995) 'Health effects of anticipation of job change and non-employment: longitudinal data from the Whitehall II study', *British Medical Journal*, vol 311, pp 1264-9.

Filakti, H. and Fox, J. (1995) 'Differences in mortality by housing tenure and by car access from the OPCS Longitudinal Study', *Population Trends*, vol 81, pp 27-30.

Goldblatt, P. (1989) 'Mortality by social class, 1971-85', *Population Trends*, vol 56, pp 6-15.

Gournay, K. and Brooking, J. (1995) 'Community psychiatric nurses in primary care', *British Journal of Psychiatry*, vol 165, pp 231-8.

Harding, S. (1995) 'Social class differences in mortality of men: recent evidence from the OPCS Longitudinal Study', *Population Trends*, vol 80, pp 31-7.

Kuh, D. and Ben-Shlomo, Y. (eds) (1997) *A life course approach to chronic disease epidemiology*, Oxford: Oxford University Press.

Kunst, A. (1997) *Cross-national comparisons of socio-economic differences in mortality*, Rotterdam: Erasmus University.

McLoone, P. and Boddy, F.A. (1994) 'Deprivation and mortality in Scotland, 1981 and 1991', *British Medical Journal*, vol 309, pp 1465-9.

Mare, R.D. (1990) 'Socio-economic careers and differential mortality among older men in the United States', in J. Vallin, S. D'Souza and A. Palloni (eds) *Measurement and analysis of mortality: New approaches*, Oxford: Clarendon Press, pp 362-87.

Marmot, M.G. and Wadsworth, M.E.J. (eds) (1997) 'Fetal and early childhood environment: long-term health implications', *British Medical Bulletin*, vol 53, no 1.

Marmot, M.G., Shipley, M.J. and Rose, G. (1984) 'Inequalities in death; specific explanations of a general pattern', *Lancet*, vol i, pp 1003-6.

Marmot, M.G., Bosma, H., Hemingway, H., Brunner, E. and Stansfeld, S. (1997) 'Contribution of job control and other risk factors to social variations in coronary heart disease incidence', *Lancet*, vol 348, pp 909-12.

Mheen, H. van de, Stronks, K., Looman, C. and Mackenbach, J.P. (1998) 'Does childhood socio-economic status influence adult health through behavioural factors?', *International Journal of Epidemiology*, vol 27, pp 431-7.

Montgomery, S., Bartley, M., Cook, D. and Wadsworth, M. (1996) 'Health and social precursors of unemployment in young men in Britain', *Journal of Epidemiology and Community Health*, vol 50, pp 415-22.

NHS Centre for Reviews and Dissemination (1998) *Review of the research on the effectiveness of health service interventions to reduce variations in health*, University of York: CRD.

Phillimore, P., Beattie, A. and Townsend, P. (1994) 'Widening inequality of health in northern England, 1981-91', *British Medical Journal*, vol 308, pp 1125-8.

Proudfoot, J., Guest, D., Carson, J., Dunn, G. and Gray, J. (1997) 'Effect of cognitive-behavioural training on job-finding among long-term unemployed people', *Lancet*, vol 350, pp 96-100.

RoSPA (Royal Society for the Prevention of Accidents) (1996) *Risk reduction for vulnerable road users*, Birmingham: RoSPA.

RoSPA (1997) *Managing occupational road risk*, Birmingham: RoSPA.

Siegrist, J. (1996) 'Adverse health effects of high effort-low reward conditions', *Journal of Occupational Health Psychology*, vol 1, pp 27-41.

Stronks, K. (1997) *Socio-economic inequalities in health: Individual choice or social circumstances*, Rotterdam: Erasmus University.

Theorell, T., Tsutsumi, A., Hallqvist, J., Reuterwall, C., Fredlund, P., Emlund, N. and Johnson, J. (1998) 'Decision latitude, job strain and myocardial infarction', *American Journal of Public Health*, vol 88, pp 382-8.

Vahtera, J., Kivimaki, M. and Pentti, J. (1997) 'Effect of organisational downsizing on health of employees', *Lancet*, vol 350, pp 1124-8.

Van Oorschot, W. (1995) *Realising rights*, London: Avebury.

Weatherall, R., Joshi, H. and Macran, S. (1994) 'Double burden or double blessing? Employment, motherhood and mortality in the longitudinal study of England and Wales', *Social Science & Medicine*, vol 38, pp 285-97.

Wunch, G., Duchene, J., Thiltges, E. and Salhi, M. (1996) 'Socio-economic differences in mortality: a life course approach', *European Journal of Population*, vol 12, pp 167-85.

4

Inequalities in health: older people

Kay-Tee Khaw

Executive summary

General

Inequalities in health that are demonstrable earlier in life continue throughout the lifespan. Inequalities in health in older people are often neglected for a number of reasons. Firstly, the relative paucity of data past retirement age often means that existence of the issue is not properly acknowledged; additionally, disability rather than mortality may be a more appropriate health outcome in elderly people but is more difficult to assess. Nevertheless, all available data indicate that inequalities persist; while the relative inequality may be similar in old age, because rates of ill-health are much greater in older people, the absolute inequalities may actually be much greater. Secondly, because of the undoubted influence of earlier life experiences on health, there is a misconception that health inequalities in elderly people are less amenable to successful intervention or remedy. However, the evidence indicates that many interventions may have substantial and direct benefits in later life. More problematic are the value judgements that reducing health inequalities in later life may be of less benefit to society and hence, of lower priority. Quite apart from issues of social justice and ethics, it could be argued that, with an ageing population, improving health in later life will contribute substantially towards supporting independence and reducing disability and dependency, with benefits for all of society.

This paper focuses on inequalities in health within the population of older people in Britain, but we should remember the widespread inequality experienced by older people as a group compared to younger age groups in many areas, including access to health services as well as policies aimed at maintaining health and well-being. Additionally, while inequalities in health within a population need remedies, in the context of international comparisons, countries which have better overall health status at older ages than Britain demonstrate what is still potentially achievable for the whole population

While there is good evidence for specific interventions and health-related outcomes, evidence that, at the policy level, a specific policy will achieve a particular end is much less clear: it is a matter of opinion and judgement, and policies themselves need critical evaluation. It would appear to be more important to focus on the main aims, as different policies may be similarly effective at achieving such aims.

Policy aims

Many of the policies to reduce inequalities for younger people will also have an impact in later life. The major aims of policies are improvement of those factors which appear to explain a substantial proportion of, and hence, that are most likely to reduce, health inequalities in older people.

Aim *Improvement of income in the poor elderly*

Two thirds of pensioners have incomes below the tax threshold. Low income and its consequences – limited access to adequate diet, housing, transport, services, and care – is a fundamental source of many of the health inequalities in older people.

Policy **Measures that ensure adequate incomes or pensions after retirement age through public or personal schemes.**

Aim *Improving factors which determine health*

Some of the adverse consequences of low income can be mitigated by ensuring equitable access to those factors which determine health. These include the following.

Aim *Equitable access to acute and long-term healthcare which is not determined by ability to pay or by geographic residence*

This includes not just hospital care but also community medical and social services such as primary healthcare and general practice, dental services, chiropody, physiotherapy and rehabilitation, attention to sight and hearing, promotion of continence.

Policy **Ensuring that access is not determined by ability to pay as is now increasingly the case; also equitable distribution of such services around the country.**

Policy **Often, those who are most likely to need care are those who are most unlikely to afford, or be eligible for, private insurance schemes (eg the poorest and frailest elderly people), and some sort of national scheme is necessary.**

Aim *Adequate and affordable diets should be available and accessible*

Policy **Policies on food taxation, pricing and subsidies which encourage intake of fresh fruit and vegetables rather than high-saturated fat and high-sodium foods; working with the food industry to reduce sodium and fat in processed foods; legislation on labelling and nutrient content of foods; advertising standards.**

Policy **Town planning should consider siting and types of shops, ensuring access and/or appropriate transport for elderly residents.**

Aim *Adequate, safe and warm housing*

Policy **Policies that encourage energy efficient housing; support maintenance and quality of housing (eg capital release schemes); planning and design of housing in communities.**

Aim *Maintenance of mobility, independence and social contact*

While acute services are important, there is a lack of investment in services in which the benefits are less obvious, but which may prevent acute events and maintain independence in the community, such as continence and mobility, home aids, etc.

Policy **Planning of housing in the community needs to consider access to local shops and facilities for elderly people.**

Policy **Affordable and accessible public transport.**

Policy **Investment in services that support independent living for elderly people.**

Policy **Information, advice and advocacy for older groups.**

Aim	*Clean environments including reduced air pollution and food safety*
Policy	**Legislation on the environment including car and industrial pollution.**

Aim	*Reduce tobacco smoking*
Policy	**Taxation and pricing, controls on advertising and sponsorship.**

Introduction

Inequalities in health that are demonstrable earlier in life continue throughout the life span to the end of life. Unfortunately, inequalities in health in older people are often neglected for a number of reasons. Firstly, there is a lack of reliable, routinely collected data on social class or proxy markers such as income or past occupation after the age of retirement, and dearth of data often means that the existence of the issue is not properly acknowledged. Nevertheless, all available data indicate that inequalities persist. While the relative inequality may be similar in old age, because rates of ill-health are much greater in older people, the absolute inequalities may actually be much greater. Secondly, there is the misconception that health inequalities in elderly people are less amenable to successful intervention or remedy; however, the evidence indicates that many interventions may have substantial benefits in later life. More problematic are the value judgements that reducing health inequalities in later life may be of less benefit to society and, hence, of lower priority. Quite apart from issues of social justice and ethics, it might be argued that, with an ageing population, improving health in later life will contribute substantially towards supporting independence and reducing dependency, with benefits for the whole of society.

This paper focuses on inequalities in health within the population of older people in Britain. Although not within the remit of this paper, we should be reminded that a crucial issue is the widespread inequality experienced by elderly people as a group compared to younger age groups in many areas,

including access to health services as well as policies aimed at maintaining health and well-being. Additionally, while inequalities in health within a population need remedies, they should also be viewed in the context of international comparisons: the international variation in the health of older people highlights the substantial potential for improving health for elderly people in Britain. For example, even people in social class I in Britain have much higher rates of coronary heart disease than the national average for the same age group in Spain or France.

Evidence of inequalities in health in older people

Good health encompasses more than simply an absence of disease and in the full sense implies social as well as physical and psychological well-being. In older cohorts, particularly, prevention of disability rather than mortality per se may be the major focus. Disability and handicap encompass functional as well as social components and may also be related to several concurrent health conditions. Therefore, disability and disease, do not directly correspond, although they are closely related (Kriegsman et al, 1997). Nevertheless, mortality statistics which are routinely available —often in the absence of better standardised data – are a good proxy indicator of overall health status and most often used. Generally, the term older people encompasses those aged 65 years and older, which is the standard work retirement age for men and now women in Britain.

The marked inequalities in health by socioeconomic status which are so clearly demonstrable in younger cohorts are not as easily identified from routine vital statistical data since there is a lack of reliable data after retirement on past occupation. Hence, social class data are not reliable. Yet all available evidence indicates that the social class inequalities apparent earlier in life persist throughout life, even post-retirement. For example, life expectancy at birth differs by three years for women and five years for men between social classes I/II and IV/V. Even at age 65 the differential between social classes I and V is two to three years (see Table 1).

Table 1: Life expectancy at birth, age 15 and age 65, by social class (1987-91)

	At birth	Life expectancy At age 15	At age 65
Men			
Social class I/II	74.9	60.5	15.0
Difference between I/II and			
IIIN	-1.3	-0.7	-0.9
IIIM	-2.5	-2.4	-1.6
IV and V	-5.2	-4.7	-2.6
Women			
Social class I/II	80.2	65.8	18.7
Difference between I/II and			
IIIN	-0.8	-0.5	-0.4
IIIM	-2.6	-2.6	-1.9
IV and V	-3.4	-3.4	-2.0

Source: Adapted from Hattersley (1997)

While identifying social class per se in persons over 65 years of age is problematic because of retirement, there are many other indicators of socio-economic status which may be used. These include residential district or region, housing tenure and access to cars (see Table 2). Table 3 shows the independent effects of social class, housing tenure and car access on Standardised Mortality Ratios in men and women in three age groups. Table 3, based on absolute rates derived from Smith and Harding (1997) also shows the relative and absolute differences; the absolute impact of the differences is greater in the older age groups where rates are higher.

Table 2: All-cause Standardised Mortality Ratios by social class, access to cars and housing tenure at the 1971 Census, women and men, all causes

	Ages					
	45-64		65-74		75+	
Social class	W	M	W	M	W	M
Non-manual social class						
With car						
Owner-occupier	70	72	71	75	81	82
Privately rented	82	83	84	89	90	82
Local authority	93	96	86	90	97	95
Without car						
Owner-occupier	91	99	84	95	90	98
Privately rented	105	129	108	111	95	102
Local authority	125	120	98	118	92	107
Manual social class						
With car						
Owner-occupier	85	82	86	83	88	93
Privately rented	100	93	91	100	100	104
Local authority	101	104	101	104	97	105
Without car						
Owner-occupier	99	101	101	103	96	102
Privately rented	128	132	110	114	104	109
Local authority	131	126	122	122	107	116

Source: Adapted from Marmot and Shipley (1996); Smith and Harding (1997)

Table 3: Age-standardised death rates per 1,000 people by housing tenure in the 1971 Longitudinal Study cohort

	Death rates per 1,000 (1981-92)		
Age at death	Death rate per 1,000	Relative risk	Absolute difference death rate/1,000
Men			
35-44 years			
Owner-occupiers	1.60	1.00	-
Private renters	2.24	1.40	0.64
LA tenants	2.51	1.57	0.91
45-59 years			
Owner-occupiers	9.99	1.00	-
Private renters	13.19	1.32	3.20
LA tenants	13.76	1.38	3.77
60-74 years			
Owner-occupiers	43.31	1.00	-
Private renters	53.20	1.23	9.89
LA tenants	57.77	1.33	14.46
75+ years			
Owner-occupiers	130.55	1.00	-
Private renters	144.73	1.11	14.18
LA tenants	153.23	1.17	22.68
Women			
35-44 years			
Owner-occupiers	0.92	1.00	-
Private renters	1.04	1.13	0.11
LA tenants	1.16	1.26	0.24
45-59 years			
Owner-occupiers	3.22	1.00	-
Private renters	4.32	1.34	1.10
LA tenants	5.07	1.57	1.95
60-74 years			
Owner-occupiers	14.65	1.00	-
Private renters	8.38	1.25	3.73
LA tenants	20.53	1.41	5.88
75+ years			
Owner-occupiers	77.83	1.00	-
Private renters	86.88	1.12	9.05
LA tenants	89.90	1.16	22.07

Note: LA = local authority.

Source: Adapted from Smith and Harding (1997)

Table 4: All-cause mortality per 1,000 person years, attributable risk and rate ratio by employment grade and age at death

	Age at death (years)		
Grade	40-64	65-69	70-89
Administrative	4.7	17.4	32.6
Professional and executive	7.3	17.3	44.8
Clerical	12.4	26.7	65.4
Other	17.6	32.1	70.9
Attributable risk			
Other versus administrative	12.9	14.7	38.3
Rate ratio			
Other versus administrative	3.12	1.73	1.86

Source: Adapted from Marmot and Shipley (1996)

5

Table 5: Life expectancy and healthy life expectancy (HLE) at age 65 in standard regions of England and Wales

	Men			Women		
	Disability rate/ 1,000	Life expectancy	HLE	Disability rate/ 1,000	Life expectancy	HLE
North	141	13.6	7.5	152	17.3	9.3
Yorkshire and Humberside	131	13.9	7.8	148	17.8	9.4
East Midlands	119	14.3	8.5	136	18.1	10.1
East Anglia	99	15.1	9.5	120	18.8	11.2
South East	95	15.0	9.5	117	18.7	11.2
Greater London	111	14.5	8.9	134	18.6	10.7
South West	104	15.1	9.5	121	19.0	11.3
West Midlands	120	14.0	8.2	140	18.0	9.9
North West	139	13.6	7.6	155	17.3	9.3
Wales	158	14.1	7.4	166	18.1	9.4

Source: Adapted from Bone et al (1995)

Not only do unfavourable circumstances in mid-life affect health outcomes in later life, but those who, in later life, lose earlier advantages also have worse health outcomes. Fletcher et al (1997), using data from the Longitudinal Study, reported that men and women in rented accommodation without access to a car had an approximately 50% higher mortality rate compared to those in owner-occupation with a car. Moving from owner-occupation to rented accommodation, loss of a spouse and, for men, loss of access to a car were all associated with increased mortality. The risk of institutional residence was much higher for women than men over the 20-year follow-up. People who had the most favourable socio-economic indicators in 1971 (owner-occupation and car access) had the lowest risk of being in an institution 20 years later, but loss of favourable indicators in retirement was still associated with an increased risk.

Longitudinal studies also provide a means of examining the impact of socio-economic factors after retirement age. A 25-year follow-up of civil servants from the first Whitehall study found that socio-economic differences in mortality persist beyond retirement age and increase with age. Social differential in mortality based on an occupational status measure seemed to decrease to a greater degree after retirement than those based on a non-work measure, suggesting that, although work itself might play an important part in generating social inequalities in health in men of working age, after retirement other factors might have a more important role (see Table 4).

Variations by residential areas or regions – which are often used as proxy indicators of socio-economic status – are as marked in those aged 65 years and over as in younger cohorts (see Table 5). Ethnic differences are also evident (Table 6). Regression analyses show the factors which explain differences in healthy life expectancy of different local authority areas and include high prevalence of low social class, as well as unemployment (Table 7).

Table 6: Synthetic estimates of life expectancy and HLE by age sex and ethnic group

	Mortality rate per 10,000	Limiting long-standing illness (%)	HLE (years)
Men			
Black			
65-74	439	37.8	6.7
75+	1,962	49.5	2.6
Indian subcontinent			
65-74	37	40.7	9.4
75+	840	40.7	9.4
White and other			
65-74	374	34.1	9.1
75+	1,054	45.7	5.2
Women			
Black			
65-74	300	42.3	7.8
75+	1,185	54.9	3.8
Indian subcontinent			
65-74	306	43.3	8.0
75+	1,111	53.6	4.2
White and other			
65-74	207	30.81	11.3
75+	803	50.6	6.2

Source: Adapted from Bone et al (1995)

Table 7: Analysis of factors affecting mean HLE rates of local authority areas

Factor	Beta coefficient	
	Men	Women
Social classes IV and V (%)	-0.29	-0.34
Unemployment rate (%) Population sparsity	-0.53	-0.40
Retirement migration (per million)	-0.14	-0.11
Non-white population (%)	0.39	0.22

Source: Adapted from Bone et al (1995)

Specific causes of mortality variations

In Britain, in men and women of working age, consistent gradients by socio-economic status can be seen for most major causes of deaths. There is a threefold variation for both stroke and ischaemic heart disease between social classes I and V for men. Diseases of the respiratory system show fivefold variation between social classes I and V, with greatest differences for chronic airway obstruction, bronchitis and emphysema. Of the cancers, lung and stomach cancer show the greatest social class differential (four- and threefold variation respectively between social classes I and V; in contrast, breast and colon cancer have little variation. Data in men and women after retirement age, while less routinely available, confirm the patterns noted in younger age groups. The widest range of mortality levels by socio-economic status are found for lung cancer and respiratory disease, as well as ischaemic heart disease and stroke (Drever et al, 1997; Harding et al, 1997, Smith and Harding, 1997).

Morbidity

Morbidity is more difficult to assess since those that rely on self-reports or doctor visits may be biased by differential thresholds for reporting or access to care by social class. Morbidity estimates based on objective measures are less likely to be biased in this way. The percentage of those reporting long-standing illness from the General Household Survey is consistently higher in manual compared to non-manual groups at all ages in women and in men aged 16 to 65 years. In men, there is no clear trend after age 65 years. In contrast, acute sickness shows no clear socio-economic trend. The prevalence of any neurotic disorder shows a marked gradient for women with increasing prevalence and decreasing social class; in men, social class I had approximately

half the rates of neurotic disorder compared to social classes II to V (Bunting, 1997).

Table 8 shows accident rates by social class, where a gradient is apparent.

Table 8: Annual accident rates per 100 by age, sex and social class

	Men		Women	
	Manual	Non-manual	Manual	Non-manual
65-74	7	10	13	16
75+	13	10	12	22

Source: Adapted form Bunting (1997)

Many measures of functional and physiological health also vary by social class; Table 9 shows prevalence of disability and Table 10 shows prevalence of low measures of respiratory function and high blood pressure by social class. The different distribution of respiratory function and blood pressure by social class are also reflected in the mortality rates for respiratory and cardiovascular disease (Prescott-Clarke et al, 1997).

Dental health also varies markedly (see Table 11). This differential is most marked in the old: in those aged 75 years and over, the percentage with total tooth loss varied from 27% in the professional class to 84% in the unskilled manual class, with gradient in between (Bunting, 1997). This is important in view of the role nutritional inequalities play in explaining health inequalities.

Table 9: Observed prevalence of disability by social class

	Social class of head of household					
	I	II	IIINM	IIIM	IV	V
Men						
Prevalence of disability						
one or more	10	15	17	21	20	29
Serious	3	2	3	5	4	8
Women						
Prevalence of disability						
one or more	10	13	22	18	23	33
Serious	2	3	5	5	6	8

Source: Adapted from Prescott-Clarke et al (1997)

Table 10: Prevalence of those with lung function below predicted level >1 sd by social class and prevalence of those with high blood pressure (BP) and mean BP by social class in men and women aged 65 years and over

	I	II	IIINM	IIIM	IV	V
Social class of head of household						
Men and women						
FEV₁ <1sd predicted level	22	23	23	34	35	32
FVC	17	19	18	28	29	25
Men 65+						
Systolic BP	147	149	150	150	150	156
Diastolic BP	80	81	80	81	81	84
% with high blood pressure	15.5	19.0	21.2	19.7	20.3	24.2
Women 65+						
Systolic BP	154	154	155	156	156	158
Diastolic BP	80	78	78	78	80	80
% with high blood pressure	21.9	20.0	23.3	24.1	25.4	26.0

Source: Adapted from Prescott-Clarke et al (1997)

Table 11: Adults with no natural teeth by socio-economic group (1993) (%)

Professional	3
Employers and managers	11
Intermediate and junior non-manual	12
Skilled manual and own account non-professional	19
Semi-skilled manual and personal services	23
Unskilled manual	33

Source: Adapted from Bunting (1997)

Health-related behaviours

The National Food Survey reported that consumption of most foods was related to income. Comsumption of cheese, fish, fruit and alcohol rose with income; consumption of milk and cream, meat, eggs, fats, sugar and preserves, vegetables, cereals and beverages increased with decreasing income. Old age pensioners showed some consumption patterns similar to the extreme of low-income groups, that is, with high consumption of fats, eggs, meat products, cereals, sugar and preserves. In particular, consumption of and expenditure on fats showed a negative relationship and fruits a positive relationship with increasing income. Intake of nutrients such vitamins (eg vitamin C, carotenoids and folate), minerals (iron, zinc, calcium, potassium and magnesium) are lower in the poor. Antioxidant intakes among the poorest fifth of families have declined dramatically over the last 15 years (Gregory et al, 1990; Bunting, 1997; Prescott-Clarke et al, 1997). Ethnic differences are also apparent: persons

of Afro-Caribbean origin have lower vitamin C intakes than Caucasians, and Asians have the lowest vitamin C levels of all. Sodium and potassium consumption also appear to vary by region and social class, although not always consistently. Williams and Bingham (1986) reported higher urinary mean excretion of sodium from men in manual social classes but little difference by social class in women. The National Dietary and Nutritional Survey reported regional differences in mean urinary excretion of sodium in men but not women, with highest levels in Scotland and the Northern region. In contrast, urinary potassium excretion is clearly associated with social class and region, with highest levels in social classes I and II and the southern regions (Prescott-Clarke et al, 1997).

Smoking prevalence shows a sharp socio-economic gradient with 16% of men and 12% of women in the professional group but 40% of men and 34% of women in the unskilled manual group reporting a smoking habit. Obesity body mass index [BMI] over 30 also increases with decreasing social class (Prescott-Clarke et al, 1997).

Physical activity patterns also differ. In those of working age within the work environment, men in the manual social classes are more than three times likely to have high physical activity than those in non-manual classes; there is no marked social class gradient for physical activity at home or by occupation for women. However, men and women in the non-manual social classes are more likely to take part in high level physical activities outside the workplace than those in manual occupations. Data by social class for those aged over 65 are not available. However, it is more likely that occupational physical activity will cease more abruptly after retirement than activity outside the workplace, so after retirement, overall levels of physical activity from walking and sports are greater in non-manual than in manual social classes.

Inequalities in access to healthcare

The socio-economic inequalities in health status in elderly people are compounded by inequalities in access to services. Numerous studies have reported age discrimination in health services for a wide range of conditions as well as variations within age groups. Seymour and Garthwaite (1996), examining inguinal hernia surgery in men and Scotland, reported inequity of referral to healthcare on the basis of age as well as inequity by deprivation category. Similar examples have been reported for a wide variety of conditions including acute medical and surgical interventions such as cancer treatment (England has the worse survival rate from many cancers compared to other European countries, and large socio-economic differences) or cardiac procedures as well as procedures such as ophthalmic surgery (there is a threefold geographical variation in over 65s across England; see Jones et al, 1996) and hip replacement. To take one example, the 10-year survival rate for breast cancer for women in the wealthiest quintile of society is much higher than the five-year survival rate for women in the poorest quintile (Schrijvers et al, 1995a, 1995b).

Functional capacity relies on sight, hearing, mobility and continence. Major causes of visual impairment in the elderly – glaucoma, cataracts and refractive problems – are amenable to treatment or amelioration, but studies have revealed substantial non-recognition of severe visual problems in particular demographic groups: old age, low socio-economic status and ethnic group (particularly being Afro-Caribbean) (Jones et al, 1996; Wormald et al, 1992). There are numerous examples of other inequalities: 90% of elderly patients in need receive no specialist treatment for incontinence (McGrother et al, 1997) and only a third of older people who might benefit from rehabilitation currently have a hearing aid (Herbst, 1996). The lack of coordination between statutory services affect the most disadvantaged and deprived sections of the community.

Summary of inequalities

Marked inequalities in health in older people can be demonstrated according to various indicators of socio-economic status including past occupational status, income, housing, car ownership, and area of residence. The specific contributors to health can be identified in terms of mortality, morbidity and disability. A large proportion of these inequalities are potentially remediable. These can be achieved through measures aimed at promoting good health by prevention of the major chronic diseases and conditions that show marked socio-economic

variations: including heart disease, stroke, respiratory diseases and many common cancers as well as dental health. While early life influences may have long-term effects, circumstances and behaviours in adult life are more likely to lie behind recent increases in inequality. Changing socio-economic status and what this entails even after retirement appears to influence health outcome. Measures include optimising diet and nutrition, mobility and ensuring adequate housing and environmental protection.

Inequalities in health also occur because of inadequate treatment and support. These include access to health and other services, for example, surgical procedures that might improve health and quality of life; appropriate support and rehabilitative care after acute hospital care; access to services for visual and hearing impairment, incontinence and mobility which may have substantial impact on independence and quality of life.

Possible interventions/policies

Maintaining health in later life

While early life experiences and health status throughout adult life influence the health of men and women when they reach older ages, there is abundant evidence that modifying life-styles and environment, or treatment of conditions at older ages have a substantial effect on elderly people's health. If anything, many interventions may in fact have greater absolute impact for elderly people. The recent increases in health inequality in the UK are mainly due to changes in circumstances and behaviour of adults rather than early life events. The major life-style influences include diet and nutrition, physical activity and cigarette-smoking habit; the environmental influences include temperature, air quality, housing and general living conditions including social support.

We already understand many of the causal factors that affect health in older people, and a substantial proportion of the socio-economic variations in health can be attributed to known variations in environmental determinants.

Diet/nutrition

Nutrition is a crucial contributor to inequalities in health at all ages, and improving nutrition provides huge potential for reducing some of the health inequalities (James et al, 1997). The relationship between nutrition and health inequalities in later life can be most clearly delineated for cardiovascular disease. Much of the three- to fourfold social class variation in coronary heart disease and stroke risk can be explained by behavioural factors including cigarette-smoking habit and diets high in sodium and saturated fat and low in antioxidants, minerals such as potassium and magnesium (derived from fruit and vegetables), and omega-3 fatty acids. These affect levels of classical risk factors such as blood pressure and cholesterol (which are higher in lower social classes) or other biological mechanisms. High intake of fruit and vegetables has been consistently demonstrated to be protective for a large number of conditions common in elderly people including cardiovascular disease, respiratory disease, many cancers, visual problems such as macular degeneration and cataracts, and variations in fruit and vegetable intake may explain some socio-economic variations. For example, the threefold regional variation in stroke rates in Britain is inversely related to fruit and vegetable consumption. Within social classes, variations exist: for example, within social class III, Standardised Mortality Ratios for coronary heart disease range from 112 for skilled workers to 54 for farmers – this may well reflect to some extent differing dietary patterns. Older people appear more sensitive to the blood pressure-elevating effects of high sodium intake and resultant stroke risk (Cappuccio et al, 1997), and cheaper processed foods are particularly high in sodium (James et al, 1997). Immune function in older people declines, predisposing to infections as well as chronic diseases. Thus, while the total calorie requirement may decline in elderly people, paradoxically, nutrient requirements may increase: nutrient-dense diets may be of particular importance in later life. Trials have shown that vitamin D and calcium supplementation in women can prevent osteoporotic fractures and that nutritional supplementation with other vitamins and minerals can improve muscle strength and immune function. Thus, good nutrition may not only prevent chronic disease in the long term, but have relatively immediate effects on functional health in elderly people. However, national nutrition surveys have demonstrated that elderly poor are particularly vulnerable to inadequate diets for many reasons. While poor dental health, which shows marked social class variation, may play a role, and is remediable, major determinants are low income and limited access.

Dowler (1997) has pointed out that most of the poor are now concentrated in inner cities, in periurban estates, and in local authority housing. In these places, small high-street food shops and street markets have more or less disappeared for a number of reasons, including changes in the food retailing sector over the past decade – superstores have increased fourfold and they are mostly outside town centres and designed for car access. The poorest urban residents do not have cars, frail elderly people cannot walk far with shopping and public transport is often inadequate. Food costs more in small stores, hence, the poorest people have to spend more because of inadequate access to cheaper food superstores. The lowest decile spend the highest proportion of their income on food (29% as opposed to 19% in the top decile) but the lowest actual amounts.

Healthy food at affordable prices has become less available for the poor and disadvantaged and desirable nutrient intakes have declined dramatically. National and local policy making must be encouraged which helps the poor to choose healthy diets and improves household access to healthy food. This includes consideration of policies on education, legislation on labelling and advertising, food subsidies and taxation, but also town planning and transport.

Cigarette-smoking habit

The adverse effects of cigarette smoking on health at all ages (including over 50 diseases) is unequivocally demonstrated. Some of the variations in health can be attributed to varying prevalence of cigarette smoking in different socio-economic groups and, again, the poor seem to be disproportionately affected. Smoking cessation, even in older people, can bring health benefits such as improved respiratory and, hence, functional capacity. Policies to end the cigarette-smoking habits are essential.

Housing and temperature

The winter excess in mortality is well documented. However, Britain has more winter excess mortality (about 20%) than many other northern countries, such as Canada or countries in Scandinavia, where winter excess mortality is approximately 7-10% despite greater variation in outdoor temperatures. Older people are more vulnerable: the winter excess increases with increasing age, with 18% excess in those aged 65-74 years and 27% excess in those aged 75 years and over. The extra risk of dying in winter is also related to socio-economic circumstances: owner-occupiers with car access have an 18% excess winter mortality rate compared to 24% in those in rented accommodation without car access. Low temperature, atmospheric pollution and influenza epidemics have been implicated in excess winter mortality (Curwen, 1997).

There is indirect evidence that indoor temperature is also important. Ambient temperature has well-documented effects on respiratory function and many cardiovascular risk factors including blood pressure and haemostasis. There is a correlation between mean indoor temperature and excess winter mortality in different countries. The poor are particularly susceptible to the effects of cold due to a combination of poor heating and energy-inefficient housing. A national survey in 1972 reported that 90% of elderly people had morning living-room temperatures below recommended levels, and 47% did not heat their homes at all. A survey of 1,000 dwellings in Scotland found mean whole-house temperatures of 14°c compared with an average of 16°c in England, 18°c in France and 21°c in Sweden (Wicks, 1978; Hunt and Gidman, 1982; Boardman, 1991; Hunt, 1997).

The poorest housing conditions are experienced by single older people living in the private-rented sector; 75% of those on the lowest incomes, living in the worst housing, are of pensionable age; approximately one million, or 22%, of households with heads aged 65 years or more live in the least energy-efficient homes; and one in five pensioners aged over 65 were found to need to spend at least 20% of their income to achieve a minimum standard of warmth (English House Condition Survey, 1991).

Affordable warmth through design and insulation of homes and adequate domestic heating is crucial. Policies must be considered that enable poorly-housed older people access to assistance to improve their homes, for example, through home improvement agencies, or equity release schemes for repairs and improvements, or to address the condition of unsatisfactory local authority housing (Harding, 1997).

Mobility, physical and mental activity and transport

The health benefits of physical activity are of particular importance in old age: not only may exercise prevent chronic disease such as cardiovascular disease, osteoporosis and diabetes, and reduce disability caused by age-related muscle weakness, and claudication, but immobility can result in increased likelihood of incontinence, deep-vein thrombosis, gravitational oedoema and skin ulceration. Immobility also leads to isolation and loneliness and continuing mental stimulation also appears to protect against dementia and depression. Men and women in non-manual social classes participate in more leisure-time physical activity. While before retirement, men in manual classes have more overall physical activity which is work-related, after retirement age, the social class pattern is likely to reverse. The causes for the differences are not known but may include living environments conducive to walking, as well as limited access to recreational activities.

Social ties have long been recognised as an important constituent of, and contributor to, health and well-being of people of all ages. Grundy (1996) has pointed out that while most older people are not socially isolated, events that are both stressful and deplete the social environment, such as bereavement, are common in later life. Both social participation as well as social support are associated with mortality and other indicators of health. Though evidence of interventions to promote social interactions are lacking, promotion of good social relationships have to be seen as self-evidently desirable. Lack of mobility may be a particular barrier to social interactions as well as maintaining mental activity in poor elderly people. Paradoxically, both urban poor and rural poor elderly groups may be disadvantaged: urban elderly through fear of crime and isolation in large housing estates, and rural poor through lack of transport. Adequate public transport for older people is a priority.

Services

There has been substantial disinvestment in many of the services that support the independent living of older people (Harding, 1997). This is manifest at many levels. Early discharge from hospital combined with lack of appropriate care on return home leads to distress for people as well as increasing emergency readmissions within 28 days of discharge, and, hence, additional costs to health services. Increased use of accident and emergency departments are a sign of inadequate care and poor home conditions.

At a different level, there are many examples of how functional capacity can be maintained or improved by appropriate care and support. These include treatments such as hip replacement, and cataract surgery, and support through visual, hearing and other living aids. Many of the inequalities in functional health and disability are due, not just to differing disease occurrence, but to demonstrably inequitable access to services and support.

Information

Many of the key national sources of statistical information on the population's health do not include people over the age of 65. This creates problems for assessing the level of health inequalities experienced by older people, for developing and planning appropriate policies and for monitoring changes over time. While available evidence indicates that inequalities in health in older people may be greater than, and just as amenable to remedy as, in younger people, the lack of information often leads to the issue being ignored or set aside. Appropriate data collection on elderly people as well as continuing research on appropriate interventions at all levels is a high priority.

References

Boardman, B. (1991) *Fuel poverty*, London: Bellhaven Press.

Bone, M.R., Bebbington, A.C., Jagger, C., Mortant, K. and Nicholaas, G. (1995) *Health expectancy and its uses*, London: HMSO.

Bunting, J. (1997) 'Morbidity and health related behaviours of adults: a review', in F. Drever and M. Whitehead (eds) *Health inequalities*, Office for National Statistics Series DS No 15, London: The Stationery Office, pp 198-221.

Cappuccio, F., Markandu, N.D., Carney, C., Stagnella, G.A. and McGregor, G. (1997) 'Double-blind randomised trial of modest salt restriction in older people', *Lancet*, vol 350, pp 850-4.

Curwen, M. (1997) 'Excess winter mortality in England and Wales with special reference to the effects of temperature and influenza', in J. Charlton and M. Murphy (eds) *The health of adult Britain 1841-1994*, London: ONS, pp 205-16.

Dowler, E. (1997) 'Nutrition and poverty in contemporary Britain: consequences for individuals and society', in B.M. Kohler, E. Feichtinger, E. Barlosius and E. Dowler (eds) *Poverty and food in welfare societies*, Berlin: Edition Sigma, pp 84-96.

Drever, F., Bunting, J. and Harding, D. (1997) 'Male mortality from major causes of death', in F. Drever and M. Whitehead (eds) *Health inequalities*, Office for National Statistics Series DS No 15, London: The Stationery Office, pp 122-42.

Fletcher, A., Slogett, A. and Breeze, E. (1997) 'Socio-economic and demographic circumstances in middle-aged and older people and subsequent health outcomes', *ONS Longitudinal Study Update*, vol 17, pp 16-23.

Gregory, J., Foster, K., Tyler, H. and Wiseman, M. (1990) *Dietary and nutritional survey of British adults*, OPCS Social Survey Division, London: HMSO.

Grundy, E. (1996) 'Social networks and support', in S. Ebrahim and A. Kalache (eds) *Epidemology in old age*, London: BMJ Publishing Group; chapter 25, pp 236-41.

Harding, S., Bethune, A., Maxwell, R. and Brown, J. (1997) 'Mortality trends using the longitudinal study', in F. Drever and M. Whitehead (eds) *Health inequalities*, Office for National Statistics Series DS No 15, London: The Stationery Office, pp 143-55.

Harding, T. (1997) *A life worth living*, London: Help the Aged.

Hattersley, L. (1997) 'Expectation of life by social class', in F. Drever and M. Whitehead (eds) *Health inequalities*, Office for National Statistics Series DS No 15, London: The Stationery Office, pp 73-82.

Herbst, K.G. (1996) 'Hearing impairment', in S. Ebrahim and A. Kalache (eds) *Epidemiology in old age*, London: BMJ Publishing Group, chapter 37, pp 344-52.

Hunt, S. (1997) 'Housing related disorders', in J. Charlton and M. Murphy (eds) The *Health of adult Britain 1841-1994*, London: ONS, pp 156-70.

Hunt, D. and Gidman, M.I. (1982) 'A national field survey of house temperature', *Building and Environment*, vol 17, pp 107-28.

James, W.T.P., Nelson, M., Ralph, A. and Leather, S. (1997) 'The contribution of nutrition to inequalities in health', *British Medical Journal*, vol 314, pp 1545-9.

Jones, H.S., Yates, J.M., Spurgeon, P. and Fielder, A.R. (1996) 'Geographical variations in rates of ophthalmic surgery', *British Journal of Ophthalmology*, vol 80, pp 784-8.

Kriegsman, D.M.W., Deeg, D.J.H., van Eijk, J.T.M., Penninx, B.W.J.H. and Boeke, A.J.P. (1997) 'Do disease specific characteristics add to the explanation of mobility limitations in patients with different chronic diseases? A study in The Netherlands', *Journal of Epidemiology and Community Health*, vol 51, pp 676-85.

McGrother, C.W., Castleden, C.M., Duffin, H. and Clarke, M. (1987) 'Do the elderly need better incontinence services?', *Community Medicine*, vol 9, pp 62-7.

Marmot, M.G. and Shipley, M.J. (1996) 'Do socioeconomic differences in mortality persist after retirement? 25 year follow up of civil servants from the first Whitehall Study', *British Medical Journal*, vol 313, pp 1177-80.

Prescott-Clarke, P., Primatesta, P., Bost, L., Dong, W., Hedges, B., Prior, G., Purdon, S. and di Salvo, P. (1997) *Health survey for England 1995*, London: The Stationery Office.

Schrijvers, C.T.M., Mackenbach, J., Lutz, J.M., Quinn, M.J. and Coleman, M.P. (1995a) 'Deprivation and survival from breast cancer', *British Journal of Cancer*, vol 72, pp 738-43.

Schrijvers, C.T.M., Mackenbach, J., Lutz, J.M., Quinn, M.J. and Coleman, M.P. (1995b) 'Deprivation at stage of diagnosis and cancer survival', *International Joutnal of Cancer*, vol 63, pp 324-9.

Seymour, D.G. and Garthwaite, P.H. (1996) 'Is there inequity of hospital referral on the grounds of age? An analysis of inguinal hernia surgery in men in Scotland', Paper presented to the British Geriatrics Society Conference, October.

Smith, J. and Harding, S. (1997) 'Mortality of women and men using alternative social classifications', in F. Drever and M. Whitehead (eds) *Health inequalities*, Office for National Statistics Series DS No 15, London: The Stationery Office, pp 168-83.

Wicks, M. (1978) *Old and cold*, London: Heinemann.

Williams, D.R.R. and Bingham, S.A. (1986) 'Sodium and potassium intakes in a representative population sample: estimation from 24h urine collections known to be complete in a Cambridgeshire village', *British Journal of Nutrition*, vol 55, pp 13-22.

Wormald, R.P.L., Wright, L.A., Courtney, P., Beaumont, B. and Haines, A.P. (1992) 'Visual problems in the elderly population and implications for services', *British Medical Journal*, vol 304, p 1226

Health inequalities: the place of housing

Richard Best

Foreword

When nearly 1,000 residents on a poor council estate in Bristol were asked 'What do you think would improve your health or the health of those who live with you?', the most common replies were 'better housing' (30%) or 'a better environment' (15%) (Ineichen, 1993). Similarly, 75% of households experiencing illness on a poor quality estate in East London felt that their ill-health had a lot to do with housing quality (Ambrose, 1996).

It may seem obvious that 'bad housing damages your health', but proving the case is not always easy. People who live in decaying, overcrowded properties are likely to be poor and face other disadvantages; the fact that they do not enjoy such good health as those in decent housing is clearly not attributable to housing conditions alone. People living in council housing are much more likely to die before the age of 65 than owner-occupiers (Goldblatt, 1990), and the incidence and severity of almost all diseases/conditions is greater for children in council housing than in owner-occupied homes (Drever and Whitehead, 1997). But it may not be the council housing that has increased the mortality and morbidity rates.

The aims of this paper are to assess the evidence for links between housing and health, and to consider what changes should be made to public policy on housing to reduce inequalities in health. The paper begins with a brief description of the types of housing problems experienced in Britain. It then reviews the latest available evidence on the link between poor housing and health. Finally, it describes and evaluates a range of policy options to improve housing in ways that should reduce inequalities in health.

Overview of housing problems

Introduction

The nation's housing problems are traditionally analysed under two headings: those of quantity and those of quality. This contribution to the debate adds a third dimension – that of location.

Shortages of affordable accommodation lead to overcrowding and homelessness. This section reviews the trends over recent years and looks ahead to the likelihood of growing shortages. The impact of overcrowding and homelessness among two key groups – single people and families – is considered.

The problems of quality are considered next. Poor conditions are manifest in the numbers of properties declared unfit for habitation or lacking in essential amenities.

Finally, in this section, the importance of location is considered: where the homes are sited may be even more important than how many are built or how good the quality is of each house or flat.

Problems of quantity

Over the last 20 years housing shortage has diminished as a national issue. Housebuilding in the private sector, and more particularly in the social (local authority and housing association) sector, has been at lower levels than in earlier decades; but a sharp decline in demolitions of existing property and relatively favourable demographic trends have meant that overall shortages have not emerged as a major issue (Figure 1).

However, during the 1990s, growth in household numbers and a muted housebuilding programme appear to point to trouble ahead. Figure 2 shows how annual output of new homes kept substantially ahead in the decades up to the 1980s; then the number of new households started to move ahead of the number of homes built and that gap has widened in the 1990s.

Figure 1: Demolitions decline dramatically (1969-93)

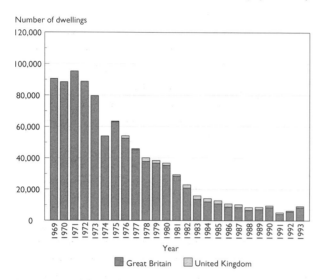

Number of dwellings

Source: Leather and Morrison (1997, Figure 7.1)

Figure 2: Annual housebuilding overtaken by household growth (1951-93)

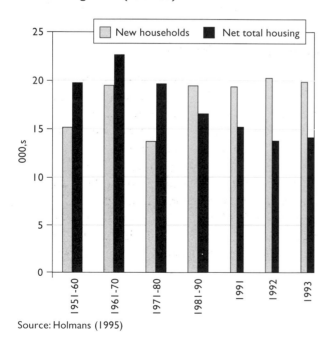

Source: Holmans (1995)

Government projections indicate that between 1991 and 2016 there will be a growth in household numbers of 4.4 million. About half of this growth (46%) comes from increased population (the second wave of 'baby boomers' growing up and having families, plus the higher number of immigrants – mostly from Europe – compared with emigrants); a third (33%) is attributable to changes in behaviour – more single-person households because of fewer marriages and more cases of divorce/separation; with most of the remainder (21%) caused by increased longevity, with homes not becoming available so quickly for the next generation (HMSO, 1996). Moreover, there is some catching up to be done with a backlog of some 500,000 households in need of accommodation at the beginning of the 1990s, because of homelessness, overcrowding or involuntary sharing (Holmans, 1995).

Assuming more homes are lost through demolitions (including of defective council estates) than are gained through conversions of one home into more, a requirement emerges for some five million new homes to be built over this 25-year period. Although this is not a high figure by comparison with earlier periods, there are new factors making it more difficult to achieve than in times past:

- Public spending constraints mean the output of subsidised housing is unlikely to return to levels of previous decades. The level of need estimated by the government for extra subsidised homes is for 60,000-100,000 pa; the numbers are put more precisely by the previous Chief Housing Economist (at the then Department of the Environment) at 90,000 homes pa for the 1990s (House of Commons Environment Committee, 1995; Holmans, 1995). But output is failing to meet even the lowest of these estimates of need (see Figure 3).

- For new homes for sale, land is more tightly constrained because (i) of resistance to building on 'greenfield' sites (by environmentalists and by local – 'NIMBY' – activists); and because (ii) the supply of desirable urban sites (which have included playing fields and open spaces) is exhausted in many areas; and because (iii) 'brownfield', recycled land is either too costly to develop or is in locations where market demand is lacking for homes for sale (Breheny and Hall, 1996).

Figure 3: Social housing falls below all assessments of need (1995/96 prices)

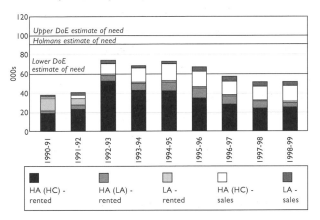

Source: Wilcox (1997)

The inhibitions on housebuilding to meet levels of need and levels of demand do not bode well for the future. If insufficient housing is built, it is those least able to exercise choice in the market-place – those who rely on subsidised housing and who are already at risk from the consequences of low incomes – who miss out. Shortages in housebuilding, even if satisfying environmental concerns to conserve the countryside, lead directly to increased overcrowding and/or homelessness: not providing the homes needed will not change the figures on numbers of new households that form (Holmans, 1995).

Homelessness: single people

Homelessness among single people is not the subject of clear recording. If this is taken to mean 'roofless', that is, people sleeping rough, a count on Census night reported relatively modest figures – 2,827 people in Great Britain (OPCS, 1991) – although the Census Office acknowledges that this is an underestimate. Nevertheless, recent audits of street homelessness indicate that the numbers of people have fallen because of the government's Rough Sleepers Initiative, which provided additional hostel and short-term rented property for people sleeping rough in central London. The London figure was down from its Census count of 1,275 to around 500 by the autumn of 1993 (Brown and Randall, 1993). However, these figures mask the true extent of shortages: a far larger number of single people are

homeless but remain hidden because they are sleeping on the floors of friends and relations, often moving from place to place. A study in the late 1980s estimated that in London alone there were at least 50,000 single people living in temporary accommodation (which might not necessarily be contrary to their wishes), or in squats or on the streets, with a further 74,000 living unwillingly as part of someone else's household (Eardley, 1989).

Surprisingly, the number of single people who are homeless in rural areas appears to be a special problem. A 1992 study for the Rural Development Commission that showed how homelessness among the statutorily defined groups had tripled in the previous four years, also indicated particular problems for young people for whom the figures are not recorded (Lambert et al, 1992).

The reasons why single people have left their previous accommodation are varied, but a study by the University of York indicated that 70% of those living rough, and 50% of those in hostels and Bed & Breakfast hotels, had previously been in some kind of institution such as a children's home, a prison or a psychiatric hospital (Anderson et al, 1993). Along with others who have left home because relationships have broken down, or are seeking work elsewhere, these single people have found that they cannot afford accommodation available on the open market.

Homelessness: families

Statistical evidence of housing shortages for families and other 'vulnerable' households is much better documented. Local authorities record the numbers of those whom they deem to have nowhere else to go, yet have not 'intentionally' made themselves homeless in order to gain priority for council housing. The number of such families showed a rapid increase from the time the statistics were first compiled in 1977 until 1991. As can be seen from Figure 4, the number of families declared homeless doubled between 1980 and 1990, but then fell in the 1990s, from its peak of about 150,000 in 1991 to around 130,000 in 1996.

Figure 4: Homelessness falls for five years

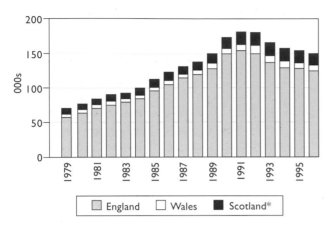

Note: * Estimated 1996 figure for Scotland.

Source: Wilcox (1997)

Figure 5: Fall in use of Bed & Breakfast accommodation (England)

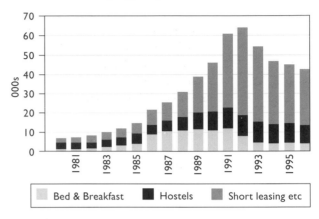

Source: Wilcox (1997)

Figure 6: Private rented growth tails off (additions to private rented stock during year in England)

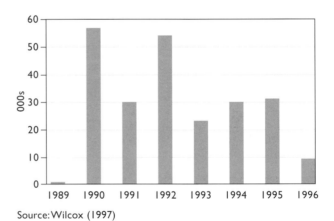

Source: Wilcox (1997)

In part, the homelessness problem was eased by a revival of the private rented sector, fuelled by Housing Benefit for those unable to pay their way. But some of this growth was attributable to the phenomenon of the 'slump landlord', the owner-occupier who let temporarily because it was not possible to achieve a sale at an acceptable price (Kemp, 1995). This source of renting seems destined to evaporate as the home ownership market picks up again (and pressure for Housing Benefit reductions squeezes profitability at the bottom end of the market).

More important than the total number of families declared homeless is the number for whom the local authority has no available housing: such households are moved into temporary accommodation which has, notoriously, often meant Bed & Breakfast hotels.

As Figure 5 shows, the number of households in Bed & Breakfast hotels – so often the least suitable accommodation – increased nearly fivefold between 1980 and 1991, but fell over the last five years. This only partly reflects the drop in the numbers accepted as homeless by local authorities: it is more to do, again, with greater use being made of accommodation in the private sector, this time through various leasing arrangements. But this switch to greater use of private renting for homeless families now looks to be coming to an end (Figure 6).

The apparently encouraging trends in homelessness – often seen as a barometer of housing shortage – need to be seen in the context of tomorrow's demographic change. Underlying shortages are beginning to accumulate when output is compared with growth in households and, with problems over the supply of suitable land and public spending constraints on social housing, there is a real danger that increased overcrowding and homelessness will follow.

Problems of quality

The quality of housing has steadily improved throughout this century. The most recent survey of stock condition is the *English House Condition Survey 1991* (EHCS) (DoE, 1993). This showed that the number of dwellings lacking basic amenities had continued its downward fall, to 1% of the stock

(205,000 homes), compared with 2.5% (463,000 homes) in 1986. But when data is drawn together from England, Northern Ireland, Scotland and Wales, the overall picture shows that one in 14 homes in the UK (rather more than 1.6 million) are unfit for human habitation (or, in Scotland, are defined as 'Below Tolerable Standard') (Figure 7). The worst problems are encountered in Wales where one in eight occupied properties are officially classified as unfit (Leather and Morrison, 1997).

Figure 7: Unfit occupied dwellings*

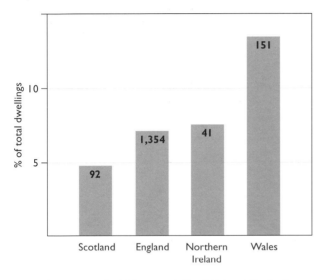

Notes: * Figures are for 1991, except Wales (1993) and Scotland are 'Below Tolerable Standard' figures.
Numbers in bars represent the total number in thousands.

Source: Leather and Morrison (1997)

Moreover, the UK has the oldest stock of homes in Europe, with one in four properties built before the end of the First World War. Yet, as shown in Figure 1, the rate at which old properties have been replaced by new homes has dropped dramatically in the past 25 years, from 91,000 to just 8,000 a year. If the present level of clearance was allowed to continue, housing in England and Wales (where clearance levels are lower than for Scotland) would theoretically have to stand for 5,600 years.

Low-income households suffer disproportionately from the state of the UK's housing. In 1991, six out of 10 households in unfit homes had incomes below £8,000 a year (roughly half the national average income). The greatest concentrations of problems were found in North East Lancashire, Manchester, Liverpool, Calderdale and cities in the Midlands. In

Scotland, poor conditions were concentrated in privately owned properties in Glasgow and in rural areas.

Older people, particularly those aged over 75, and younger people just starting their housing careers, are the groups most likely to live in poor conditions. In both England and Scotland, households where the head is from a minority ethnic community were generally more likely to live in poor conditions (Leather and Morrison, 1997).

In terms of the resources available to tackle poor housing conditions, low-income households have depended on local authority grants. However, these are no longer mandatory and, from reaching a peak in 1982-83 (when over 300,000 grants were provided across the UK), provision has slumped to about 60,000 pa in England with a similar cut in Scotland and Northern Ireland (but in Wales the decline from the mid-1980s has been less pronounced).

Grant aid for equipment and adaptations – so that frail and disabled people need not move out – after falling in the early 1990s, rose to new peaks in the mid-1990s (at rather more than £100m pa) but are now at only one third this level (Figure 8).

Figure 8: Grants for home improvements at local levels

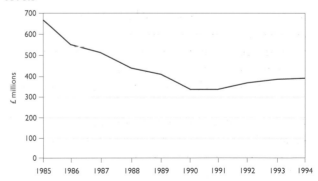

Source: Heywood and Smart (1996)

Owner-occupiers' own spending on repairs and improvements fell during the years of housing recession but may be picking up again now. Regrettably, research indicates that many people invest principally in more cosmetic types of work – such as new kitchen units – rather than in essential repairs.

In summary, this country's housing stock is ageing and needs constant investment to deal with disrepair. Low-income households have been very dependent upon local authority grants, yet these are not available in many cases. The Department of Environment, Transport and the Regions (DETR) has estimated that about 500,000 poor owners qualify for means-tested grants which are not available from their local authorities. Alternative measures to encourage private owners and landlords to carry out renovation are now needed to prevent an unwelcome deterioration in the stock.

One hopeful sign is the growth of local home improvement agencies – 'Staying Put' projects and 'Care and Repair' schemes – which help people to remain independently in their own homes, by organising necessary renovation work for them, facilitating any grants that are available and exploring ways in which the equity in the home can be released without occupiers having to sell the property and move. Some 24,000 people were helped with building work and twice as many were helped with advice, by some 224 home improvement agencies in England and Wales in 1994/95 (Leather and Rolfe, 1995). An extension of this form of support – diagnosing the problem, obtaining estimates from reliable builders, ensuring the work is carried out properly, etc – could be immensely valuable, particularly in those areas (such as the South West and Yorkshire, where little is happening at present).

On the local authority side, renovation of council housing in the 1990s was running at three times the level in the private sector: activity peaked in 1994 with almost 300,000 dwellings being the subject of renovation. This has followed from the tight budgets and restrictions on capital spending which has shifted the emphasis of housing departments away from new building toward renovation of their existing stock. But the picture is patchy, both at the regional level and between individual local authorities. Even at the simple level which ignores the wider context in which a council home is sited, substantial investment remains needed. Calculations based on the average injection of extra resources for 'catch-up repairs' for the stock transferred so far from councils to new ownership suggests that bringing all council housing to a similar standard would cost some £22bn – perhaps spread over a decade (Wilcox, 1997).

Problems of location

No home exists in a vacuum. The quality of life for its occupiers may be affected more by its environs than its condition. Occupiers may worry more about their neighbours than about the physical state of their property.

The English House Condition Survey (EHCS) says little about the environment in which individual properties are located. The EHCS statistics are blind to the conditions on a council or housing association estate, outside the front door, yet some of the greatest anxieties for residents relate to insecurity and low quality of the estate's environment.

We now know – not least from research on the characteristics of the locations where civil disorder erupted to the point of being classified as 'riots' in the 1990s – that modernising the physical strategies on a housing estate is no protection where there are concentrations of unemployed young men (Power and Tunstall, 1997).

A substantial study by Professor Brian Robson and colleagues at the University of Manchester, on the impact of government investment in some of our worst urban neighbourhoods (Robson, 1994) has shown that physical improvements are not enough. Heavy spending on the bricks and mortar can leave untouched the wider malaise affecting an area. Such investment is seldom followed by significant improvements in the statistics for crime, educational achievement, employment or health.

Over recent years, central government policy has shifted from straightforward housing goals to wider policies that seek regeneration on a broader front. Programmes such as City Challenge and support through the Single Regeneration Budget administered by Government Regional Offices, have taken a more holistic approach, seeing the improvement of housing as part of a broader strategy.

Alongside this shift in policy there have been marked changes in *where those in different income bands are living*. Broadly, population has shifted outwards from inner London and the centres of metropolitan cities, and to a lesser extent from other major urban areas, to market towns, seaside towns, villages and more remote rural areas (Champion, 1996). At the same time, those occupying rented housing provided by local authorities and housing associations have exhibited much higher levels of poverty than in the past: people moving in have tended to be families with children living on the lowest incomes (with disproportionate numbers of single parents) while those moving out have been older, with higher incomes and fewer children (Burrows, 1997). This enhanced concentration of those on the lowest incomes in particular, defined locations – estates which are usually physically distinct from owner-occupied streets – has been a major contributor to the phenomenon of 'social exclusion', that is, of sections of the population becoming segregated and separated from the mainstream, not sharing in the fruits of economic growth and increasingly cut off from the opportunities available to the majority.

The danger of the concentration of disadvantaged households on particular estates, or in confined neighbourhoods, is that local services can be overloaded with consequent increases in crime, school exclusions and, indeed, health problems which relate to social conditions. Good neighbourliness can be overwhelmed if there are too many people with problems, and too few with the economic independence, social skills or personal security to help.

It is not the case that all the unpopular estates comprise high-rise blocks or low quality prefabricated buildings. Even new estates built by housing associations have quickly become stigmatised (Page, 1993). This is particularly so where the new homes are adjacent to existing council estates (Crook, 1996). Problems have been compounded by a financial regime which has allowed (and sometimes compelled) housing associations to raise rents to levels which only those families in receipt of Housing Benefit find affordable; high rents, matched by high benefits, have then deterred the potentially economically active from taking jobs.

New measures to tackle social exclusion – centred on the government's Social Exclusion Unit – will target those 1,360 council estates where lack of opportunity is most concentrated. If the locational aspect of bad housing is to be addressed, and inner city and peripheral urban areas are not to be confined to those unable to leave, solutions must be pursued that enhance education and training, bend mainstream

programmes to address the *welfare-to-work* agenda, and build up the capacity of communities to look after their own affairs (Best, 1997a).

Links between housing and health

Introduction

The link between health and housing was clearer a hundred – or even fifty – years ago. The drive to replace slums with new homes was based on a recognition that more sanitary conditions would improve public health. Indeed, up to the time of the Second World War, the Minister of Health was responsible for the nation's housing. Today, following the eradication of epidemics spread by a lack of sanitation and clean water, we may not see the health and housing connections so clearly.

One recent study – admittedly of relatively extreme conditions – has looked carefully at housing and health connections. A survey published in November 1996 of two estates in the London Borough of Tower Hamlets, largely occupied by Bangladeshi families, included the following findings:

- over 50% of the population were sleeping in damp bedrooms;
- over one third of households suffered some infestation;
- 69% of households said the heating did not keep everyone warm enough;
- over the 150-days survey, the sample of 107 households experienced 280 illness episodes; a well-housed sample in Paddington, in contrast, had only 14% of the illness rate;
- 75% of episodes required a visit to the doctor and 65% required prescriptions;
- commonest symptoms were coughs and colds, aches and pains, asthma and bronchial problems, diet and digestive problems, stress and depression; the 20 households in the worst housing had the worst health records;
- 73% of households felt their ill-health had a lot to do with housing quality (85% mentioning damp and cold);
- GPs and health visitors saw clear connections between bad housing and ill health. (Ambrose, 1996)

It is not hard to conclude that on estates like these, investment in housing would pay dividends in reduced healthcare costs.

Two books published in 1993 – *Homes and health* by Ineichen and *Unhealthy housing* edited by Burridge and Ormandy – pull together an impressive array of evidence to explain how housing and health interact. In addition, *Health, housing and social policy* by Arblaster and Hawtin (1993) summarises the case for reducing health inequalities by improving housing conditions. Together, these studies make the case for accepting that 'bad housing damages your health'.

This section reviews the available evidence about housing and health. First, it considers the impact of homelessness on people's health. Second, it looks at the health problems caused by damp and cold housing. Next it considers how poor housing can result in fires, accidents and infestations which damage health. It then reviews the evidence more generally about the impact of housing on individuals' mental health. Finally, it looks at the centrality of housing to the success of 'Care in the Community' policies.

Homelessness and health

Few would need convincing that the extreme conditions of homelessness of sleeping rough, are bound to affect health. A 1989 study found that 25% of the people sleeping rough and in supportive housing projects reported an inpatient hospital stay in the previous year, compared with 9% of the population as a whole (Stem et al, 1989). Bronchitis, tuberculosis, arthritis, skin diseases and infections, as well as alcohol/drug related problems and psychiatric difficulties, are all more prevalent among single people who are homeless (Barry et al, 1991).

More recent research indicates that chronic chest conditions or breathing problems were three times as high among people sleeping rough as in the general population; for single people in hostels and Bed & Breakfast hotels the figure was twice that of the general population. Much the same results were discovered in relation to frequent headaches, musculoskeletal problems and difficulties in seeing (although heart problems were consistently lower among people who were homeless). The study also shows that many young people recently made

homeless do not have adequate access to healthcare. All people who are homeless are at a particular disadvantage unless special service provision is designed for them (Bines, 1994).

Families living in temporary accommodation of the Bed & Breakfast kind face a range of hazards, even if the hotel is in relatively good condition.

It is difficult to maintain hygiene while washing, eating and sleeping in one overcrowded room. High levels of gastroenteritis skin disorders and chest infections have been reported. Kitchen facilities are often absent or inadequate, so people are forced to rely on foods from cafes and take-aways, which is expensive and may be nutritionally unsatisfactory. The stress of hotel life undermines parents' relationships with each other and their children. Normal child development is impaired through lack of space for safe play and exploration. High rates of accidents to children have been reported, probably due to a combination of lack of space and hazards such as kettles at floor level. (BMA, 1987, pp 13-14)

Cold and damp homes

Perhaps the clearest evidence that poor housing has an impact on health relates to the effects of inadequate heating and dampness.

Obviously, hypothermia is related to inadequate levels of warmth. It is clear from the higher proportion of deaths in winter than in summer (and the further increase in deaths when the winter is very cold) that many older people who die as a result of respiratory disease, heart disease or a stroke have had their illness exacerbated by the cold. A survey of older people in 1988 found that 25% were not using as much heat as they would have liked because of the cost (Savage, 1988). Unmodernised older properties have far higher heating costs – mostly because of low standards of insulation – than improved and newer homes. (On a scale from 0 to 10, new homes will typically have a national home energy rating of 7-8, whereas an unmodernised Victorian house might only score 2-3 on the scale.)

Dampness in the home very clearly contributes to respiratory illness.

The house dust mite and flinal spores both thrive in damp housing conditions. The debris of that house dust mite, particularly its faecal pellets, act as an allergen and can cause chest problems such as wheezing.

Condensation, which is almost pure water, unlike penetrating or rising damp where the water contains salts, encourages the growth of fungal spores. These can cause allergies such as asthma, a runny nose (rhinitis), and inflammation of the lungs (alveolitis). (Arblaster and Hawtin, 1993, p 17)

A study in Edinburgh found that children living in homes affected by damp and mould were twice as likely to have wheezing and chesty coughs as those who slept in dry rooms. This was unrelated to smoking in the household (Strachan, 1988). In a survey of housing in Glasgow, Edinburgh and London, Platt and colleagues (1989) found higher levels of a whole range of symptoms for both children and adults in damp and mouldy houses against dry dwellings. There appeared to be a dose-response relationship, with the number of symptoms increasing with the number of housing problems. Again, the relationship was independent of smoking and socio-economic factors.

Housing and accidents

Forty per cent of all fatal accidents in the UK happen in the home; home-related accidents are the most common cause of death in children aged over one year, and almost half of all accidents to children are associated with architectural features in and around the home (DTI, 1991). Households in disadvantaged circumstances are likely to be the worst affected by such accidents (Constantinides, 1988).

Those living in high-rise buildings are more prone to serious accidents, such as falling from windows and balconies. Coroners' records for England and Wales show that in 1973-76 children living above the first floor were 57 times more likely to be killed by falling than children in accommodation on the ground and first floors. Moreover, the danger of fire spreading through tower blocks is well known to fire brigades.

The Child Accident Prevention Trust has noted that families living in temporary accommodation are particularly likely to suffer accidents in the home: accommodation in Bed & Breakfast hotels and similar housing is notoriously ill-designed, ill-equipped and ill-maintained (CAPT, 1989).

Construction techniques and health

The industrialised building techniques of the early 1960s and 1970s have left a legacy – sometimes compounded by poor maintenance which will create problems for years to come. As well as damp and condensation – from buildings that were poorly insulated and are difficult to heat economically – the construction of this era has proved particularly prone to infestation by cockroaches, which thrive in warm, wet conditions. The risk to tenants from such infestation comes from germs transferred from house to house, from allergy (caused by the bodies of dead cockroaches remaining in ducting), from the use of pesticides to kill the cockroaches, and from stress caused by the infestation (Freeman, 1993).

The descriptions given in Box A of system-built tower blocks – frequently constructed with low-quality materials and poor workmanship – in Belfast and Manchester could be applied in a hundred other towns and cities.

> **Box A: Divis Estate in Belfast**
>
> Cracks in the cladding, poorly constructed joints, ill-fitting windows, cold bridging between slabs, and poor insulation made the flats cold and damp. Flat roofs encouraged penetrating damp. Asbestos had been widely used for insulation, including blue asbestos rope around the window panels. Calcium chloride had been added to the cement to speed the drying time, and when the concrete later cracked water-penetrated and chloride ions attacked the steel supporting beams. There were problems with the sewerage system, and flooding was common. Rats and cockroaches colonised cracks in the structure. (Lowry, 1990, p 390)
>
> **Hulme Estate in Manchester**
>
> The ducts, heated by the hot water pipes, became warm, moist environments, often contaminated with sewage, as soil pipes began

to develop leaks. These conditions of high temperature and humidity are ideal for cockroach development, reproduction and movement and soon immense populations of German cockroaches built up.... The local authority was eventually forced to carry out whole-block saturation pesticide application....

... the health effects of this cockroach infestation ... should be considered. The tenants suffered the risk of pathogens carried on to food by the cockroaches. They also suffered the possibility of cockroach allergy ... considerable stress and inconvenience and will have been subjected to pesticide exposure....

... a cockroach infestation which is now merely controlled, eradication not being possible, has caused, and will continue to cause, danger to the health of occupants.

Housing and environmental factors

The quality of the environment affects all of us. Where housing is built will influence levels of traffic congestion and pollution, the likely levels of car use (to schools, jobs, services). How houses are built will have varying impacts on the levels of natural resources that are used – particularly from non-sustainable sources – and the amount of mineral extraction and manufacturing required for the materials. The building process will also expose the workforce to differing levels of harmful chemicals.

Design will greatly influence energy efficiency, leading to varied levels of carbon dioxide emissions, as well as affecting the cost to occupiers of their heating. Use of solar energy, large glazed windows facing south, levels of roof/floor/wall insulation, the efficiency of heating systems, will all make a difference. Decisions will be taken by housebuilders and providers on whether building materials should achieve low maintenance, whether conversions of existing property (including buildings previously occupied by commercial or industrial uses) will take precedence over new development, on the amounts of water which will be used by the building's systems, on the provision of facilities for separation of waste and the energy-efficiency of any white goods installed: all these factors will affect the housing's

long-term impact on the environment, and therefore, ultimately on the health of the planet.

Other volumes address issues of sustainability and energy conservation in new and existing homes; this paper simply notes this link between housing and health (Rudlin and Falk, 1995; EDAW, 1997).

Housing and stress

Statistics are less helpful in establishing a clear link between housing and stress-related illness. Nevertheless, there are good grounds for believing that the many aspects of poor housing listed above create anxiety and mental suffering when endured for prolonged periods. Poor sound insulation between neighbouring homes, as well as a lack of privacy and overcrowding, are all likely to contribute to mental health problems. In an analysis of housing and health in Edinburgh, Glasgow and London, Hunt (1990) found that indicators of emotional stress were much more common for both adults and children in the presence of adverse housing conditions.

Since women spend more time in the home, bad housing affects them to a greater degree. Interviews with women over many years have noted the relationship between their mental health and overcrowding, neighbourhood noise and poor structural conditions (Gabe and Williams, 1993).

Housing and care

Residents of nursing homes, residential care and specialist hostels fall outside the definition of 'housing' used for this paper. (Although some social housing landlords provide accommodation in institutional settings as well as in self-contained homes and many are seeking ways of breaking down barriers between the two, for example, through providing sheltered housing, residential care and nursing within the same premises.) However, the work of housing and health professionals intertwines in the context of community care and the meeting of so-called 'special needs' in straightforward housing.

The government White Paper, *Caring for people*, acknowledged that "housing is a vital component of community care and it is often the key to independent living" (DoH, 1989, p 25); policies for care in the community depend upon suitable home environments. Here the connection between health and housing relates to the role of the home in avoiding the need for a disruptive move away from familiar surroundings or from informal carers, and/or contributing to recovery, and/or supporting the process of a move to independent living.

Increasingly people with health problems are expected to live and be cared for in their homes. This might mean an older person being discharged from hospital much earlier than in the past; the concept of 'nursing at home' is being tested more widely. Closures of psychiatric hospitals have also moved people into ordinary housing where care and support can be delivered (as well as into specialist, shared housing and hostels, which are beyond the scope of this paper).

Sometimes the motivation for a general policy of keeping people out of residential care or psychiatric hospitals has been purely financial. But the belief that community care is always a cheap option is misguided. The foundation for policies which encourage independent living must be the knowledge that most people – including those with physical disabilities and learning difficulties – *want* to live outside institutions.

The problem is that suitable accommodation may simply be unavailable: problems of quantity (shortages of affordable homes), quality (adequate space/accessibility) and location (unsupportive environments) apply keenly to this ingredient in the housing–health debate.

Accessibility

Housing that is not suitable for people with mobility problems, because of its space standards and its external and internal design, will mean disabled people who want to live there must look elsewhere, friends and relatives with disabilities will not be able to visit, those who suffer accidents or illness which leads to mobility problems will be forced to move out (or may become prisoners in their own homes if they cannot negotiate stairs and steps), those ready to leave hospital may not be able to go home, and elderly people may be forced to move into residential accommodation prematurely.

The problems of inaccessible housing can be overcome in two ways: either homes can be built which, from the outset, are equipped to meet almost any circumstance which may arise later; or attempts can be made to carry out adaptations – which will not always be possible because of the design of the building – when needs arise. The first of these options is greatly to be preferred since designing for accessibility and adaptability costs very little at the outset, while remodelling the house at a later date can prove extremely expensive (or unachievable).

Over recent years, the Joseph Rowntree Foundation has been pressing the case for *Lifetime homes* which incorporate 16 design features to ensure that housing is flexible, adaptable and accessible (JRF, 1995a; Brewerton and Darton, 1997). The *Lifetime homes* standards include level access from car-parking to entrances, and over the threshold, with internal space in hallways and circulation areas for wheelchairs, together with a downstairs toilet, switches/sockets at a height useable by all, and the opportunity to fit a stairlift or houselift later. These features can be applied to virtually all new homes at very little additional cost, as has been proved by the housing associations which have adopted the *Lifetime homes* principles. (Extra costs work out at less than £300 for a three-bedroom home, compared with far higher sums for fitting unsightly ramps and handrails and redesigning interiors.)

In several European countries – not least in response to concerns about civil rights for disabled people – building regulations require housebuilders to adopt standards of accessibility similar to those in *Lifetime homes*. Steps in this direction are expected shortly in the UK. They will revolutionise the design of new homes for the future and, over the longer term, save individuals and the state substantial sums. From the outset, they will be more convenient to all households, making life easier for those who are pregnant, pushing buggies or carrying heavy shopping. With a requirement for another five million homes over the next 20 years or so, at the same time as the population is ageing, building regulations could achieve substantial improvements to the quality of life for increasing numbers.

Adaptations

Changes of design will come too late for the majority. Many people with disabilities and mobility difficulties require existing accommodation to be adapted. In recent years, the number of requests for help with adaptations from social services departments has risen sharply (15% per year from 1990 to 1995) (Heywood and Smart, 1996). These requests do not reveal the full extent of the need for adaptations since many potential applicants are unwilling to apply or lack information and advice.

Most of the costs of adaptations come from housing budgets (about 86% in 1993/94), with social services budgets making up most of the rest. As noted above, housing budgets have been squeezed although disabled tenants in local authority and housing association homes have been able to obtain some priority within confined budgets: average expenditure on adaptations more than doubled between 1990 and 1994. The problem is that the burden of increased demand is becoming too great for many housing departments who are looking for help from community care budgets (including through Joint Finance to which the NHS contributes) for the future.

The most common adaptation needs have been to facilitate bathing (which can be particularly expensive if the building of an extension on the ground floor is necessary), toilet adaptations and the provision of stair lifts; items of growing importance include hoists (following regulations on lifting, introduced in 1993) and alarms/door answering devices which are regarded as increasingly important for older people wanting to remain in their own home (Heywood and Smart, 1997).

Most worrying are the delays in getting help, by those who need adaptations. The average wait from request to completion for a grant-funded application is 52 weeks, but in the worst cases waiting times are reported of 148 weeks; this can, of course, mean that elderly applicants may not live to benefit from this support. Variations in practice, often revolving around degrees of cooperation between different statutory agencies, are a source of anxiety. And the means-test – the 'Test of Resources' – is widely regarded as unfair (Heywood and Smart, 1996).

Particular problems have been noted by the Family Fund Trust (FFT) which provides grant aid from the Department of Health to families caring for a disabled child in their own home (to a level of some £22m in 1996). The FFT notes that delays created by problems of coordination between services are particularly harmful to the development of the disabled child: a suitable home environment in the early years is crucial to the development of the child's senses, motor ability and social skills. Since delays of two to four years are commonplace, severely disabled children can miss out on crucial stages of development and become far more dependent as adolescents and adults. This has cross-sector implications in costs to health, education and social services (and, of course, there are implications for the health of parents too). The Trust reports more direct requests for help because money from social services departments (including funds to top-up the Disabled Facilities Grant or to help where parental contributions arising from the Test of Resources are set at unrealistically high levels) is not available. It may well be important for health authorities to recognise the value of directing some of their resources to meeting these needs (Mattingly, 1997).

Location

Wherever decent housing is scarce, those being moved from psychiatric hospitals or other institutions may end up in conditions which are more insecure and more stressful than those they leave. The use of 'hard-to-let' properties on unpopular council estates for the housing of people with psychiatric problems, or with problems of drug and alcohol abuse, can expose them to hostility from neighbours, crime and violence. Where 'the community' is already suffering from problems of poverty and disadvantage, it is unlikely to offer sanctuary to those with special needs. A move toward independent living requires sensitivity on the part of those placing residents, but also the availability of adequate accommodation in relatively desirable environments.

Housing and play/fitness

A survey by the Chartered Society of Physiotherapy in 1995 noted that: "Many of today's children lack stamina, are short of breath after the simplest of exercise; have poor posture leading to lower back pain; are not interested in exercise or sport; are tired and lethargic ... and seem reluctant to walk anywhere."

Where housing is situated and how it is designed are major determinants in the amount of exercise children take. Building new homes in places that necessitate car journeys to school, as well as to work and to shops and services, reduces the number of children who walk or cycle regularly. Design of new housing estates which gives priority to the car, and fails to incorporate formal and informal areas for play, confines more children to the home.

The range of a nine-year-old child today is equivalent to that of a six-year-old in 1970: the nine-year-old's accessible environment has been reduced to a ninth of the 1970 area (Wheway, 1995). In 1971 80% of seven- and eight-year-old children were allowed to go to school without adult supervision; by 1990, this figure had fallen to just 9% (Hillman, 1988). Girls and children from minority ethnic groups are likely to be the most restricted, because of parental fears of abduction, abuse or harassment (Millward, 1989).

Parents are encouraged to help their children adopt healthier, more active life-styles, but the general increase in car use, and the accompanying dangers from traffic, join with fears of 'stranger danger', bullying and bicycle theft to undermine this message. Housing providers have a role to play in reversing the unhealthy trend toward life-styles which decrease mobility, with detrimental effects on fitness and the establishing of physical activity patterns in childhood which are likely to carry forward to adulthood.

Research for the Joseph Rowntree Foundation shows how play can be facilitated on new – and existing – housing developments. Better estate design can liberate children to move about more freely as well as reducing road accidents near the home. Design features to reduce traffic levels and speeds can involve: small groups of houses and cul-de-sac; short roads; 'sleeping policemen'; different surfaces, ramps and tight turns to encourage people to drive slowly; and very low speed limits (Wheway and Millward, 1997).

The provision of play space has increasingly been the victim of cost-cutting, not least with land at a

premium. Formal play areas require ongoing expenditure in their supervision and maintenance, and can be seen as a source of nuisance (diminishing property values or arousing hostility between residents). But when properly handled, the freedom and opportunity for children to play out of doors can enhance the lives of all those living in the area: the natural energies of children can only be suppressed to a certain extent and if no thought is given to locations for play, vandalism and destructive behaviour elsewhere can result.

An important finding from the Joseph Rowntree Foundation research is that the concept of small, formal 'safe areas' for play is unduly restrictive: at least as important are the opportunities for informal play, with children having the space to play near their homes in front or back gardens and on roads and pavements. Children are keen to walk or cycle between different places, developing creative and social skills as well as taking exercise.

Policy change: the context

Introduction

The evidence above appears to demonstrate that the housing and health connections are important: bad housing is dangerous to health; good housing prevents and promotes good health and supports objectives of health services. It follows that tackling housing problems should reduce inequalities in health. The remainder of this paper considers how this might be done.

Before launching into a 'wish list' of housing policies, the realities of public expenditure constraints must be acknowledged. First, this section considers the level of public expenditure devoted to housing. It then reviews how public money is spent on subsidies to homeowners and on the provision of social housing. It discusses the policy changes required in both of these areas to remove inequalities and expand the quantity and quality of homes available. Finally, it examines the role of the housing sector in combating social exclusion, in area regeneration, and in stimulating the economy as a whole.

Government investment in housing

Efforts over recent years to curb public expenditure have led to substantial cuts in the capital budget for housing. As Figure 9 shows, in contrast to spending on health, social security, personal social services, law and order and so on, housing has suffered a sharp decline.

Figure 9: Spending on housing cut disproportionately (% of real change: 1980/81 to 1996/97)

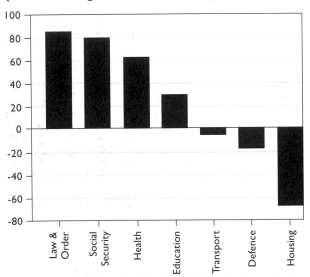

Source: Wilcox (1997; update to table in JRF *Housing Finance Review 1994/95*)

Simultaneously, the sale of council houses has been contributing very substantial sums to ease the government's funding problems. So far, sales under the 'Right to Buy' have returned over £26bn to the Exchequer (about the same as the proceeds from privatising the Gas, Water and Electricity utilities together); sales through the transfer of council estates to new or existing housing associations have nearly doubled this contribution. Council housing can, therefore, claim to be taking the strain disproportionately on two counts.

Housing associations have been the favoured agencies for providing new, subsidised homes since the beginning of the 1980s. Since 1988, they have been enabled to borrow from private lenders so that only their capital grants are counted as public expenditure: through progressive cuts to grant levels (from an average of over 75% to an average of about 50%, over the decade from 1988) the government investment has been stretched (although the price has been paid in higher rents).

The programme of housing associations, fuelled by the combination of public and private funding, expanded in the 1990s. But as Figure 10 shows, government concerns about the Public Sector Borrowing Requirement have hit the housing associations hard in recent years.

Figure 10: Rise and fall in housing association investment in England

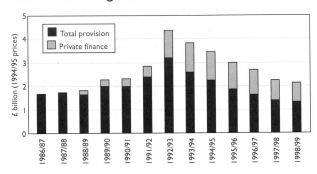

Source: Wilcox (1997)

The incoming Labour government of 1997 accepted the constraints on public expenditure set by its predecessor. This has confined plans for public spending within very tight ceilings. But the decision was accompanied by a commitment to the phased release over the next five years of capital receipts accumulated by local authorities from sales but not yet spent – estimated at £5bn.

Figure 11: Receipts soften impact of council investment cuts

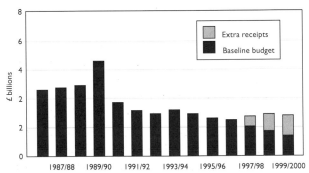

Source: Wilcox (1997)

Figure 11 shows how the use of capital receipts will compensate, in part, for recent and planned cuts. But overall spending is set to remain at levels markedly below those of the early 1990s. This overarching constraint necessitates a search for a more effective use of existing levels of government support.

Subsidies to homeowners

The *Inquiry into British housing*, chaired by the Duke of Edinburgh, which produced its first report in 1985 (National Federation of Housing Associations, 1985) and its second in 1991 (JRF, 1991), was keen to see a phasing-out of tax relief on mortgages: this subsidy created an 'uneven playing field' between renting and owning and provided support disproportionately to those who were better off. The Inquiry believed that the savings achieved should be recycled to boost rented provision, and also to finance personal subsidies to cover mortgage costs for homeowners facing financial problems (a 'mortgage benefit', similar to Housing Benefit); this 'needs-related housing allowance' would also be available to poorer owner-occupiers who were struggling with the maintenance costs for their home (JRF, 1991).

During the 1990s, the (previously unthinkable) policy of phasing out Mortgage Interest Relief At Source (MIRAS) was adopted by successive Chancellors. Instead of allowing relief for top tax rates, the figure was reduced to 25p (1993), to 20p (1994), to 15p (1995) and will go down by another 5p in 1998. Over recent years, the falls in mortgage interest rates have more than offset the loss of this concession for homeowners. Next year the cost of Mortgage Interest Relief At Source (MIRAS) will stand at about £1.8bn – compared with £7.8bn (in today's prices) in 1990/91.

But the extra revenue for the Exchequer is not finding its way into supporting those owners who fall on hard times. Indeed, owners have seen a parallel withdrawal of subsidy available through Income Support for Mortgage Interest (ISMI) arrangements (which cover payments during periods of unemployment). This protection has also been substantially withdrawn and the government's plan has been for owner-occupiers to take out private Mortgage Payment Protection Insurance (MPPI) to substitute for the government's safety net. In reality, those facing the greatest employment risks are unable or unwilling to take out a MPPI policy which leaves growing numbers of new purchasers vulnerable to a down-turn in the economy and/or to rises in mortgages rates (Ford and Kempson, 1997).

The absence of a safety net for homeowners revealed a major flaw in the policies of the 1980s which promoted home ownership so heavily (Wilcox, 1993a). As is shown in Figure 12, the growth of repossessions and mortgage arrears produced a startling change in the housing scene, with over 500,000 households going through the traumas of losing their home from 1990 to 1996.

Figure 12: Repossession and long-term arrears (UK)

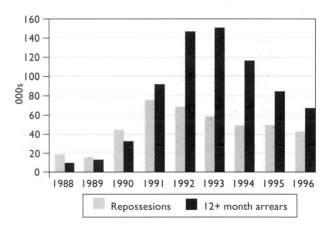

Source: Wilcox (1997)

The extra exposure to the risk of arrears/repossessions now that ISMI has been cut back and MPPI is not taking its place points to problems if interest rates rise rapidly again or job opportunities deteriorate.

Helping less fortunate homeowners would not absorb all the savings from phasing out tax relief. The Inquiry believed that the remainder should go to boosting the quantity and quality of rented housing, both through modest tax concessions to stimulate the private sector and through direct support to the housing associations and local authority landlords.

In the event, housing subsidies have been redirected away from these objectives and into higher payments for Housing Benefit, caused by higher rent levels for those in social housing which followed reductions in support for social landlords and by poorer people paying market rents to private landlords. The result is that Housing Benefit – that is, rent rebates for social housing tenants and rent allowances for private sector tenants – has absorbed virtually all the savings from MIRAS reductions and from cuts in grants (Figure 13).

Figure 13: Increases in Housing Benefit costs (£bn 1994/95 prices)

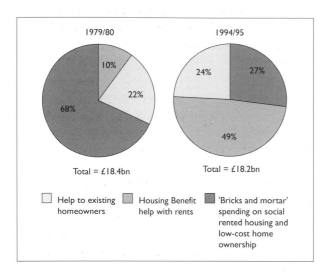

Source: DoE (1995) – Crown Copyright is reproduced with the permission of the Controller of Her Majesty's Stationery Office

Raising finance for social housing

The reduction in the role of council housing has been driven partly by hopes of a more competitive, market-orientated system. To achieve this, housing associations (or 'Registered Social Landlords') have been propelled into the development role previously assumed by local authority housing departments. After the 1998 Housing Act, public investment in housing associations were stretched by reducing levels of grant paid for each extra home, and leaving associations to borrow the balance from the private sector (repaying the extra loans by charging higher rents).

Because current counting conventions dictate that housing associations lie outside the public sector, the money they borrow from private sources is not counted within the PSBR. Thus if a housing association builds a new home, only the grant element – three quarters of the cost in 1989 but down to about 45% in 1997 – counts as public spending; if the same homes were provided by local authority, 100% of its costs would be regarded as public expenditure, achieving only half as many new homes for the same level of 'public expenditure'.

These accounting conventions have stimulated greater interest in the idea of local authorities passing their properties out of direct ownership into the

hands of newly created organisations (often using the same staff). Such voluntary transfers have now shifted over 200,000 homes out of the public sector. This trend seems likely to continue, and may generate the extra resources which are so badly needed to rectify deficiencies in local authority stock. Council housing is valued conservatively at £40bn, but the outstanding debt is only about half this figure: so if the properties were in the hands of a housing association – or a local housing company, as suggested in a joint publication by the Joseph Rowntree Foundation and the Institute of Housing (Wilcox, 1993b) – a further £20bn could be borrowed against these assets. This would provide the investment needed to renew the worst estates and improve their environments.

Economic side-effects from housing policies

Housing policies have implications for the wider economy and the nation's overall prosperity.

Work for the Joseph Rowntree Foundation by Geoff Meen at Oxford Forecasting Centre has shown how extra capital spending on housing of £1bn could increase the numbers of people employed in construction and related industries, at a net cost (after receipt of tax, rental returns etc) of approximately half a billion pounds in the following year (Meen, 1993).

This has much relevance to the government's *welfare-to-work* New Deal: jobs in construction are of particular value for the groups hardest hit by changes in the job market – men who lack skills and want manual work. The 'intermediate labour market' organisations who are tackling the problems of unemployed men – for example, the WISE Group which acts as the intermediary between the unemployed and employers in Scotland, East London and the East Midlands – have found that the best chances for training and work come from contracts from local authority housing departments and housing associations (McGregor et al, 1996).

Investment in rented housing would assist those who need to move for job reasons but who are currently tied down by the lack of alternatives to home ownership. Younger, more affluent people need the opportunity for mobility that the private sector can bring. And the cost of incentives for private renting could be offset by the gains not only from the same households not claiming tax relief as homeowners but from benefits to the UK's international competitiveness (Maclennan, 1995).

There are also wider economic implications that flow from the way grants are paid to the social housing sector. Providing bricks-and-mortar grants to keep rents within the reach of those in low-paid employment, without forcing them into reliance on Housing Benefit, has important effects on the national economy. Conversely, cutting the producer subsidies and raising rents has been shown to be inflationary and counterproductive. This is because two thirds of those in housing association and local authority homes already get Housing Benefit, so the substantial increases in their rents over recent years simply means the money going round in a circle (with high administrative costs in the middle). Rents rising at a far higher rate than earnings is inflationary, encouraging wage claims at higher levels which hinders competitiveness; it also leads indirectly to higher government pay-outs on benefits linked to the Retail Price Index (RPI) (because rent levels are taken into account in calculating the RPI). Housing policies which produce higher rents, therefore, can end up costing the government more, as shown in Figure 14 (Meen, 1994).

Figure 14: Higher rents have economic consequences

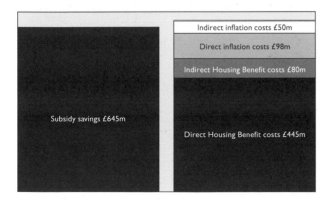

In addition, a regime of high rents, coupled with high Housing Benefit, reduces incentives to earn more. Very little is gained by a family on low wages when earnings rise from £50 per week to £230 per week, because of the corresponding withdrawal of Family Credit, free school meals, Council Tax Benefit

and, biggest of all, Housing Benefit (Wilcox, 1993b). Yet staying at home, unable to improve one's standard of living by working, can undermine self-respect and is likely to contribute to individual health problems, as well as making little sense economically.

Policy change: the remedies

Change through regulation

Some changes could be achieved by regulation rather than government spending. If the nation has deep-seated reasons for wanting greater energy efficiency or for requiring accessible housing from now on, then the producers can be compelled to behave differently.

Building regulations have ushered in higher standards of insulation over the last decade. But residential buildings still account for higher carbon dioxide emissions than industry (and three quarters as much as for all road transport): if government commitment to a 20% overall reduction is to be met by 2010, further regulation seems inevitable (May, 1997).

In relation to accessibility, the Conservative government announced its intention to reform Part M of the building regulations which relate to access to public and commercial buildings, so that residential buildings would also be affected. The new government – not least because of a concern for the civil rights of disabled people – is likely to enforce regulations which will alter the design of all new homes, at minimal extra building costs with substantial longer-term savings and expenditure on adaptation.

At the local level, planning authorities are being encouraged to place additional requirements on the producers of new homes: provision for amenities and protection of natural environments may follow the current opportunities for planners to require a proportion of new homes on larger sites to be 'affordable'.

Insofar as regulations of all these kinds lead to higher production costs, it does not follow that the consumer necessarily pays more (or that private housebuilders see their profits reduced). Instead, the costs may be reflected in the price paid for land – the residual factor when developers work out the difference between the cost of building and the value of the completed home on the open market. Landowners, therefore, may have to absorb the extra costs of complying with new regulations (although they may exercise the option of not selling at all if the price reductions seem too severe) (JRF, 1995b).

Meanwhile, regulation may also be the mechanism for tackling poor conditions in Houses in Multiple Occupation (HMOs) at the bottom end of the private sector. Existing arrangements have not always prevented breaches of health and safety requirements; new proposals for licensing of such premises seem likely to be cost-effective (although not cost-free since supervision through the Environmental Health Service is essential) (Beacock, 1995).

Changes to the process

The way services are structured and delivered often works against the holistic approach in which housing and health (and other issues) are tackled together. Separate central and local government departments – often in competition for resources and prestige – have responsibilities for different pieces of the jigsaw; separate professions jealously guard their own spheres of interest. Citizens – the service users, the customers, the clients, the patients, the tenants, the consumers – do not see their lives as falling neatly into the compartments devised by government.

Where health and housing services come together, the obstacles to coordination for effective delivery sometimes look insuperable. Although interagency working is recognised as important, in practice lack of time and resources constrain it. Tensions can emerge over funding arrangements and issues of public accountability (should health funds be spent on housing? should housing funds be spent on health?). Significant gaps have been noted, for example, for single people with mental health problems and in health provision to support domiciliary care (with efficiency indices for health providers acting as a disincentive to achieving a change in treatment and care for people away from hospitals). Responsibility for housing lies with the lowest tier of local government; social services are

located in the same body only for unitary authorities (and, of course, even then cooperation is not guaranteed); national health services lie outside all tiers of local government; and further layers of complexity follow from the substantial role of voluntary bodies. At the same time, there has been substantial organisational restructuring, often with changes in personnel, which also undermine efforts at long-term planning (Goss and Kent, 1995).

Better interagency working can lead to substantial cost savings as well as improved outcomes for those with problems at the interface of housing and health. There are now good examples of joint commissioning groups, of joint care planning teams, of consortia which sometimes have a housing association at the centre, and of many individual projects – sometimes centring on closure of long-stay institutions, or advice services for users – which show the way forward.

At a higher tier, the creation of Regional Development Agencies, building on the broader approach which Regional Government Officers have adopted to the funding of an area's regeneration needs, may hold one key to ensuring a more holistic approach for the future. But it is uncertain how the different services will be incorporated within this regional approach.

Finally, in the context of the processes for effecting change, it is worth reflecting that housing providers can pay a pivotal role:

- as the owners of much of the property (including community buildings and shops) on the estates where problems are concentrated – they are in the front line;
- they can act as the catalysts in organising greater involvement by residents in tackling estate-based problems;
- they have a direct interest in the effects of crime and vandalism, as owners of the property;
- housing providers are well placed to engineer local partnerships, not least since they have to work with the private sector to obtain funding;
- these providers spend substantial sums on building and maintenance, landscaping, gardening and caretaking: they offer opportunities for training and employment through which it may be possible to tackle underlying problems;

- in common with health providers, calling upon their support does not lead to the sense of stigma or insecurity which may come from drawing in the social services department or the police.

Housing would appear to be well placed to play a central part in the processes of regeneration and community effort to tackle local problems.

More investment

As noted above, more and better housing could be provided if existing housing subsidies were spent to greater effect. The MIRAS subsidies to owner-occupiers continue to be curtailed and the remaining subsidy (some £1.8bn pa in 1988/89) could be redirected, both for protecting homeowners in need and through stimulating the production of affordable, good-quality homes for rent. Borrowing against the hidden assets in the council sector – through transfers of stock to newly created or existing owners outside PSBR constraints – could unlock the resources to tackle the disrepair on council estates.

Targeted investment in new and improved housing would also improve health by reducing the risks of accident and fire, as well as overcrowding and cold, damp conditions. Without the need for homeless families to live in substandard Bed & Breakfast hotels, not only are fire and safety hazards reduced but, in the longer term, less public money is spent on meeting housing needs.

There are also ways of funding the improvement of substandard owner-occupied housing, where often the homeowner is an older person. Frequently there is equity tied up in the home (since mortgages have been repaid) which could be released to finance building works. Advice and information, provided through home improvement (Care and Repair) agencies or the local authority, may make a major difference in encouraging anxious owners to get much-needed work done to their home. And new techniques for extracting some of the personal assets of the 'capital rich, income poor' tied up unhelpfully in their homes, could unlock hidden resources (King, 1995). Higher levels of improvement grant are not the only answer here (Leather and Mackintosh, 1994).

In trying to maximise value for money, targeting public expenditure on better insulation and heating systems (combined with adequate ventilation) may give the best returns. Not only does the consequent reduction in cold and damp improve health, but it also reduces fuel bills which are disproportionately burdensome to poorer households (Markus, 1993). In rented property landlords also benefit from lower maintenance costs that follow from reductions in condensation, mould growth and the deteriorating effects of dampness. At the same time, expenditure here has global benefits by reducing emissions of CO_2 (greenhouse) gases (Haylock, 1993), and because the work requires relatively unskilled, manual labour, it is a high priority for meeting training and employment objectives.

The other form of targeting of public investment which seems likely to pay the highest dividends would follow from a reversal of the reduction in bricks-and-mortar capital subsidies to the providers of social housing: capital subsidies have been out of favour in recent years, but the concentration on personal subsidies to the individual (Housing Benefit) has now proved so expensive that a change seems essential. Lower rents from increased capital subsidies to providers would remove the disincentives for individuals to take up employment – without a substantial increase overall in government expenditure because of the resulting reduction in Housing Benefits. Recent policy statements indicate that there is now an understanding that the availability of sufficient, decent housing is not the only consideration: the homes must also be affordable.

Targeting disadvantaged neighbourhoods

The determinants of health include the social and community networks that surround the individual. Strengthening such networks can provide emotional support, which reduces stress and alleviates isolation. In turn, this can improve the health of people in disadvantaged circumstances.

Investment in community development – paying for common facilities, funding individuals on estates who can coordinate activities, as well as securing environmental improvements – can reduce crime/ fear of crime, stress and mental illness. Supervised play facilities can allow children to take exercise in safety, thereby reducing accidents. If the physical regeneration of an area involves the residents the gains are multiplied: employment is generated, there are opportunities for training in new skills, and the capacity of those in disadvantaged neighbourhoods is enhanced. The marked improvement that follows from community-led development is illustrated on the Meadowell estate in North Tyneside (Gibson, 1993). And a recent overview of experiences in eight cities in the UK and Germany shows the importance of integrating physical and economic initiatives with social renewal, in improving multiply-deprived neighbourhoods (Thake and Staubach, 1993). Also, a roundup of 33 research reports on renewing the quality of life on council estates, concluded that involvement of residents in the process – 'unleashing the potential' – was the key to success (Taylor, 1995).

Investment in disadvantaged neighbourhoods can also tackle the problems of social exclusion where problems have followed the concentration and segregation of poorer households. Neighbourhoods, and individual new estates, need some mix of people in employment alongside those who are unemployed; of households without children as well as those with children (reducing overall child density); of homeowners (or shared owners) among properties for rent; and of different age groups. This balance of income groups, tenures and ages can provide role models of working adults, increase financial resources on an estate and prevent the creation of 'welfare housing': otherwise there seems an inevitable overload on good neighbourliness and on services – the least, education, as well as health – from the isolation of those suffering the greatest disadvantages. The ghettos of American cities – characterised by 'wave upon wave of violence and crime' – provide stark evidence of what happens when public housing becomes the 'housing of last resort' and areas face a breakdown of normal social controls (Carr, 1993; Kasarda, 1993; Newman, 1993).

The concept of Health Action Zones recognises that concentrating resources in a particular place can have disproportionate benefits. This approach could target resources, based on a geographical understanding of marginalised communities, which achieves the greatest results for the sums invested.

Conclusion

Tackling inequalities in housing also addresses health inequalities. National investment in new and improved housing, particularly when targeted on improving disadvantaged neighbourhoods, also has important impacts on the wider issues of health and well-being. These links can be seen, for example, in heavy expenditure on reducing cold and damp conditions on a council estate: this will not only reduce illness among residents but can also be the catalyst for community development – bringing residents together in ways that make the estate more neighbourly, more secure and less stressful – as well as generating the opportunity for jobs and skill-building, with spin-offs in reducing the crime and anguish associated with poverty.

Good housing and good health go together: this paper suggests that the health of the nation depends on recognising this connection.

References

Ambrose, P. (1996) *Housing and health on the Limehouse Fields and Ocean Estates in Stepney*, Brighton: Centre for Urban and Regional Research, University of Sussex.

Anderson, I., Kemp. P. and Quilgars, D. (1993) *Single homeless people*, London: HMSO.

Arblaster, L. and Hawtin, M. (1993) *Health, housing and social policy*, London: Socialist Health Association.

Barry, A., Carr-Hill, R. and Glanville, J. (1991) *Homelessness and health: What do we know? What should be done?*, Discussion Paper 84, York: Centre for Health Economics, University of York.

Beacock, N. (1995) 'Improving houses in multiple occupation', in G. Randall et al.

Best, R. (1997a) 'Unlocking the doors that cause the divide', *Housing Today*, no 52, 25 September, p 11.

Best, R. (1997b) 'Making a crowded island habitable', *Parliamentary Monitor*, vol 5, no 6, pp 3-5.

Bines, W. (1994) *The health of single homeless people*, Housing Research Finding No 128, York: JRF.

BMA (British Medical Association) (1987) *Deprivation and ill-health*, London: BMA Board of Science and Education Discussion Paper.

Breheney, M. and Hall, P. (1996) *The people: Where will they go?*, London: Town and Country Planning Association.

Brewerton, J. and Darton, D. (1997) *Designing lifetime homes*, York: JRF.

Brown, S. and Randall, G. (1993) *Permanent homes for people living in short-life housing*, Housing Research Findings No 81, York: JRF.

Burridge, R. and Ormandy, D. (1993) *Unhealthy housing: Research, remedies and reform*, London: E & FN Spon.

Burrows, R. (1997) *The changing population in social housing in England, contemporary patterns of residential mobility in relation to social housing in England*, York: Centre for Housing Policy, University of York.

CAPT (Child Accident Prevention Trust) (1989) *Basic principles of child accident prevention*, London: CAPT.

Carr, J. (1993) *Housing Research News*, vol 2, no 1, Washington: Office of Housing Research, Fannie Mae Foundation.

Champion, A. (1996) ESRC Discussion Paper on internal migration, Newcastle: University of Newcastle.

Constantinides, P. (1988) 'Safe at home? Children's accidents and inequality', *Radical Community Medicine*, Spring, pp 31-3.

Crook, A. (1996) *A new lease of life? Housing association investment on local authority housing estates*, Bristol: The Policy Press.

DoE (Department of the Environment) (1993) *English House Condition Survey 1991*, London: HMSO.

DoE (1995) *Our future homes – Opportunity, choice, responsibility*, London: HMSO.

DoH (Department of Health) (1989) *Caring for people: Community care in the next decade and beyond*, Cm 849, London: HMSO.

Drever, F. and Whitehead, M. (1997) *Health inequalities*, ONS, London: The Stationery Office, p 119

DTI (Department of Trade and Industry) (1991) *Home and leisure accident research: Twelfth annual report, 1988 Data*, London: DTI Consumer Safety Unit.

Eardley, T. (1989) *Move-on housing*, London: Single Homeless in London/National Federation of Housing Associations.

EDAW (1997) *Living places: Sustainable homes, sustainable communities*, London: National Housing Forum.

Ford, J. and Kempson E. (1997) *The impact of changes to the social security safety net for mortgagors, Bridging the gap? Safety nets for mortgage borrowers*, York: Centre for Housing Policy, University of York.

Freeman, H. (1993) 'Mental health and high-rise housing', in R. Burridge and D. Ormandy, *Unhealthy housing: Research, remedies and reform*, London: E & FN Spon, pp 168-90.

Gabe, J. and Williams, P. (1993) 'Women, crowding and mental health', in R. Burridge and D. Ormandy, *Unhealthy housing: Research, remedies and reform*, London: E & FN Spon, pp 191-208.

Gibson, T. (1993) *Meadowell community development*, Telford: Neighbourhood Initiatives Foundation.

Goldblatt, P. (1990) *Longitudinal study: Mortality and social organisation, 1971-1981*, London: OPCS Series LS No 6, London: HMSO.

Goss, S. and Kent, C. (1995) *Health and housing: Working together?*, Bristol: The Policy Press.

Haylock, B. (1993) *Responding to the challenge of fuel poverty*, Report of Joseph Rowntree Foundation Seminar, September, York: JRF.

Heywood, F. and Smart, G. (1996) *Funding adaptations*, Bristol: The Policy Press.

Hillman, M. (1988) 'Foul play for children: a price of mobility', *Town and Country Planning*, vol 56.

HMSO Green Paper (1996) *Household growth – Where shall we live?*, London: HMSO for the DoE.

Holmans, A. (1995) *Housing demand and need in England 1991-2011*, York: JRF (unpublished supplement, 1997).

Hunt, S. (1990) 'Emotional distress and bad housing', *Health and Hygiene*, vol 11, pp 72-9.

Ineichen, B. (1993) *Homes and health: How housing and health interact*, London: E & FN Spon.

JRF (Joseph Rowntree Foundation) (1991) *Inquiry into British housing, Second Report June 1991*, chaired by HRH The Duke of Edinburgh KB KT, York: JRF.

JRF (1995a) *Inquiry into planning for housing*, Chaired by Dame Rachel Waterhouse, York: JRF.

JRF (1995b) *Lifetime homes*, York: JRF.

Kasarda, J. (1993) *Inner city concentrated poverty in neighbourhood distress*, USA: University of North Carolina.

Kemp, P. (1995) *The future of private renting*, York: JRF.

King, N. (1995) *Equity release shared ownership*, Housing Research Summary No 9, York: JRF.

KPMG (1996) *Investing in urban housing: Options for attracting private investment into urban public housing through voluntary stock transfer*, York: JRK.

Lambert, C., Jeffers, S., Burton, P. and Bramley, G. (1992) *Homelessness in rural areas*, London: Rural Development Commission.

Leather, P. and Mackintosh, S. (1994) *Renovation grants and the condition of older housing*, Housing Research Findings No 104, York: JRF.

Leather, P. and Morrison, T. (1997) *The state of UK housing: A factfile on dwelling conditions*, Bristol: The Policy Press.

Leather, P. and Rolfe, S. (1995) *Improving efficiency of the housing repair and maintenance industry*, Bristol: The Policy Press.

Lowry, S. (1990) 'Getting things done', *British Medical Journal*, vol 300, pp 390-2.

Maclennan, D. (1995) *A competitive UK economy*, York: JRF.

Markus, T. (1993) 'Cold, condensation and housing poverty', in R. Burridge and D. Ormandy, *Unhealthy housing: Research, remedies and reform*, London: E & FN Spon, pp 141-67.

Mattingly, R. (1997) *Aids and adaptations and The Family Fund Trust*, Unpublished paper.

May, R. (1997) quoting from *Report from intergovernmental panel on climate change*, London: HMSO.

McGregor, A., Ferguson, Z., Fitzpatrick, I., McConnachie, M. and Richmond, K. (1996) *Bridging the jobs gap: An evaluation of the WISE Group and the intermediate labour market*, York: JRF.

Meen, G. (1993) 'Housing and the economy: an over-reliance on interest rates', in S. Wilcox, *Higher rents and work disincentives*, Housing Research Findings No 93, York: JRF.

Meen, G. (1994) *Impact of higher rents*, Housing Research Findings No 109, York: JRF.

Millward, A.M. (1989) *Children, nature and the city*, Birmingham (unpublished).

National Federation of Housing Associations (1985) *Inquiry into British housing*, Report chaired by HRH The Duke of Edinburgh KG KT, London: National Federation of Housing Associations.

Newman, S. (1993) *Last in line: Housing assistance for households with children*, Baltimore: Johns Hopkin University.

OPCS (1991) *1991 Census, local base statistics*, Crown Copyright.

Page, D. (1993) *Building for communities: A study of new housing association estates*, York: JRF.

Platt, S., Martin, C., Hunt, S. and Lewis, C. (1989) 'Damp housing, mould growth and symptomatic health state', *British Medical Journal*, vol 298, pp 1673-8.

Power, A. and Tunstall, R. (1997) *Dangerous disorder: Riots and violent disturbances in 13 areas of Britain 1991-92*, York: JRF.

Robson, B. (1994) *Assessing the impact of urban policy*, University of Manchester, London: DoE/HMSO.

Rudlin, D. and Falk, N. (1995) *Building to last*, London: URBED.

Savage, A. (1988) *Warmth in winter: Evaluation of an information pack for elderly people*, Cardiff University of Wales College of Medicine Research Team for the Care of the Elderly.

Stern, R., Stilwell, B. and Heuston, J. (1989) *From the margins to the mainstream: Collaboration in planning services with single homeless people*, London: West Lambeth Health Authority.

Strachan, D. (1988) 'Damp housing and childhood asthma: validation of reporting of symptoms', *British Medical Journal*, vol 297, pp 1223-6.

Taylor, M. (1995) *Unleashing the potential: Bringing residents to the centre of regeneration*, York: JRF.

Thake, S. and Staubach, R. (1993) *Investing in people: Rescuing communities from the margin*, York: JRF.

Wheway, R. (1995) *Streets for all children and for the total child*, Paper to 'Play in the Streets' Conference, London.

Wheway, R. and Millward, A.M. (1997) *Child's play*, Coventry: Chartered Institute of Housing.

Wilcox, S. (1993a) *Housing Finance Review 1993*, York: JRF.

Wilcox, S. (1993b) *Higher rents and work disincentives*, Housing Research Findings No 93, York: JRF.

Wilcox, S. (1995) *Local housing companies: New opportunities for council housing*, York: JRF.

Wilcox, S. (1997) *JRF Housing Finance Review 1997/98*, York: JRF.

6

The social environment[1]

Richard Wilkinson

There have been numerous independent observations (17 in all – see Box 1) suggesting that countries with narrower income differences between rich and poor tend to have lower mortality rates (three examples of the relationship are shown in Figures 1-3). The only negative finding is based on data held by the Luxembourg Income Study (Judge et al, 1996), and even in this data a relationship has been shown after allowing for the differences in the response rates to surveys of household income in different countries (McIsaac and Wilkinson, 1997).

Box 1: Papers reporting a statistical association between income distribution and health

1. Rodgers, G.B. (1979) 'Income and inequality as determinants of mortality: an international cross-section analysis', *Population Studies*, vol 33, pp 343-51.

2. Flegg, A. (1982) 'Inequality of income, illiteracy, and medical care as determinants of infant mortality in developing countries', *Population Studies*, vol 36, pp 441-58.

3. Wilkinson, R.G. (1986) 'Income and mortality', in R.G. Wilkinson (ed) *Class and health: Research and longitudinal data*, London: Tavistock.

4. Le Grand, J. (1987) 'Inequalities in health: some international comparisons', *European Economic Review*, vol 31, pp 182-91.

5. Waldmann, R.J. (1992) 'Income distribution and infant mortality', *Quarterly Journal of Economics*, vol 107, pp 1283-302.

6. Wilkinson, R.G. (1992) 'Income distribution and life expectancy', *British Medical Journal*, vol 304, pp 165-8.

7. Wennemo, I. (1993) 'Infant mortality, public policy and inequality – a comparison of 18 industrialised countries 1950-85', *Sociology of Health & Illness*, vol 15, pp 429-46.

8. Wilkinson, R.G. (1994) 'Health, redistribution and growth', in A. Glyn and D. Miliband (eds) *Paying for inequality: The economic cost of social injustice*, London: Rivers Oram Press.

9. Kaplan, G.A., Pamuk, E., Lynch, J.W., Cohen, R.D. and Balfour, J.L. (1996) 'Income inequality and mortality in the United States: analysis of mortality and potential pathways', *British Medical Journal*, vol 312, pp 999-1003.

10. Kennedy, B.P., Kawachi, I. and Prothrow-Stith, D. (1996) 'Income distribution and mortality: cross sectional ecological study of the Robin Hood Index in the United States', *British Medical Journal*, vol 312, pp 1004-7.

---

[1] Corrected January 1999.

11. Steckel, R.H. (1983) 'Height and per capita income', *Historical Methods*, vol 16, pp 1-7. See also Steckel, R.H. (1994) 'Heights and health in the United States', in J. Komlos (ed) *Stature, living standards and economic development*, Chicago, IL: University of Chicago Press.

12. Ben-Shlomo, Y., White, I.R. and Marmot, M. (1996) 'Does the variation in the socioeconomic characteristics of an area affect mortality?', *British Medical Journal*, vol 312, pp 1013-14.

13. Davey Smith, G. and Egger, M. (1996) 'Commentary: understanding it all – health, meta-theories, and mortality trends', *British Medical Journal*, vol 313, pp 1584-5.

14. Wilson, M. and Daly, M. (1997) 'Life expectancy, economic inequality, homicide, and reproductive timing in Chicago neighbourhoods', *British Medical Journal*, vol 314, pp 1271-4.

15. Fiscella, K. and Franks, P. (1997) 'Poverty or income inequality as predictors of mortality: longitudinal cohort study', *British Medical Journal*, vol 314, pp 1724-8.

16. Lynch, J., Kaplan, G.A., Pamuk, E.R., Cohen, R.D., Heck, K.E., Balfour, J.L. and Yen, I.H. (1998) 'Income inequality and mortality in metropolitan areas of the United States', *American Journal of Public Health*, vol 88, pp 1074-80.

17. Kawachi, I., Kennedy, B.P. and Lochner, K. (1997) 'Long live community. Social capital as public health', *The American Prospect*, November-December, pp 56-9.

Figure 1: Life expectancy (male and female) and Gini coefficients of post-tax income inequality (standardised for household size)

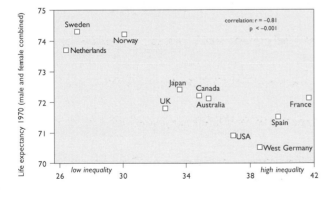

Source: Data from Sawyer (1976, Table 11, pp 3-36) and World Bank

Figure 2: The annual rate of change of life expectancy in 12 European Community countries and the rate of change in the percentage of the population in relative poverty (1975-85)

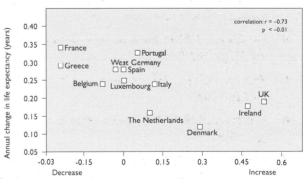

Source: Data from O'Higgins and Jenkins (1990)

Figure 3: Life expectancy (1991-93) and income inequality in post-transition Eastern Europe

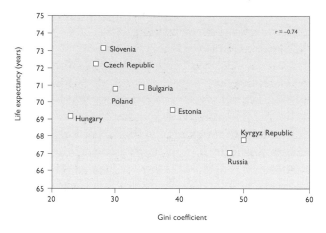

Source: Davey Smith and Egger (1996)

After having been reported in different international data sets – both cross-sectionally and in changes over time – the relationship was then tested on separate data covering the 50 states of the USA (Figure 4) and, most recently, on data for the 282 Standard Metropolitan Areas in the USA (Lynch et al, 1998). In both cases correlations of 0.6 or 0.7 were found. The difference in mortality between states in the most and least egalitarian quartiles of the income distribution was equivalent to the combined loss of life from lung cancer, diabetes, motor vehicle crashes, HIV infection, suicide and homicide (Lynch et al, 1998).

Figure 4: Age-adjusted mortality rates (male and female) per 100,000 population and 'Robin Hood Index' of income inequality in the 50 states of the United States (1990)

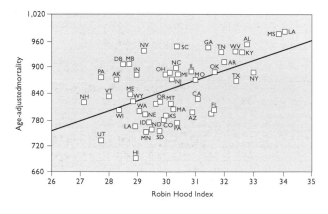

Source: Kennedy et al (1996)

Because of the number of times this relationship has been reported it cannot be regarded as a product of chance. The only way it might occur without some causal significance is if income distribution and mortality were both powerfully determined by some underlying variable. However, no plausible intervening variables have been suggested which would explain why this relationship has been found in so many different contexts (cross-sectionally and in changes over time, between countries and within countries, in developed and less developed countries) but also why it has withstood controlling for average incomes, absolute poverty, expenditure on medical care, and smoking. It is implausible that there could be some other underlying factor which is simultaneously such a powerful determinant of both income distribution and mortality in such different contexts. Even if no one had controlled for expenditure on medical care, the accumulated evidence does not suggest that medical care is a sufficiently powerful determinant of population mortality rates, and there is, of course, no suggestion that it affects income distribution.

In addition, there are two important pieces of evidence which lend strong support to the view that the amount of income inequality is a powerful determinant of mortality. The first indicates that health in the developed world is more closely related to relative than to absolute income. Although there are steep mortality gradients related to income (and other measures of material standards) *within* developed countries, clear gradients are not found when you look at mortality in relation to the income differences *between* developed societies. Thus, among OECD countries in 1993, there was no cross-sectional association between each country's average income and mortality (see Figure 5). Similarly, changes in GDP per capita over a 23-year period showed only a weak correlation (r=0.3 not significant) with changes in life expectancy (Figure 6).

Figure 5: Relation between GDP per capita and life expectancy among OECD countries (1993)

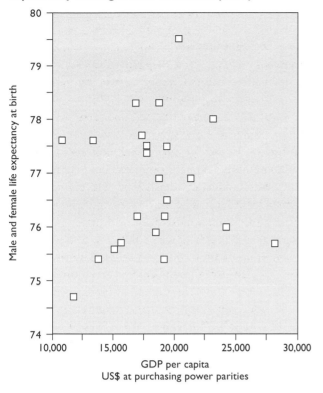

Source: Data from OECD (1996) and World Bank (1996)

Figure 6: Relation between % change in GDP per capita and years increase in life expectancy (1970-93)

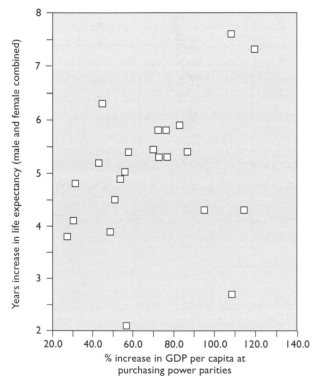

Source: Data from OECD (1996) and World Bank (1996)

The possibility that closer relationships between health and material living standards may be obscured by national differences in culture and diet cannot explain why a closer relationship is not found among the 50 states of the USA (Figure 7) despite smaller cultural differences as people shop at the same chain stores offering much the same range of goods. The median income of one state can be twice as high as another without benefit to its mortality rates. Indeed, when the correlation of -0.26 between median state incomes and mortality rates is controlled for income distribution, instead of revealing a stronger underlying relation, it disappears altogether (partial r=-0.06).

Figure 7: Age-adjusted mortality per 100,000 (male and female combined) 1989-91 in relation to median income in 1990 among the 50 US states

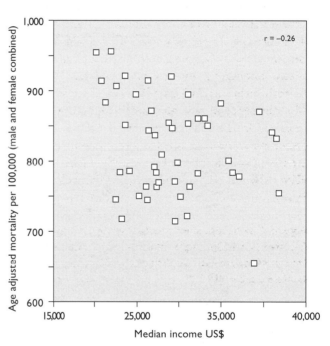

Source: Drawn from data kindly supplied by J. Lynch (personal communication)

That the strong relationships between mortality and material standards found within countries should contrast so sharply with the weak relationship found between countries, suggests that within countries we are dealing with relative income. Where income differences are indicative of differences in social status (as they are within countries or US states) they are also closely related to health; but where (as with the differences in average incomes between countries) they have no significance for social status, they are not closely related to health. In other words, we are dealing with a relationship between health and relative income or social status, rather with one between absolute income and health. (Wilkinson [1994] has suggested that the epidemiological transition marks the point in economic development beyond which further rises in absolute material standards have much less significance for improvements in health.)

Although based on wholly independent evidence, these indications that health is related to relative income rather than to absolute material circumstances is highly consistent with the evidence of a relationship between income distribution and population mortality rates. However, evidence of the mechanism involved provides further confirmation that the relationships between income distribution and mortality has causal significance. The link between them seems to be provided by social cohesion.

At first there was only qualitative evidence to suggest that societies which were unusually egalitarian and unusually healthy were also more socially cohesive (Wilkinson, 1996). Illustrative examples included Britain's experience during the two world wars when income differences narrowed dramatically under the combined impact of the virtual disappearance of unemployment, a narrowing of earnings differences and a sharp rise in higher tax rates as the government sought to show that the burden of war was equally shared. The effect of this narrowing of income differentials and of the sense of unity in the face of a common enemy contributed to the well-known wartime sense of camaraderie. Exceptionally rapid improvements in mortality rates (two or three times faster than usual) took place in both of the decennial periods in which the wars occurred.

Another example is Japan which achieved the highest life expectancy in the world and narrowest income distribution of any country reporting to the World Bank. It is also known to be an unusually cohesive society. On a much smaller scale, the Italian-American community of Roseto in Pennsylvania attracted the attention of epidemiologists in the 1960s because it had much lower death rates than surrounding towns (Bruhn

and Wolf, 1979). After finding no explanation in terms of nutritional and behavioural risk factors, its good health was attributed to the remarkably close knit nature of the community and the lack of outward indications of differences in wealth between people. During the next decades Roseto lost these characteristics and, as had been predicted, it also lost its health advantage (Egolf et al, 1992).

Eastern Europe in the 1970s and 1980s also provides an example of the damaging health effects of a loss of social cohesion. Until the late 1960s, and despite being poorer, several Eastern European countries — such as East Germany, Hungary and Bulgaria — had better health than several Western European countries and were known to be more egalitarian. However, from about 1970 onwards mortality rates ceased to improve throughout Eastern Europe — in sharp contrast to the continued improvements in Western Europe. The evidence suggests that the standards of social life and public conduct deteriorated in Eastern Europe. The bureaucracies became cynical and the societies more atomised, with accompanying rises in death rates particularly from violence and alcohol related causes (Wilkinson, 1996).

In addition to this kind of circumstantial evidence that social cohesion may mediate between narrower income differences and lower mortality rates, Kawachi et al (1997) have recently shown statistical evidence that social cohesion may provide the link between the two. The proportion of people in each American state who felt that other people could not be trusted and would take advantage of them was strongly related to both income inequality ($r=0.7$) and to mortality ($r=0.8$). Path analysis suggested that almost all the relationship between income inequality and mortality was mediated by these measures of 'social trust' which could perhaps be regarded as indicators of how hostile or hospitable was people's experiences of their social environment.

Although Putnam et al's (1993) analysis of social cohesion in the regions of Italy did not extend to health, they did note that their measure of the strength of 'civic community' was closely correlated with income distribution ($r=0.8$). After surveying opinions in each region, Putnam et al said: "Citizens in more civic regions, like their leaders, have a pervasive distaste for hierarchical authority patterns" (p 104). "Political leaders in the civic regions are more enthusiastic supporters of political equality than their counterparts in less civic regions" (p 102). Talking more about a social ethos of equality rather than of income distribution itself, they concluded "Equality is an essential feature of the civic community" (p 105).

Finally, a powerful indicator of the association between income inequality and social cohesion comes from studies of violent crime. A meta-analysis of some 34 papers concluded that, like mortality, violent crime is related to income inequality (Hsieh and Pugh, 1993).

The epidemiological evidence that more socially integrated individuals enjoy better health lends credibility to the view that social cohesion may mediate between income distribution and mortality on the societal scale. Studies showing two- and threefold differences in mortality rates between people with high and low levels of social integration have been reviewed by House et al (1988) and by Berkman (1995). Most recently Cohen et al (1997) reported the results of an experiment in which people were given nasal drops containing cold viruses. People with friends in few areas of their lives were over four times as likely to develop colds as people with friends in more areas of life. The relationship showed a dose-response gradient and was unaltered by statistical controls for prechallenge virus-specific antibody, virus type, age, sex, season, body mass index, education, and race. Although smoking, poor sleep quality, alcohol abstinence, low dietary intake of vitamin C, elevated catecholamine levels, and being introverted were all associated with greater susceptibility to colds, they could only partially account for the relation between social networks and susceptibility to colds.

The hypothesis that the extent of income inequality affects health by changing the nature of the social fabric is supported by data on homicide and violent crime. Homicide has been shown to be closely related to income inequality and to mortality from all other causes at both the state and the neighbourhood level in the United States (correlations ranging from r=0.7 and r=0.9) (Kaplan et al, 1996; Wilson and Daly, 1997; Wilkinson et al, 1998). A relationship between income distribution and homicide has also been reported internationally

(Braithwaite and Braithwaite, 1980; Krohn, 1976). As mentioned above, a meta-analysis of 34 aggregate data studies concluded that violent crime was related to income inequality (Hsieh and Pugh, 1993). Among the American states, the variance in homicide almost exactly covers the covariance between income inequality and all non-homicide mortality – so much so that it suggests that the social milieu which gives rise to violence is also a social milieu which gives rise to higher death rates from other causes of death. This pattern is specific to homicide and violent crime: property crime has a different distribution (Wilkinson et al, 1998).

The literature on violence, including the autobiographies of violent men, shows that a powerful component comes from people feeling that they are denied respect. Gilligan (1996), who was a prison psychiatrist in US prisons for 25 years before becoming Director for the Centre for the Study of Violence at Harvard, said: "I have yet to see a serious act of violence that was not provoked by the experience of feeling shamed and humiliated, disrespected and ridiculed, and that did not represent the attempt to prevent or undo this 'loss of face' – no matter how severe the punishment." (p 110).

McCall (1994), who was himself imprisoned for violence, gives much the same picture:

Some of the most brutal battles I saw in the streets stemmed from seemingly petty stuff…. But the underlying issue was always respect. You could ask a guy, 'Damn, man, why did you bust that dude in the head with a pipe?' And he might say, 'The motherfucka disrespected me!' That was explanation enough. It wasn't even necessary to explain how the guy had disrespected him. It was universally understood that if a dude got disrespected, he had to do what he had to do. It's still that way today. Young dudes nowadays call it 'dissin'. (McCall, 1994, p 52)

If violence is often related to feelings of not being respected, it is easy to see why it should be more common where income differences are wider: the wider they are the more people are excluded from the normal sources of status and respect and the less likely they are to be treated as equals.

Although deaths in most of the main causal categories (infections, cardiovascular diseases, respiratory diseases, cancers etc) seem to be more common where income differences are greater, the ones which show the biggest percentage differences related to differences in inequality are alcohol related deaths, accidents and violence (McIsaac and Wilkinson, 1997). But instead of regarding homicide as a form of behaviour which is discontinuous with all other social behaviour, we should perhaps regard it as the visible tip of a shift in the nature of social relations to more conflictual and less nurturing interactions. Rose (1992) showed that for many risk factors (such as raised blood pressure, alcohol consumption, cholesterol levels etc), the proportion of people above some level of risk in each society reflects a societal continuum of exposure to that risk factor. In this light we should perhaps see homicide and violent crime rates as indicative of general differences in social relations throughout a society. This is suggested not only because other forms of violent crime show similar but weaker relations with income inequality as those found for homicide, but also because at the other end of the spectrum of social behaviour we have the relationship with social trust which Kawachi et al (1997) identified. The correlation between social trust and homicide among US states was 0.82, suggesting that these measures are indeed part of a social continuum (Wilkinson et al, 1998).

In countries, or US states, with wider income differences and therefore more relative deprivation, what we seem to be seeing – at least in the deprived areas – is a shift towards a less supportive, less trusting and more aggressive social environment. Whether this is confined to life on the streets or extends, as seems likely, to school playgrounds and perhaps into more conflictual family life and childrearing, is still a matter for speculation. The impression that greater inequality is associated with a more 'macho' culture and high risk life-style is also suggested by the experience of Eastern Europe as social cohesion declined during the 1970s and 1980s (Wilkinson, 1996). During those decades deaths associated with alcohol and violence increased and the rises in mortality were particularly pronounced among single rather than married people and were greater among men than women (Watson, 1995; Hajdu et al, 1995). In the upheavals since 1989 the same patterns have been even more accentuated.

If more unequal societies do tend to have less supportive and more conflictual pattern of social relations, then the work on social support, friendship patterns and wider social involvement would lead one to expect large differences in health to result (House et al, 1988; Berkman, 1995; Cohen et al, 1997). In addition to the effects of social networks, Shively suggests that low social status is itself a direct source of "low intensity social stress" (Shively et al, 1997, p 871). In terms of the plausibility of some of these and other psychosocial influences on health, it is perhaps worth pointing out that the pathways through which the psychosocial becomes biological are rapidly becoming clearer. There are now a number of useful summaries of what is known (Sapolsky, 1993, 1998; Chrousos et al, 1995; Lovallo, 1997; Martin, 1997).

References

Berkman, L.F. (1995) 'The role of social relations in health promotion', *Psychosomatic Research*, vol 57, pp 245-54.

Braithwaite, J. and Braithwaite, V. (1980) 'The effect of income inequality and social democracy on homicide', *British Journal of Criminology*, vol 20, no 1, pp 45-53.

Bruhn, J.G. and Wolf, S. (1979) *The Roseto story*, Norman, OK: University of Oklahoma Press.

Chrousos, G.P., McCarty, R., Pacak, K., Cizza, G., Sternbery, E., Gold, P.W. and Kvetnansky, R. (eds) (1995) *Stress: Basic mechanisms and clinical implications, Annals of the New York Academy of Sciences*, vol 771, New York.

Cohen, S., Doyle, W.J., Skoner, D.P., Rabin, B.S. and Gwaltney, J.M. (1997) 'Social ties and susceptibility to the common cold', *Journal of the American Medical Association*, vol 277, pp 1940-4 .

Davey Smith, G. and Egger, M. (1996) Commentary: 'Understanding it all – health, meta-theories and mortality trends', *British Medical Journal*, vol 313, pp 1584-5.

Egolf, B., Lasker, J., Wolf, S. and Potvin, L. (1992) 'The Roseto effect: a 50-year comparison of mortality rates', *American Journal of Public Health*, vol 82, pp 1089-92.

Gilligan, J. (1996) *Violence: Our deadly epidemic and its causes*, New York, NY: GP Putnam.

Hajdu, P., McKee, M. and Bojan, F. (1995) 'Changes in premature mortality differentials by marital status in Hungary and England and Wales', *European Journal of Public Health*, vol 5, pp 529-64.

House, J.S., Landis, K.R. and Umberson, D. (1988) 'Social relationships and health', *Science*, vol 241, pp 540-5.

Hsieh, C.C. and Pugh, M.D. (1993) 'Poverty, income inequality, and violent crime: a meta-analysis of recent aggregate data studies', *Criminal Justice Review*, vol 18, pp 182-202.

Judge, K., Benzeval, M. and Mulligan, J.A. (1996) 'Income inequality and population health among rich industrial nations', *Journal of Epidemiology and Community Health*, vol 50, no 5, p 580.

Kaplan, G.A., Pamuk, E., Lynch, J.W., Cohen, R.D. and Balfour, J.L. (1996) 'Inequality in income and mortality in the United States: analysis of mortality and potential pathways', *British Medical Journal*, vol 312, pp 999-1003; see also Kaplan, G.A. (1996) 'Correction: inequality in income and mortality in the United States: analysis of mortality and potential pathways', *British Medical Journal*, vol 312, p 1253.

Kawachi, I., Kenedy, B.P, Lochner, K. and Prothrow-Stith, D. (1997) 'Social capital, income inequality and mortality', *American Journal of Public Health*, vol 87, pp 1491-8.

Kennedy, B.P., Kawachi, I. and Prothrow-Stith, D. (1996) 'Income distribution and mortality: cross sectional ecological study of the Robin Hood Index in the United States', *British Medical Journal*, vol 312, pp 1004-7; see also Kennedy, B.P., Kawachi, I. and Prothrow-Stith, D. (1996) 'Important correction. Income distribution and mortality: cross sectional ecological study of the Robin Hood Index in the United States', *British Medical Journal*, vol 312, p 1194.

Krohn, M.D. (1976) 'Inequality, unemployment and crime', *Sociological Quarterly*, vol 17, pp 303-13

Lovallo, W.R. (1997) *Stress and health: Biological and psychological interactions*, London: Sage Publications.

Lynch, J., Kaplan, G.A., Pamuk, E.R., Cohen, R.D., Heck, K.E., Balfour, J.L. and Yen, I.H. (1998) 'Income inequality and mortality in metropolitan areas of the United States', *American Journal of Public Health*, vol 88, pp 1074-80.

McCall, N. (1994) *Makes me wanna holler. A young black man in America*, New York, NY: Random House.

McIsaac, S.J. and Wilkinson, R.G. (1997) 'Income distribution and cause-specific mortality', *European Journal of Public Health*, vol 7, pp 45-53.

Martin, P. (1997) *The sickening mind*, London: Harper Collins

OECD (1996) *OECD National Accounts*, Paris: OECD.

O'Higgins, M. and Jenkins, S.P. (1990) 'Poverty in the EC', in R. Teekens and B.M.S. van Praag (eds) *Analysing poverty in the European Community*, Luxembourg: EUROSTAT, pp 187-209.

Rose, G. (1992) *The strategy of preventive medicine*, Oxford: Oxford University Press.

Putnam, R.D., Leonardi, R. and Nanetti, R.Y. (1993) *Making democracy work: Civic traditions in modern Italy*, Princeton, NJ: Princeton University Press.

Sapolsky, R.M. (1993) 'Endocrinology alfresco: psychoendocrine studies of wild baboons', *Recent Progress in Hormone Research*, vol 48, pp 437-68.

Sapolsky, R.M. (1998) *Why zebras don't get ulcers. A guide to stress, stress-related disease and coping*, New York, NY: WH Freeman.

Sawyer, M. (1976) 'Income distribution in OECD countries', *OECD Economic Outlook*, *Occasional Studies*, Paris, pp 3-36.

Shively, C.A., Laird, K.L. and Anton, R.F. (1997) 'The behavior and physiology of social stress and depression in female cynomolgus monkeys', *Biological Psychiatry*, vol 41, pp 871-82.

Watson, P. (1995) 'Explaining rising mortality among men in Eastern Europe', *Social Science & Medicine*, vol 41, pp 923-34.

Wilkinson, R.G. (1994) 'The epidemiological transition: from material scarcity to social disadvantage?', *Daedalus (Journal of the American Academy of Arts and Sciences)*, vol 123, no 4, pp 61-77.

Wilkinson, R.G. (1996) 'Health and civic society in Eastern Europe before 1989', in C. Hertzman, S. Kelly and M. Bobak (eds) *The East-West life expectancy gap in Europe*, Dordrecht: Kluwer, pp 195-209.

Wilkinson, R.G., Kawachi, I. and Kennedy, B. (1998) 'Mortality, the social environment, crime and violence', *Sociology of Health & Illness*, vol 20, no 5, pp 578-97.

Wilson, M. and Daly, M. (1997) 'Life expectancy, economic inequality, homicide, and reproductive timing in Chicago neighbourhoods' *British Medical Journal*, vol 314, pp 1271-4.

World Bank (1996) *World tables*, Oxford: Oxford University Press.

7

Poverty across the life-course and health

George Davey Smith

Introduction: poverty, inequality and health

Since the appearance of the Black Report much of the focus of research into socio-economic differentials in health has related to the continuous gradient of improving health from the bottom to the top of the socio-economic hierarchy (Davey Smith et al, 1990a; Macintyre, 1994; Marmot, 1994). This focus on inequality and health represents a move from an earlier focus on poverty and health (M'Gonigle and Kirby, 1936; Titmuss, 1943), in which the poor health status of the most socially disadvantaged was the major concern. Consider, for example, the near-linear association between median family income for area of residence and all-cause mortality demonstrated for a large cohort of white men in the US, shown in Figure 1 (Davey Smith et al, 1996). It is clear that the men in the moderately high income categories are not deprived in any absolute sense, although they have elevated mortality rates in comparison with the men in the highest income category. In this population, if all men had experienced the same death rate as the highest income category the overall mortality rate would be reduced by a quarter. This is an underestimate of the deaths which can be attributed to socio-economic position, since the use of an ecological indicator will lead to attenuation of the underlying associations.

In Table 1 the proportion of deaths attributable to socio-economic position which occur in the bottom of the income spectrum are presented for different cut-offs. As can be seen, only a small proportion (less than 10%) of attributable deaths occur in the very poor (lowest 3% of the income distribution) group

and nearly a half of attributable deaths occur in the upper two thirds of the income distribution. This is analogous to the situation seen with factors like blood pressure and cholesterol concentration where, as Geoffrey Rose has elegantly demonstrated, only a small proportion of attributable deaths occur among people with greatly elevated levels of these risk factors (Rose, 1992).

Figure 1: Mortality by zip code of area of residence among over 300,000 white men screened for the MRFIT study

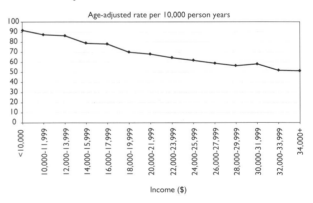

Source: Adapted form Davey Smith et al (1996)

Table 1: The proportion of deaths attributable to socio-economic position which occur in lower income groups

	% of population	Proportion of excess deaths
Bottom	1	0.03
Bottom	3	0.08
Bottom	9	0.19
Bottom	18	0.34
Bottom	31	0.54

The graded relationship between socio-economic position and health, which has been shown in numerous studies and in relation to morbidity as well as mortality, have been taken to indicate that the psychological consequences of inequality and of subordinate positions in a social hierarchy – rather than the consequences of material deprivation – are the key factors (Wilkinson, 1996). An alternative (though not mutually exclusive) interpretation is that lifetime experiences of economic hardship will differ between the highest and middle income groups. A greater proportion of people in middle income groups will have experienced material deprivation in earlier life than is the case for the highest income groups (Goldthorpe, 1987). The usual indicators of social position in health studies – single measures of socio-economic circumstances in adulthood – are an inadequate marker of social circumstances across the life-course. Several studies have demonstrated that lifetime social circumstances are strongly related to morbidity and mortality in adulthood (Mare, 1990; Davey Smith et al, 1997a; Lynch et al, 1997). For example, Figure 2 demonstrates that cumulative social class (indexed by the number of occasions from childhood to adulthood an individual was in a manual social class location) together with the deprivation level of current area of residence are powerful predictors of mortality risk. Childhood and adulthood social circumstances make independent contributions to the risk of dying. Cumulative experience during adult life is also important. Individuals with average or higher income who experience fluctuating reductions to low income levels have higher mortality rates than those who remain on average or high incomes (McDonough et al, 1997). The highest mortality rates by a considerable degree are seen among those with persistently low incomes.

Figure 2: Mortality according to cumulative social class and deprivation level of area of residence

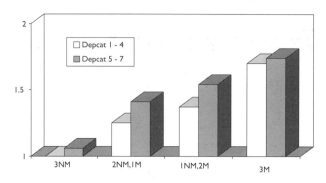

Depcat	Deprivation category
3NM	Social class non-manual during 3 periods (childhood, early adulthood and middle age)
2NM, 1M	Social class non-manual during 2 periods, manual during 1
1NM, 2M	Social class non-manual during 1 period, manual during 2
3M	Social class manual during all 3 periods

Deprivation at different stages of the life-course and health: aetiological considerations

Socio-economic inequalities in health should be considered against the background of broad secular changes and international differences in health status and mortality risk. Over the 20th century there have been very sizeable declines in mortality in most industrialised countries, with infant mortality rates in the 1990s being only 5% of those at the turn of the century in England and Wales, for example. For one- to four-year-olds the situation is even more dramatic – mortality rates for the 1990s are 2% of those at the turn of the century. Even among the middle-aged there have been substantial reductions, with end of the 20th-century mortality rates being around one fifth to one third the rates seen at the beginning of the century (Charlton and Murphy, 1997). It is likely that the factors which have contributed to the sizeable reductions in mortality are also those which contribute to the current differentials in mortality between socio-economic groups.

If our understanding of the factors generating socio-economic differentials in health is to be advanced we need to consider the particular factors which contribute to international differences, secular trends and socio-economic differentials in particular causes of ill-health. Some illustrative cases are given here. Internationally, stomach cancer is a major cause of mortality, being one of the most common cancers seen in developing countries and in earlier times in developed countries. Stroke mortality shows a similar geographical and temporal distribution to stomach cancer mortality and also has declined dramatically over this century. Among middle-aged men and women in England and Wales stroke mortality at the beginning of the 20th century was up to seven times higher than at the end of the century (Charlton and Murphy, 1997). The declines in stroke and stomach cancer in England and Wales contributed to the declines in mortality among post-childhood age groups. The risk of these diseases seems to be established to a sizeable extent in childhood. People migrating from high to low stomach cancer areas after childhood take with them the risk of stomach cancer of the place they have migrated from (Coggon et al, 1990). Cohort effects can be seen in the mortality trends, in support of this conclusion (Hansson et al, 1991). Data from a large prospective study in Scotland (Davey Smith et al, 1997a, 1997b) demonstrates that stomach cancer and stroke risk is associated with parental socio-economic position – and hence socio-economic circumstances in childhood – more strongly than to socio-economic position in adult life. It is suggested that the material conditions of existence at the time people who are currently dying of stomach cancer and stroke were born are important factors underlying current risk for these conditions. Adverse socio-economic circumstances in childhood favour *Helicobacter pylori* (Mendall et al, 1992) acquisition and *Helicobacter pylori* infection appears to be an important cause of stomach cancer (Forman et al, 1991). Declining rates of *Helicobacter pylori* infection have accompanied improving social conditions over the century (Banatvala et al, 1993) and thus may underlie the falling rates of stomach cancer mortality. Infections acquired in childhood may also be important factors in the production of risk of stroke in adult life. Thus current morbidity and mortality patterns for these conditions are related directly to poverty-associated factors such as overcrowding and hygiene practices acting in early life.

For other important causes of morbidity and mortality in adulthood socially patterned exposures acting in early life appear to interact with or accumulate with later life exposures. Thus morbidity and mortality from respiratory disease in adulthood is related to housing conditions and infections acquired in childhood. Smoking and occupational exposures in later life then influence disease risk, in association with these earlier life factors (Mann et al, 1992). In the case of diabetes, hypertension and coronary heart disease, low birthweight – which is strongly socially patterned and related to intergenerational experiences as well as maternal nutrition – interacts with obesity in later life (increasingly prevalent among people in unfavourable social circumstances) to produce elevated disease risk (Phillips et al, 1994; Leon et al, 1996; Frankel et al, 1996; Lithell et al, 1996). Large differences in relative and absolute risk for various forms of morbidity can be demonstrated when groups are defined by clusters of socially-patterned adverse exposures acting throughout life. These exposures include health-related behaviours and the effects of psychosocial exposures such as job insecurity.

Poverty can influence health through a broad range of factors acting over the life-course. This includes such embodied features as low birthweight, height, obesity and lung function. There is increasing evidence of intergenerational influences on these attributes and the influence of nutrition (Gunnell et al, 1996) and infection in early life should be given more attention. The extent to which health-related behaviours, such as dietary patterns and smoking, are constrained by structural factors should be acknowledged when considering the underlying determinants (rather than proximal mechanisms) of health inequalities (Graham, 1988; Davey Smith and Brunner, 1997). Parsimonious explanations would consider broad secular changes in biologically plausible aspects of the material conditions of people's existences to underlie the broad secular changes in health, the substantial differences in health status between countries and the socio-economic differentials in health within countries. Alternative explanations should be sought when it is apparent that such material conditions of existence fail to account for health differentials. It is clear that biologically plausible mechanisms linking the experience of poverty to many particular health problems exist (of which only illustrative examples are given above, due to space limitations) and that the proportion of disease and ill-health in a population which may be attributable to poverty-related exposures is likely to be considerable.

Poverty across the life-course in Britain

Any consideration of how the cumulative experience of poverty across the life-course can influence health requires an operational definition of poverty. It is sometimes stated that poverty no longer exists in Britain, generally on the grounds that consumer durable ownership is now high even among the lowest income groups (see Table 2) (Goodman et al, 1997). This fails to acknowledge that technological change and innovation can both generate the availability of such durables and lead to them becoming necessities for meaningful participation in society (Gordon and Pantazis, 1997). If video ownership is taken to refute the existence of poverty (as, famously, it was by Peter Lilley) then we are forced to consider that 100% of the population was in poverty in the 1930s. As overall communication and personal transportation facilities improve then the need to have access to them for social participation, for being able to compete in the labour market, and for fulfilling domestic obligations is increased. The notion that an inability to meet the needs, material and social, which are recognised as essential within a society is a meaningful definition of poverty allows for the distinction between poverty and inequality to be made. The EC has produced a definition of poverty (see Box 1) which is broadly in line with this reasoning.

Table 2: Access to consumer durables of the bottom decile income group (%)

Percentage of individuals in household with access to a:	1962-63	1972-73	1982-83	1992-93
Telephone	8	20	58	78
Washing machine	–	54	79	89
Fridge or fridge-freezer	–	52	95	99
Car	–	26	44	56
Video cassette recorder	–	–	–	68
Central heating	–	20	46	73

Source: Goodman et al (1997) by permission of Oxford University Press

Box 1: EC definition of poverty

... the poor shall be taken to mean persons, families and groups of persons whose resources (material, cultural and social) are so limited as to exclude them from the minimum acceptable way of life in the Member State in which they live. (EEC, 1995)

In the UK the pioneering *Breadline Britain* surveys of 1983 and 1990 (Gordon and Pantazis, 1997) obtained data on the perception of a sample of the general public of social necessities (Table 3). Not being able to meet three or more of the items which over 50% of the public consider to be social necessities due to a lack of resources was taken to indicate being in poverty. By this definition the *Breadline Britain* survey estimated that 20% of households (approximately 11 million people) fell below the poverty line in 1990. Attempts to make similar estimates for previous periods suggested that there is a continuing decline in relative poverty between the 1930s and 1970s which then reversed and was followed by substantial increases over the 1980s and 1990s. This accords with researchers who have been able to examine trends in low-income families (defined by those falling below the Supplementary Benefit or Income Support level) between 1961 and 1993 (Figure 3) (Goodman et al, 1997). The *Breadline Britain* estimates of the prevalence of poverty in 1990 closely approximates to estimates based upon the numbers on or below the Supplementary Benefit and Income Support level and proportion of the population at below 50% of the national average income. All three methods give estimates of between 11 and 14 million people falling below these cut-offs.

Poverty is, of course, distributed very unevenly across the population. The highest prevalence is seen among lone parents, of whom 41% fall below the poverty line. For other families with children 23% fall below the line, whereas for other non-pensioner households the equivalent figure is 14%. Similar figures are seen when percentage of family types with incomes below half the national average is examined (Table 4). Furthermore it is families with children who are most likely to remain in the lowest income category over time and experience persistent poverty (Table 5). Women are over-represented among those experiencing poverty, with 24% falling below the threshold in the *Breadline Britain* survey in contrast to 17% of men (Gordon and Pantazis, 1997). Examining life-course experiences of poverty demonstrates that women are particularly likely to be in poverty when they are responsible for bringing up children. Because of this unequal distribution of poverty between household types and across the life-course, 33% of children in Britain were living in households below the poverty line in 1993-94. This has increased from 10% in 1979. The British situation with respect to child poverty and income inequality is particularly poor (Figures 4 and 5) (Lynch and Kaplan, 1997). If we consider that the concomitants of poverty – poor nutrition; over-crowded, damp or inadequately heated housing; an increased risk of infections; appropriate psychosocial stimulation and the ability to maintain cleanliness – are of particular importance during prenatal, infant and childhood life then the current distribution and trends in poverty bode ill for health trends in the future.

Figure 3: Percentage of the population below 50% of national average income (using income before housing costs deducted)

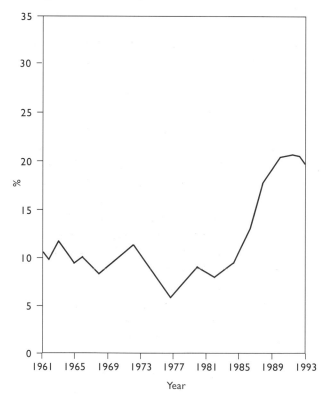

Source: Goodman et al (1997) by permission of Oxford University Press

Table 3: The perception of necessities: 1983 and 1990 compared

Standard-of-living items in rank order	% claiming item as necessity	
	1990 (n=1,831)	1983 (n=1,174)
A damp-free home	98	96
Heating to warm living areas in the home if it's cold	97	96
An inside toilet (not shared with another household)	97	97
Bath, not shared with another household	95	94
Beds for everyone in the household	95	94
A decent state of decoration in the home	92	–
Fridge	92	77
Warm waterproof coat	91	87
Three meals a day for children	90	82
Two meals a day for adults	90	64
Insurance of contents of dwelling	88	–
Daily fresh fruit and vegetables	88	–
Toys for children eg dolls or models	84	71
Bedrooms for every child over 10 of different sexes	82	77
Carpets in living rooms and bedrooms	78	70
Meat/fish (or vegetarian equivalent) every other day	77	63
Two pairs of all-weather shoes	74	78
Celebrations on special occasions	74	69
Washing machine	73	67
Presents for friends/family once a year	69	63
Child's participation in out-of-school activities	69	–
Regular savings of £10 a month for 'rainy days'	68	–
Hobby or leisure activity	67	64
New, not second-hand, clothes	65	64
Weekly roast/vegetarian equivalent	64	67
Leisure equipment for children eg sports equipment	61	57
A television	58	51
A telephone	56	43
An annual week's holiday away, not with relatives	54	63
A 'best outfit' for special occasions	54	48
An outing for children once a week	53	40
Children's friends round for tea/snack fortnightly	52	37
A dressing gown	42	38
A night out fortnightly	42	36
Child's music/dance/sport lessons	39	–
Fares to visit friends four times a year	39	–
Friends/family for a meal monthly	37	32
A car	26	22
Pack of cigarettes every other day	18	14
Holidays abroad annually	17	–
Restaurant meal monthly	17	–
A video	13	–
A home computer	5	–
A dishwasher	4	–

Source: Gordon and Pantazis (1997)

Table 4: Percentages of family types with incomes below half the contemporary mean

	Before housing costs			
	1979	1992-93	1979	1992-93
Pensioner couple	16	25	21	26
Single pensioner	16	25	12	36
Couple with children	7	20	8	24
Couple without children	4	10	5	12
Single with children	16	43	19	58
Single without children	6	18	7	22
All family types	8	20	9	25

Source: Goodman et al (1997) by permission of Oxford University Press

Table 5: Characteristics of individuals remaining in the bottom income quintile over three years and of individuals escaping from the bottom income quintile at some point over three years

Family type	Of those permanently in bottom quintile (%)	Of those who escaped at some point (%)
Couple pensioner	11	10
Single pensioner	14	14
Couple with children	40	38
Couple, no children	4	13
Single with children	24	12
Single, no children	6	13
Total	100	100

Source: Goodman et al (1997) by permission of Oxford University Press

Figure 4: Changes in child poverty rates between 1967 and 1992

Increases in child poverty rate, 1967-1992	
More than 30%	UK, USA
10-15%	Norway
5-10%	Netherlands, Belgium, Germany
Around 0%	Australia, Spain, France
Decreases	Sweden, Denmark, Finland, Canada, Italy

Source: Reprinted by permission of Sage Publications Ltd from Lynch and Kaplan (1997)

Figure 5: Changes in income inequality between 1967 and 1992

Increases in income inequality, 1967-1992	
More than 30%	UK
16-29%	USA, Sweden
10-15%	Australia, Denmark
5-10%	Norway, Netherlands, Belgium
Around 0%	Spain, France, Finland, Canada, Germany
Decreases	Italy

Source: Reprinted by permission of Sage Publications Ltd from Lynch and Kaplan (1997)

Another dramatic change in the distribution of poverty has been the rapid growth of the long-term sick and disabled among those receiving Income Support (Goodman and Webb, 1991). It is probable that this reflects a disguised form of unemployment, where individuals are encouraged to acquire this category as it allows for more reasonable treatment by the benefit system. The effects of such self-labelling have not been investigated, but could clearly be detrimental to the psychosocial functioning of individuals. This hidden unemployment also draws attention to the influence of insecurity at work on health, where a wide range of subjective and objective health measures are seen to deteriorate during periods of job insecurity (Ferrie et al, 1995). Incomes are also becoming subject to considerably greater uncertainty than was previously the case and income, as well as job, insecurity may be detrimental to health (McDonough et al, 1997).

Which policies could reduce the burden of ill-health attributable to poverty?

The current fashion in policy making in the health arena is for 'evidence-based' recommendations. While these are highly appropriate for clinical interventions targeting individuals, with regard to population health a demand for randomised or experimental evidence leads to the inappropriate directing of recommendations to individual-based strategies (Frankel and Davey Smith, 1997). Thus the research review commissioned for the 'Variations in health' subgroup of the Chief Medical Officer's Health of the Nation Working Group in 1995 (Arblaster et al, 1995) applied evidence-based medicine principles to the issue of socio-economic inequalities in health and therefore failed to recognise that inequalities in health are determined by economic and social conditions and not by the inadequate implementation of results from randomised controlled trials (RCTs).

In this regard consider the major indicators of mortality and morbidity risk in industrialised countries: gender, poverty, smoking and constitution (including genetic profile). Life expectancy differences between men and women are 5.6 years; between social class I and social class V 5.2 years in men and 3.4 years in women (differences would be greater if more refined socio-economic categories were used – Davey Smith et al, 1990b); and between smokers and never smokers around 5 years. Life expectancy differences generated by genetic and other constitutional factors have not been formally estimated, but are likely to be substantial (Sorensen et al, 1988). In none of these cases have RCTs demonstrated their importance with respect to life expectancy (and in the case of gender and genetic factors this would not be possible). The only unifactorial RCT of smoking cessation strategies found no significant effect on mortality (Rose and Colwell, 1992), yet the response to the lack of RCTs evidence in this case has, rightly, not been to abandon serious efforts to reduce smoking. The same should be the case with efforts to reduce the health burdens of poverty and inequality.

There are two legitimate responses to the evidence on socio-economic inequality, poverty and health differentials. The first is to accept that widening income inequalities and increasing proportions of (especially) children living in poverty generate increasing socio-economic health differentials and threaten to arrest future secular improvements in health, but to argue that large income inequalities are necessary for economic growth – through, for example, the incentives of large increases in income for those already on high incomes leading to improved productivity and overall economic performance. In this case the health effects of widening disparities in income and the increasing prevalence of poverty may be considered an unfortunate – but necessary – price to pay for national prosperity, which itself will ultimately lead to an improved health profile. While the evidence suggests that inequality is not necessary for economic growth – indeed it points the other way (see Figure 6) (Glynn and Miliband, 1994; Hutton, 1996; Davey-Smith et al, 1998) – this position can be advanced and the economic evidence disputed. The second legitimate response is to implement a fiscal programme aimed at arresting and reversing the increasing trend in income inequalities, in order to decrease socio-economic health differentials and remove the threat of future cessation in secular improvements in health. A third option – to intimate that there is serious concern with inequalities in health and that concerted efforts will be made to reduce such inequalities, without being

willing to implement necessary fiscal reforms – is not a legitimate response.

Figure 6: Income inequality around 1980 and labour productivity growth between 1979 and 1990

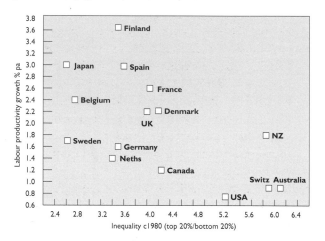

Source: Davey Smith et al (1998)

Examples of policy options are here grouped under three headings.

Policies aimed at reducing the proportion of children born into and living in poverty

Such policies require guaranteed incomes for households with children. One randomised controlled trial (of complex design) in the US suggested that income maintenance for poor women led to a reduction in low birthweight (Kehrer and Wolin, 1979). Unfortunately there has apparently been no replication of this pioneering study (a systematic review of health effects of income maintenance is currently being carried out by Anthony Rodgers and colleagues in New Zealand and should be available soon). The fact that very few controlled studies of the effects of fiscal policy on health have been carried out means that suggesting that only 'evidence-based' recommendations are acceptable is, in effect, excluding the potentially most important area of intervention from consideration.

- It is essential for reducing inequalities in child health that all pregnant women are able to afford an adequate diet. Budget Standards research at the University of York would indicate that the current maternity allowance is insufficient to achieve this aim. The abolition of the universal maternity allowance was also a retrograde step. Maternity entitlements need to be increased, particularly for women dependant on Income Support and in low paid jobs.

- A third of all children are born into and live in families dependant on Income Support. The level of Income Support is therefore one of the key factors underlying the amount of child poverty in Britain. These are currently so low that families with children will eventually sink into poverty if they become dependent on Income Support for any length of time. Additional benefits are required to support families with children.

- Children born to young mothers are particularly vulnerable. The decision to exclude 16- and 17-year-old mothers from benefit provision should be reversed.

- Means-tested benefits are a costly and inefficient method of alleviating poverty as they rarely can achieve better than 80% take-up rate. Universal Child Benefit rates should therefore be increased.

- The lone parent premium should not be abolished – indeed we should be discussing by how much it should be increased. The long-term health consequences of being born into poor single-parent families has not been examined (indeed the low prevalence of such families prior to 1970 would make this difficult) but in the future this could become an important indicator of a disadvantaged early start in life and the health sequelae of this.

- The rent limit on Housing Benefit needs to be raised for families with children and increased building of social housing is required to end the need for Bed & Breakfast accommodation. Accepting that past rents have already paid many times over for the cost of previous building it should now be possible to reduce real rent levels.

- Nutritional standards for school meals should be reintroduced and new technology (eg smart cards) should be employed to remove the stigma from free school meals. Free school meals entitlement should be extended to families receiving Family Credit and free school milk provision should again be made mandatory. School breakfast schemes should be examined, and where successful be extended.

- An educational campaign needs to be introduced to reduce teenage pregnancies.

- The imprisonment of parents for non-payment of debt should be avoided. Changes to the legal aid system are likely to increase the degree to which families living in poverty cannot protect themselves against challenges to their rights and liberty.

Policies aimed at reducing inequalities in income more generally

Such policies will reduce the proportion of the population living in poverty. As well as reducing inequality between individuals these policies could redistribute income across the life-course. Currently individuals tend to live in the poorest circumstances they will experience in life in their early years and in old age. Growing evidence on the persistent health effects of early life exposures suggests that the redistribution of income across the life-course could itself produce health gain. Examples of such policies include the following.

- Various measures should be implemented to reverse the increasing inequalities in income and to direct wealth differentials towards a more equitable plane. These measures would also reduce levels of poverty. They include continuing reductions in MIRAS; reducing the tax-free savings threshold; removing charitable status from private education and private healthcare; block the tax loopholes inherent in company car provision; extending windfall profit taxation; ensuring the collection of inheritance tax (and increase the rate of such taxation); abolishing the upper earnings limit for National Insurance; reversing legislation relating to trade unions and wages councils which have precipitated increasing income inequalities; and introducing a national minimum wage at a reasonable level.

- Benefit levels and pensions should be linked over time to earnings rather than to prices.

- Subsidised childcare and after-school care places are needed to enable parents to take up paid work.

- The supposition that people aged less than 25 require less benefit than those over 25 should be re-examined urgently.

- Non-take-up of benefits to which people are entitled should be combated with educational campaigns and specific initiatives like benefit counsellors in general practices and health centres.

- Benefit disqualifications and limits to mortgage assistance that apply in the early weeks of unemployment should be removed.

Specific policies targeting areas of particular concern

A substantial influence on overall socio-economic differentials in health will only follow from broad fiscal policies. However, in several particular areas where inequalities are substantial specific policies which could be implemented with relative ease could be introduced. Examples include the following.

- Pedestrian child deaths and injury due to road traffic accidents have a steep socio-economic gradient (greater than fivefold gradient from social class I to social class V – Roberts and Power, 1991). An immediate and ridged enforcement of the speed limits in residential areas would be a rapid and inexpensive means of reducing inequalities in health. The law needs to be enforced and the technology to achieve this (traffic calming measures, speed cameras, etc) is both readily available and relatively cheap. Speed traps might well prove to be income generating.
- Accidental childhood deaths due to fires show a 14-fold gradient from social class I to social class V (Roberts and Power, 1996). The free distribution of smoke alarms has been shown in a randomised trial (Mallonee et al, 1996) to reduce injuries due to fires and should be given serious consideration.
- Smart cards giving date of birth could be introduced as a method of making underage purchase of cigarettes and alcohol more difficult, with a requirement that these cards are checked for any individual who may be underage.

References

Arblaster, L., Entwistle, V., Lambert, M., Froster, M., Sheldon, T. and Watt, I. (1995) 'Review of the research on the effectiveness of health service interventions to reduce variations in health', CRD Report 3, York: NHS Centre for Reviews and Dissemination.

Banatvala, N., Mayo, K., Megraud, F., Jennings, R., Deeks, J.J. and Feldman, R.A. (1993) 'The cohort effect and *Helicobacter pylori*', *The Journal of Infectious Diseases*, vol 168, pp 219-21.

Charlton, J. and Murphy, M. (1997) *The health of adult Britain 1941-1994*, 2 volumes, London: The Stationery Office.

Coggon, D., Osmond, C. and Barker, D.J.P. (1990) 'Stomach cancer and migration within England and Wales', *British Journal of Cancer*, vol 61, pp 573-4.

Davey Smith, G. and Brunner, E. (1997) 'Socio-economic differentials in health: the role of nutrition', *Proceedings of the Nutrition Society*, vol 56, pp 75-90.

Davey Smith, G., Bartley, M. and Blane, D. (1990a) 'The Black Report on socioeconomic inequalities in health 10 years on', *British Medical Journal*, vol 301, pp 373-7.

Davey Smith, G., Morris, J.N. and Shaw, M. (1998) 'The Independent Inquiry into Inequalities in Health', *British Medical Journal*, vol 317, pp 1465-6.

Davey Smith, G., Shipley, M.J. and Rose, G. (1990b) 'The magnitude and causes of socio-economic differentials in mortality: further evidence from the Whitehall study', *Journal of Epidemiology and Community Health*, vol 44, pp 265-70.

Davey Smith, G., Hart, C., Blane, D. and Hole, D. (1997b) 'Adverse socioeconomic conditions in childhood and cause-specific adult mortality: prospective observational study', *British Medical Journal*, vol 316, pp 1631-5.

Davey Smith, G., Neaton, J.D., Wentworth, D., Stamler, R. and Stamler, J. (1996) 'Socioeconomic differentials in mortality risk among men screened for the Multiple Risk Factor Intervention Trial: I. White men', *American Journal of Public Health*, vol 86, no 4, pp 486-96.

Davey Smith, G., Hart, C., Blane, D., Gillis, C. and Hawthorne, V. (1997a) 'Lifetime socioeconomic position and mortality: prospective observational study', *British Medical Journal*, vol 314, pp 547-52.

EEC (1995) *On specific community action to combat poverty* (Council Decision of 19 December 1984), Official Journal of the EEC, 85/8/EEC, pp 2-24.

Ferrie, J.E., Shipley, M.J., Marmot, M.G., Stansfeld, S. and Smith, G.D. (1995) 'Health effects of anticipation of job change and non-employment: longitudinal data from the Whitehall II study', *British Medical Journal*, vol 311, pp 1264-9.

Forman, D., Newell, D.G., Fullerton, F., Yarnell, J.W.G., Stacey, A.R., Wald, N. and Sitar, F. (1991) 'Association between infection with *Helicobacter pylori* and risk of gastric cancer: evidence from a prospective investigation', *British Medical Journal*, vol 302, pp 1302-5.

Frankel, S. and Davey Smith, G. (1997) 'Evidence-based medicine and treatment choices', *Lancet*, vol 349, p 571.

Frankel, S., Elwood, P., Sweetnam, P., Yarnell, J. and Davey Smith, G. (1996) 'Birthweight, body mass index in middle age, and incident coronary heart disease', *Lancet*, vol 348, pp 1478-80.

Glynn, A. and Miliband, D. (1994) *Paying for inequality: The economic cost of social justice*, London: Rivers Oran Press.

Goldthorpe, J.H. (1987) *Social mobility and class structure in modern Britain*, 2nd edn, Oxford: Oxford University Press.

Goodman, A. and Webb, S. (1991) 'Why are there so many long term sick in Britain?', *Economic Journal*, vol 101, pp 252-62.

Goodman, A., Johnson, P. and Webb, S. (eds) (1997) *Inequality in the UK*, Oxford: Oxford University Press.

Gordon, D. and Pantazis, C. (eds) (1997) *Breadline Britain in the 1990s*, Aldershot: Ashgate Publishing Limited.

Graham, H. (1988) 'Women and smoking in the United Kingdom: the implications for health promotion', *Health Promotion*, vol 3, pp 371-82.

Gunnell, D.J., Davey Smith, G., Frankel, S.J., Nanchahal, K., Braddon, F.E.M. and Peters, T.J. (1996) 'Childhood leg length and adult mortality – follow up of the Carnegie survey of diet and growth in prewar Britain', Abstract in *Journal of Epidemiology and Community Health*, vol 50, pp 580-1.

Hansson, L.-E., Bergström, R., Sparén, P. and Adami, H.-O. (1991) 'The decline in the incidence of stomach cancer in Sweden 1960-1984: a birth cohort phenomenon', *International Journal of Cancer*, vol 47, pp 499-503.

Hutton, W. (1996) *The state we're in*, London: Vintage.

Kehrer, B.H. and Wolin, C.M. (1979) 'Impact of income maintenance on low birth weight: evidence from the Gary experiment', *Journal of Human Resources*, vol 14, pp 434-62.

Leon, D.A., Koupilova, I. and Lithell, H.O., Berglund, L., Mohsen, R., Vagers, D., Lithell, V.B. and McKeigue, P.M. (1996) 'Failure to realise growth potential in utero and adult obesity in relation to blood pressure in 50 year old Swedish men', *British Medical Journal*, vol 312, pp 401-6.

Lithell, H.O., McKeigue, P.M., Berglund, L., Mohsen, R., Lithell, U.-B. and Leon, D.A. (1996) 'Relation of size at birth to non-insulin dependent diabetes and insulin concentrations in men aged 50-60 years', *British Medical Journal*, vol 312, pp 406-10.

Lynch, J.W. and Kaplan, G.A. (1997) 'Understanding how inequality in the distribution of income affects health', *Journal of Health Psychology*, vol 2, pp 297-314.

Lynch, J.W., Kaplan, G.A. and Shema, S.J. (1997) 'Cumulative impact of sustained economic hardship on physical, cognitive, psychological and social functioning', *New English Journal of Medicine*, vol 387, pp 1889-95.

McDonough, P., Duncan, G.J., Williams, D. and House, J. (1997) 'Income dynamics and adult mortality in the United States, 1972 through 1989', *American Journal of Public Health*, vol 87, pp 1476-83.

Macintyre, S. (1994) 'Understanding the social patterning of health: the role of the social sciences', *Journal of Public Health Medicine*, vol 16, pp 53-9.

Mallonee, S., Istre, G.R., Rosenberg, M., Reddish-Douglas, M., Jordan, F., Silverstein, P. and Tunell, W. (1996) 'Surveillance and the prevention of residential fire injuries', *New England Journal of Medicine*, vol 335, pp 27-31.

Policy	**Expand the public health and collaborative capacity of health authorities to promote equity in health and healthcare**
Benefits	• Improved capacity to tackle the broader determinants of health inequalities.
	• Improved capacity to address the healthcare needs of disadvantaged populations.
	• Improved continuity of care across health and social care sectors.
Evidence	The main determinants of health inequalities lie beyond the immediate control of the healthcare sector. Hence, the health service must work collaboratively with other agencies to tackle them. A systematic review of effective intersectoral collaborations showed that healthcare systems can influence other agencies' agendas to reduce health inequalities.

Introduction

The NHS has long failed to take the issue of health inequalities seriously in two ways. First, the NHS has not placed sufficient emphasis on ensuring that there is equitable access to healthcare in England. Second, its potential to work with other agencies to tackle the broader determinants of health inequalities has not been fully exploited. The purpose of this paper is to demonstrate how the NHS has failed to take equity seriously, to provide evidence of resulting inequalities in the health services, and to suggest ways in which these can be tackled.

The nature of the problem

There are four areas within the NHS in which mechanisms for ensuring equity are inadequate. These are:

• strategic planning for equity in health and healthcare;
• resource allocation;

• appropriate services for disadvantaged groups;
• intersectoral partnerships to address the broader determinants of health.

Strategic planning for equity in health and healthcare

National policy framework

Equity of access to healthcare by need has been a fundamental principle of the NHS since it was established (Benzeval et al, 1995). However, with the exception of resource allocation policies described below, this principle has not been translated into explicit policy goals at the national level. Moreover, the scope of the NHS has never been defined in terms of rights to specific ranges and levels of service except in a limited number of areas codified within the *Patient's Charter* (Harrison and New, 1996). This means, for example, that there is considerable variation in the level and quality of service provided by different authorities (Le Grand et al, 1997) and the extent of user charges for domiciliary care (Harrison and New, 1997).

The health services' responsibility to address the broader determinants of health is a more recent policy goal, articulated in two policy initiatives launched in the 1990s. First, health promotion payments were introduced as part of the 1990 GP contract, which were subsequently revised due to criticism in 1993 and again in 1996 (Gillam et al, 1996; Florin, 1996). Second, a national strategy for health – the *Health of the nation* White Paper (DoH, 1992) – was published in 1992. Both of these led to a narrow interpretation of health promotion, emphasising health education and individual life-style change (Blackburn, 1993; Moran, 1996; Daykin and Naidoo, 1997) rather than a broad range of policies necessary to promote health (Whitehead, 1995), and neither emphasised equity in health. In response to this problem the *Variations in health* report (DoH, 1995) made policy recommendations about what the NHS should do to improve equity, but no accountability mechanisms were established to ensure that these were implemented (Benzeval, 1997).

Performance management of commissioning

The introduction of the purchaser/provider split and the development of a national health strategy created the potential for purchasers to refocus their activities towards equity and promoting health. However, despite the articulation of equity goals in purchasing plans and health strategies (Redmayne, 1995) and a greater emphasis on *Health of the nation* priority areas (Redmayne et al, 1993), such documents have had little influence over the commissioning process for several reasons (Milner and Meeking, 1996):

- purchasing is dominated by the contracting process, which is driven by acute sector issues (Øvretveit, 1995; Milner and Meeking, 1996);
- purchasers often do not have the specialist knowledge necessary (Harrison and New, 1997) or the power to enforce guidelines and standards on how specific services should be provided. Decisions are therefore left to clinicians, which results in medical practice variations;
- the NHSE *Priority and planning guidance* (NHSE, 1993, 1994, 1995, 1996), although mentioning the importance of equity of access to healthcare and the need to take account of 'variations in health', have not developed explicit objectives in relation to them;
- the accountability of purchasers is not linked to health or equity goals but to such targets as the efficiency index and objectives within the *Patient's Charter*. It is hardly surprising that most purchasers monitor efficiency rather than equity (Majeed and Pollock, 1993).

During the 1990s there has been a dramatic growth in sub-district purchasing including fundholding, GP or locality commissioning, and total purchasing (Mays and Dixon, 1996). There is concern that this could lead to the fragmentation of a strategic approach to commissioning (Benzeval et al, 1995). In addition, fundholding has been criticised for creating a two-tier system (Le Grand et al, 1997), although this problem is currently being addressed (Dobson, 1997).

Monitoring equity in health and healthcare

The NHS has no specific reporting requirements to assess equitable access to health services. Recording postcodes and more recently ethnicity on hospital and community medical records would allow some analyses to be conducted, although the data are incomplete and do not cover primary care.

The annual *On the state of public health* report and some local public health reports have, from time to time, addressed broader health inequalities. However, there is no requirement to do so and the quality of the reports is variable.

Resource allocation

Revenue resources for health and related social care are allocated to local areas by three separate funding streams, none of which take into account the distribution of resources in the other two, which is likely to exacerbate inequalities (Judge and Mays, 1994).

General Medical Services (GMS)

As the majority of expenditure on GMS is paid directly to GPs through a negotiated system of fees and allowances, the distribution of GPs is crucial to equitable access to primary care. The Medical Practices Committee (MPC) aims to equalise list sizes between areas, but does not take account of variations in need in any systematic way. This has resulted in substantial inequalities in access to GPs between areas (Benzeval and Judge, 1996; Bloor and Maynard, 1996). To attract GPs to disadvantaged areas, the government established the GP deprivation payment system, which, while welcome in principle, has been criticised both for its methodology (Carr-Hill and Sheldon, 1996) and for its failure to compensate GPs adequately for the extra workload in deprived areas (Worrall et al, 1997).

The MPC and Advisory Committee for Resource Allocation have set up two joint committees to examine the distribution of workforce and resources for primary care (Eccles, 1997). In the meantime the MPC has announced that it will weight list sizes in relation to the receipt of deprivation payments in the area (MPC, 1997), and the Department of Health has given health authorities £4m to develop a salaried GP scheme to improve access to healthcare in underserved areas (Milburn, 1997). This and other cash-limited GMS – for practice staff, cost rent schemes and computers – are allocated to health authorities on the basis of the needs-weighted capitation formula (NHSE, 1997). However, the need measure has not been empirically derived and many authorities are substantially under target (NHSE, 1997).

Hospital and Community Health Services (HCHS)

Over the last 20 years much effort has gone into developing a formula to allocate HCHS resources in relation to need (Mays, 1995; Sheldon, 1997). The current version weights populations for differences in age, structure, need – measured by proxies including morbidity, mortality and socio-economic factors – and differences in the costs of inputs (NHSE, 1997). The development of the needs indicators has been much criticised (Mays, 1995; Sheldon, 1997; Bevan, 1997). For example, they do not account for unmet need (Sheldon, 1997; Bevan, 1997) and the statistical models do not incorporate the extra costs of delivering healthcare to specific populations, such as minority ethnic groups (Smith, 1997).

At sub-district level, resource allocation was not attempted in any systematic way nor received much policy attention until the introduction of fundholding (Bevan, 1997). Difficulties in developing a capitation formula for fundholders led to their being funded on the basis of historic spending patterns, which exposed considerable local inequities both in favour and against fundholding practices (Le Grand et al, 1997). The expansion of sub-district commissioning is likely to exacerbate these problems, unless a clear mechanism for allocating resources to localities is developed (Bevan, 1997).

Personal Social Service (PSS) expenditure on community care

Although community care is not directly financed or provided through the NHS, it is crucial to the development of good quality healthcare, and therefore its distribution should be considered

alongside that of NHS resources (Judge and Mays, 1994). The main element of finance for community care is allocated to local authorities on the basis of the Standard Spending Assessments, which are derived from models of past utilisation (Judge and Mays, 1994). There is little clear evidence about whether or not this is done effectively or equitably. Moreover, this money is not ring-fenced and hence local authorities have the autonomy to spend more or less than the designated amount on these areas of care (Harrison and New, 1997).

Appropriate services for disadvantaged groups

People from disadvantaged backgrounds and members of some minority ethnic groups face particular cultural, economic and geographical barriers to accessing healthcare that should be addressed if services are to meet their needs (Benzeval, 1995).

Particular problems occur when users and professionals have different social and cultural backgrounds. For example, communication problems and cultural differences can reduce the quality of maternity care (Bowler, 1993), the appropriateness and uptake of domiciliary care (Boneham et al, 1997) and the quality of GP consultations (Rudat, 1994) among minority ethnic groups.

The distance from health facilities affects utilisation (Bentham and Haynes, 1985) and may affect clinical outcomes for emergency care (Harrison and Prentice, 1996). Geographical access can be a particular problem for people living in poverty or in rural areas, as well as older people and people with disabilities without ready means of transport (Benzeval, 1995). The increasing trend to centralise services to exploit economies of scale or concentrate expertise to improve the quality of care may directly conflict with promoting equity of access to services (Benzeval, 1995).

Evidence suggests that user charges for sight tests, dentistry, prescriptions and community care services, while modest in Britain compared with those of most other countries, may inhibit the use of services for those least able to pay. For example, a survey of adults over 60 found that people in non-manual occupations were more likely to have had a sight test than manual workers (RNIB, 1997).

Perhaps more important is the high opportunity cost of using health services experienced by some people. For example, workers in relatively low-status occupations may be reluctant to attend clinics during normal opening hours if they consequently lose income (Benzeval, 1995). More significantly, people who are homeless or living in poverty may have so many pressing demands on their time that making an effort to obtain healthcare is not a priority for them (Graham, 1987; Conway, 1993).

Intersectoral partnerships

To date, national cross-government measures to improve health through broader public policies have been noticeable by their absence (Benzeval, 1997). Although the *Health of the nation* White Paper proposed a Ministerial Cabinet Committee for Health and policy guidance on health impact assessments, neither appear to have been implemented effectively nor do they have a specific remit to address inequalities in health.

At a more local level, many health authorities have always had small-scale projects to improve the health of disadvantaged communities and have worked with other agencies for this purpose (Ashton, 1992; Allen, 1992; Laughlin and Black, 1995; DoH, 1995). However, such intersectoral action is fraught with difficulties, which, with notable exceptions (Benzeval et al, 1995; Birmingham Public Health Department, 1995; ELCHA, 1996), have substantially limited progress in this area. Barriers to interagency collaborations identified in a number of local studies (Nocon, 1993; Higgins et al, 1994; Moran, 1996; Higginbottom and Simpson, 1996; Costongs and Springett, 1997) include: conflicting models of health; constant internal organisational changes; lack of understanding of the roles of others; limited or no resources devoted to such activities; and lack of senior support and unclear goals.

The extent of the problem

There is mixed evidence of inequalities in access to healthcare, outlined below. Unfortunately, it is impossible to demonstrate the precise consequences of the health services' failure to work with other agencies to tackle the broader determinants of health, since its potential to do so has never been fully developed or assessed.

Overall healthcare

There have been few attempts (and none by the NHS itself) to assess the overall success of the NHS in ensuring equity of access to healthcare. Three studies have been published using the General Household Survey to examine the extent to which NHS expenditure has been delivered in relation to need across different social groups. A study using 1970s data found that the NHS favoured the middle classes (Le Grand, 1978). However, using data from the 1980s and a different approach to assessing need, a second study (O'Donnell and Propper, 1991) found that the NHS was 'pro poor'. Similarly, using data from 1984-91 a third study (Smaje and Le Grand, 1997) found that, with the exception of the Chinese, different ethnic groups received broadly similar care in relation to need.

The General Household Survey has also been used to assess the equity of use of specific services. A study (Whitehead et al, 1997) in the 1990s found that GP utilisation, but not outpatient care, favours people in manual occupations after accounting for differences in gender, age and health status. In relation to community care, a study in the 1980s found gender bias in the provision of domiciliary care (Bebbington and Davies, 1993) while a 1990s study found that disadvantaged groups used home helps more intensively than affluent groups (Evandrou and Falkingham, 1997). However, such macro studies run counter to a plethora of small-scale studies which suggest that there are considerable problems for access to care for some social groups.

Preventive care

There is some evidence that untargeted preventive care can widen inequalities in uptake (Reading et al, 1994), as people in deprived circumstances are less likely to use preventive services such as immunisation (Marsh and Channing, 1987; Reading et al, 1993), screening (Coulter and Baldwin, 1987; Majeed et al, 1994), health checks (Waller et al, 1990) and health promotion clinics (Gillam, 1992) than more affluent groups. Similarly, other studies have found lower uptake of screening among specific ethnic groups (McAvoy and Raza, 1988).

Primary and community health services

As mentioned above, evidence suggests that the distribution of GPs across England is not related to need (Benzeval and Judge, 1996; Bloor and Maynard, 1996) and that deprivation payments fail to provide adequate compensation for unequal workloads (Worrall et al, 1997). Some studies show that practices in disadvantaged areas face difficulties in recruiting GPs (MPC, 1997). Indicators of the quality of primary care services – such as the number of single-handed GPs, GPs over the age of 65, premises below minimum standards or practices without training status – are worse in disadvantaged localities (Johnstone et al, 1996; Boyle and Hamblin, 1997), and are a particular problem in London (Tomlinson, 1992; Boyle and Hamblin, 1997). A number of studies have shown differential referral rates (Cummins et al, 1981; Blaxter, 1984), use of diagnostic tests (Hartley et al, 1984) and prescribing behaviour (Cockburn, 1997) between different social groups, although they do not examine the appropriateness of the decisions. Some local evidence also suggests that the distribution of practice nurses, community practitioners and health visitors varies by area and is unrelated to need (Johnstone et al, 1996; Boyle and Hamblin, 1997).

Hospital care

The methodology for linking hospital usage and quality of care by need is in its infancy. Some studies demonstrate inequalities in cardiovascular (Ben-Shlomo and Chaturvedi, 1995; Johnstone et al, 1996; Payne and Saul, 1997) and orthopaedic interventions (Johnstone et al, 1996), and cancer survival rates by socio-economic group (Carnon et al, 1994; Schrijvers et al, 1995, 1997). Isolated studies also suggest that there are inequalities in cardiovascular treatment by gender (Kee et al, 1993; Petticrew et al, 1993; Majeed and Cook, 1996). By contrast, Hospital Episode Statistics data suggests that waiting times and usage of hospital services do not appear markedly unequal by socio-economic group (Steele and Willmer, 1997). However, most studies in this area do not adequately control for need, or examine the appropriateness of the care received.

Policy options

To ensure that the NHS takes inequalities in health more seriously in the future, new policies are required to: develop a framework for equity in health and healthcare; improve resource allocation by need; provide appropriate services for disadvantaged groups; and expand the public health and collaborative capacity of health authorities.

Develop a framework for equity

Strategic planning is required across a range of issues to make equity a reality within the NHS.

Central government action

The Department of Health and the Minister for Public Health need to develop cross-government mechanisms to tackle inequalities in health and to monitor their progress. These include:

- developing an appropriate methodology to assess the impact on health inequalities of government policies and publishing the results;
- using the Cross-Cabinet Health Committee to promote social policies that improve equity in health and to tailor or stop those that are likely to harm it (for example, the abolition of one-parent family benefit). The Committee should be accountable to the appropriate parliamentary review procedures.

National strategy for equity

A strategy needs to be developed for promoting equity in health and healthcare at all levels of the health system. It should comprise: a national policy for tackling inequalities in health (Benzeval et al, 1995), and a constitution for the NHS, which explicitly sets out the underlying aims and principles of the NHS and the range and standard of services that citizens, wherever they live, might expect of it (King's Fund Policy Institute, 1997). Both policies should be linked to performance management targets.

Local performance management

Commissioners should be held accountable for promoting equity in health and healthcare. For example, performance management targets should be developed to cover:

- the development of a joint health strategy with local authorities;
- the implementation of procedures for equity audits of healthcare and health impact assessments of both local authority and NHS activities;
- improving the uptake of healthcare by disadvantaged groups, especially for preventive health services;
- reducing social inequalities in health outcomes that are amenable to local action, for example, childhood accidents and teenage pregnancies.

Audit and monitoring mechanisms

The NHS should publish regular national and local reports on its progress in tackling health inequalities and promoting access to healthcare. In addition, independent audits of the health service could be broadened to cover equity issues. To meet these goals, data collection mechanisms need to be improved. Specifically:

- the requirement to record postcode and ethnic information should be extended to all healthcare records. More effective systems should be developed to ensure accurate and comprehensive coding;
- comparative equity data needs to be fed back to purchasers and providers in order for them to review their relative positions and take appropriate action;
- specific studies need to be conducted to develop a better understanding of the stages in the process of care which contribute most to inequalities in access.

Improve resource allocation

Primary care

GMS resources need to be allocated more directly in relation to need. First, an accurate assessment should

be made of the need for primary care resources across the country. Second, means of expanding and developing primary care resources in underserved areas need to be developed, for example, by providing incentives for primary care staff to work in disadvantaged areas by using cash-limited GMS funding in innovative ways. The government has recently announced new funds to promote salaried GPs; such activities should be encouraged and expanded (Milburn, 1997).

Localities

With the continued expansion of locality/GP commissioning, clear guidance on the allocation of resources in relation to need within health authorities needs to be developed. One useful approach has been developed by Bevan (1997), which combines national needs-weighted formula with local information.

Health and social care

The close interdependence between care provided in primary, hospital and community settings should be taken into account in funding decisions (Benzeval et al, 1995). An analysis of the relationship between funding in each of the three streams should be assessed. Mechanisms then need to be developed to support those areas that are poorly served across all funding systems. In the long term, the three funding systems could be brought into line. In addition, there needs to be some scope for virement between the different funding streams to promote innovative methods of providing integrated health and social care. Current government policy (NHSE, 1997) on this matter should be reviewed and developed.

Provide appropriate services for disadvantaged groups

Improve primary care

Community practitioners, particularly health visitors, are in a unique position to identify the underlying causes of ill-health and to work with the community to tackle them (Doyle and Thomas, 1996). To achieve this a more team-based approach to the provision of primary and community care needs to be developed, with an emphasis on the needs of the community as well as of individual clients

(Blackburn, 1993; Daykin and Naidoo, 1997). Many initiatives in the primary care White Papers (DoH, 1996a, 1996b) could help to develop this, although emphasis must be placed on promoting equity.

Promote effective interventions

Several reviews have identified effective interventions to promote the health of disadvantaged groups (Bunton et al, 1994; Gepkens and Gunning-Schepers, 1996; Arblaster et al, 1997); commissioners should be encouraged to employ such initiatives as appropriate. Some illustrative initiatives are shown in Box 1. New initiatives should take into account developing knowledge about what works best with such groups. Key characteristics of effective services already identified include: empowerment and support of disadvantaged groups; intensive and sensitive services; effective targeting and outreach; and, multidisciplinary and multifaceted approaches (Shorr, 1988; Benzeval et al, 1995; Gepkens and Gunning-Schepers, 1996). In addition, rigorous methods must be applied to the evaluation of interventions for equity (DoH, 1995; Gepkens and Gunning-Schepers, 1996).

Box 1: Interventions to improve health among disadvantaged groups

A systematic review of interventions to improve the health of disadvantaged groups was undertaken and is regularly updated by the NHS Centre for Reviews and Dissemination (Arblaster et al, 1997). This evidence should be disseminated widely and used to inform and audit programmes seeking to reduce health inequalities. Examples of interventions include:

- GP reminder systems to improve the uptake of preventive services, such as smoking cessation, cervical screening and hypertensive treatment, by relatively deprived groups;

- home visiting by health visitors, GPs and trained community peers to reinforce preventive health measures;

- NHS provision of nicotine replacement therapies;

- the use of anti-hypertensive medication for primary and secondary prevention of cardiovascular disease events;

- widening access to contraceptive services and the use of folic acid and calcium supplementation before and during pregnancy;

- employing bilingual health advocates to promote the use and quality of consultations in primary care;

- providing benefits advice in community settings, such as general practice clinics.

Reform professional education

Professional education needs to encourage multidisciplinary approaches to providing healthcare (Blackburn, 1993; Doyle and Thomas, 1996) and to ensure that practitioners are capable of responding to underlying social causes of ill-health (Blackburn, 1993; Daykin and Naidoo, 1997). These two objectives could be achieved by promoting multidisciplinary education (Blackburn, 1993; Doyle and Thomas, 1996) and by developing core courses that cover public health and broader health promotion issues (Blackburn, 1993; Daykin and Naidoo, 1997). The communication skills of professionals also need to be improved (Audit Commission, 1994), with particular emphasis on cultural sensitivity (Yee, 1997). One way of achieving these goals might be to establish a common foundation course for all health professionals (Schofield, 1996).

Expand the public health and collaborative capacity of health authorities

Public health in the NHS needs to be strengthened to enable it to meet the health and healthcare needs of the population (Jacobson et al, 1991). Health authorities should become public health agencies to develop effective intersectoral collaborations capable of tackling underlying causes of health inequalities, and to ensure that the local healthcare system meets population's needs in an equitable manner. Evidence suggests that community participation is required to achieve both these objectives (Gilles, 1997). More specifically, studies (Nocon, 1993; Higgins et al, 1994; Higginbottom and Simpson, 1996; Costongs and Springett, 1997) have identified a number of key features for effective collaboration, including:

- clarity of purpose and benefit for each partner;
- dedicated project leadership and senior commitment from all organisations;
- the development of mutual respect through interagency team-building balanced with achieving tangible benefits in the short term to maintain enthusiasm;
- clear management structures and delineation of responsibilities;
- dedicated resources.

Building these features into partnerships between local agencies and the community will provide a firm foundation from which to tackle health inequalities at the local level.

Acknowledgements

We are grateful to a number of colleagues who helped us develop our ideas or commented on an earlier draft of this paper, in particular: Nick Black, Mildred Blaxter, Sean Boyle, Jacky Chambers, Jennifer Dixon, Frances Drever, Chris Ham, Anthony Harrison, Iona Heath, Bobbie Jacobson, Lucy Johnson, Ken Judge, Amanda Killoran, Julian Le Grand, Nick Mays, Jo-Ann Mulligan, Diane Plamping, Alex Scott-Samuel, Peter Steele, Margaret Whitehead, Richard Willmer, Ian Wylie.

In addition, we gratefully acknowledge the submissions to the Inquiry into Inequalities in Health that helped to inform this report.

References

Allen, P. (1992) *Off the rocking horse: How councils can promote your health and environment*, London: Green Print.

Arblaster, L., Entwistle, V., Fullerton, D., Glanville, J., Forster, M., Lambert, M., Sheldon, T., Sowden, A. and Watt, I. (1997) *A review of the effectiveness of health promotion interventions aimed at reducing inequalities in health*, York: NHS Centre for Reviews and Dissemination, University of York.

Ashton, J. (1992) *Healthy cities*, Milton Keynes: Open University Press.

Audit Commission (1994) *What seems to be the matter? Communication between hospitals and patients*, London: HMSO.

Bebbington, A. and Davies, B. (1993) 'Efficient targeting of community care: the case of the home help service', *Journal of Social Policy*, vol 22, no 3, pp 373-91.

Ben-Shlomo, Y. and Chaturvedi, N. (1995) 'Assessing equity in access to health care provision in the UK: does where you live affect your chances of getting a coronary artery bypass graft?', *Journal of Epidemiology and Community Health*, vol 49, pp 200-4.

Bentham, C.G. and Haynes, R.M. (1985) 'Health, personal mobility and the use of health services in rural Norfolk', *Journal of Rural Studies*, vol 1, no 3, pp 231-9.

Benzeval, M. (1995) 'Health care for all? How to take equity seriously', in A. Harrison and S. Bruscini (eds) *Health care UK 1994/95*, London: King's Fund, pp 67-71.

Benzeval, M. (1997) 'Health', in A. Walker and C. Walker (eds) *Britain divided: The growth of social exclusion in the 1980s and 1990s*, London: CPAG, pp 153-69.

Benzeval, M. and Judge, K. (1996) 'Access to health care in England: continuing inequalities in the distribution of GPs', *Journal of Public Health Medicine*, vol 18, no 1, pp 33-44.

Benzeval, M., Judge, K. and Whitehead, M. (1995) 'The role of the NHS', in M. Benzeval, K. Judge and M. Whitehead (eds) *Tackling inequalities in health: An agenda for action*, London: King's Fund, pp 95-121.

Bevan, G. (1997) *Resource allocation within health authorities: Lessons from total purchasing sites*, London: King's Fund.

Birmingham Public Health Department (1995) *Closing the gap: Ten benchmarks for equity and quality in health*, Birmingham: Birmingham Public Health Department.

Blackburn, C. (1993) 'Making poverty a practical issue', *Health & Social Care in the Community*, vol 1, pp 297-305.

Blaxter, M. (1984) 'Equity and consultation rates in general practice', *British Medical Journal*, vol 288, pp 1963-7.

Bloor, K. and Maynard, A. (1996) *Equity in primary care*, York: Centre for Health Economics, University of York.

Boneham, M., Williams, K., Copeland, J., McKibbin, P., Wilson, K., Scott, A. and Saunders, P. (1997) 'Elderly people from ethnic minorities in Liverpool: mental illness, unmet need and barriers to service use', *Health & Social Care in the Community*, vol 5, no 3, pp 173-80.

Bowler, I. (1993) '"They're not the same as us": midwives' stereotypes of South Asian descent maternity patients', *Sociology of Health and Illness*, vol 15, no 2, pp 157-78.

Boyle, S. and Hamblin, R. (1997) *The health economy of London: A report to the King's Fund London Commission*, London: King's Fund.

Bunton, R., Burrows, R., Gillen, K. and Muncer, S. (1994) *Interventions to promote health in economically deprived areas: A critical review of the literature. A report to the Northern Regional Health Authority*, Newcastle upon Tyne: NHSE Northern and Yorkshire.

Carnon, A., Ssemwogerere, A., Lamont, D., Hole, D., Mallon, E., George, D. and Gillis, C. (1994) 'Relation between socioeconomic deprivation and pathological prognostic factors in women with breast cancer', *British Medical Journal*, vol 309, pp 1054-7.

Carr-Hill, R. and Sheldon, T. (1996) 'Designing a deprivation payment for general practitioners: the UPA(8) wonderland', *British Medical Journal*, vol 302, pp 393-6.

Cockburn, J.P.S. (1997) 'Prescribing behaviour in clinical practice: patients expectations and doctors perceptions of patients expectations – a questionnaire study', *British Medical Journal*, vol 315, pp 520-3.

Conway, J. (1993) 'Ill-health and homelessness: the effects of living in bed and breakfast accommodation', in R. Burridge and D. Ormandy (eds) *Unhealthy housing: Research remedies and reform*, London: E & FN Spon, pp 283-300.

Costongs, C. and Springett, J. (1997) 'Joint working and the production of a city health plan: the Liverpool experience', *Health Promotion International*, vol 12, no 1, pp 9-19.

Coulter, A. and Baldwin, A. (1987) 'Survey of population coverage in cervical cancer screening in the Oxford region', *Journal of the Royal College of General Practitioners*, vol 37, pp 441-3.

Cummins, R., Jarman, B. and White, P. (1981) 'Do general practitioners have different "referral thresholds"?', *British Medical Journal*, vol 282, pp 1037-9.

Daykin, N. and Naidoo, J. (1997) 'Poverty and health promotion in primary health care: professionals perspective', *Health & Social Care in the Community*, vol 5, no 5, pp 309-17.

Dobson, F. (1997) *Fairness and equity for hospital treatment: End of 'two-tier' NHS in sight*, London: DoH Press Release 97/169.

DoH (Department of Health) (1992) *The health of the nation: A strategy for health in England*, London: HMSO.

DoH (1995) *Variations in health: What can the Department of Health and NHS do?*, London: DoH.

DoH (1996a) *Choice and opportunity: Primary care: The future*, Cm 3390, London: The Stationery Office.

DoH (1996b) *Primary care: Delivering the future*, Cm 3512, London: The Stationery Office.

Doyle, Y. and Thomas, P. (1996) 'Promoting health through primary care: challenges in taking a strategic approach', *Health Education Journal*, vol 55, pp 3-10.

Eccles, L. (1997) *Briefing note – capitation funding*, London: DoH (unpublished).

ELCHA (East London and the City Health Department) (1996) *Health in the East End. Annual Public Health Report 1995/96*, London: ELCHA.

Evandrou, M. and Falkingham, J. (1997) 'The personal social services', in H. Glennerster and J. Hills (eds) *The state of welfare*, 2nd edn, Oxford: Oxford University Press, pp 189-255.

Florin, D. (1996) 'Barriers to evidence based policy: health promotion in primary care changes again', *British Medical Journal*, vol 313, pp 894-5.

Gepkens, A. and Gunning-Schepers, L.J. (1996) 'Interventions to reduce socioeconomic health differences: a review of the international literature', *European Journal of Public Health*, vol 6, no 3, pp 218-26.

Gillam, S.J. (1992) 'Provision of health promotion clinics in relation to population need: another example of the inverse care law?', *British Journal of General Practice*, vol 42, pp 54-6.

Gillam, S.J., McCartney, P. and Thorogood, M. (1996) 'Health promotion in primary care: even less coherent than before', *British Medical Journal*, vol 312, pp 324-5.

Gilles, P. (1997) *Review and evaluation of health promotion: The effectiveness of alliances or partnerships for health promotion*, London: Health Education Authority.

Graham, H. (1987) 'Women smoking and family health', *Social Science and Medicine*, vol 25, no 1, pp 47-56.

Harrison, A. and New, B. (1996) 'Commentary', in A. Harrison (ed) *Health care UK, 1995/96: An annual review of health care policy*, London: King's Fund, pp 55-90.

Harrison, A. and New, B. (1997) 'Main events', in A. Harrison (ed) *Health care UK 1996/97: The King's Fund annual review of health policy*, London: King's Fund, pp 1-68.

Harrison, A. and Prentice, S. (1996) *Acute futures*, London: King's Fund.

Hartley, R., Charlton, J., Harris, C. and Jarman, B. (1984) 'Influence of patient characteristics on test ordering in general practice', *British Medical Journal*, vol 289, pp 735-8.

Higginbottom, G. and Simpson, C. (1996) 'Developing alliances for health: principles and practice', *Health Visitor*, vol 69, no 5, pp 108-9.

Higgins, R., Oldman, C. and Hunter, D. (1994) 'Working together: lessons for collaboration between health and social services', *Health & Social Care in the Community*, vol 2, pp 269-77.

Jacobson, B., Smith, A. and Whitehead, M. (1991) *The nation's health: A strategy for the 1990s*, London: King's Fund.

Johnstone, F., Lucy, J., Scott-Samuel, A. and Whitehead, M. (1996) 'Deprivation and health in North Cheshire: an equity audit of health services', Liverpool Public Health Observatory: EQUAL.

Judge, K. and Mays, N. (1994) 'Allocating resources for health and social care in England', *British Medical Journal*, vol 308, pp 1363-6.

Kee, F., Gaffney, B., Carrie, S. and O'Reilly, D. (1993) 'Access to coronary catheterisation: fair shares for all?', *British Medical Journal*, vol 307, pp 1305-7.

King's Fund Policy Institute (1997) 'A new constitution for the NHS', in A. Harrison (ed) *Health care UK, 1996/97 the King's Fund annual review of health policy*, London: King's Fund, pp 138-54.

Laughlin, S. and Black, D. (1995) *Poverty and health: Tools for change*, Birmingham: Public Health Trust.

Le Grand, J. (1978) 'The distribution of public expenditure: the case of health care', *Economica*, vol 45, pp 125-42.

Le Grand, J., Mays, N., Mulligan, J., Goodwin, N., Dixon, J. and Glennister, H. (1997) *Models of purchasing and commissioning: Review of the evidence: A report to the Department of Health*, London: King's Fund, mimeo.

McAvoy, B. and Raza, R. (1988) 'Asian women: (i) contraceptive knowledge, attitudes and usage (ii) contraceptive services and cervical cytology', *Health Trends*, vol 20, pp 11-17.

Majeed, F. and Cook, D. (1996) 'Age and sex differences in the management of ischaemic heart disease', *Public Health*, vol 110, pp 7-12.

Majeed, A. and Pollock, A. (1993) 'Health authorities should monitor equity of service', *British Medical Journal*, vol 306, p 1689.

Majeed, F., Chaturvedi, N., Reading, R. and Ben-Shlomo, Y. (1994) 'Monitoring and promoting equity in primary and secondary care', *British Medical Journal*, vol 308, pp 1426-9.

Marsh, G. and Channing, D. (1987) 'Narrowing the health gap between a deprived and an endowed community', *Archives of Disease in Childhood*, vol 62, pp 392-6.

Mays, N. (1995) 'Geographical resource allocation in the English National Health Service, 1971-1994: the tension between normative and empirical approaches', *International Journal of Epidemiology*, vol 24, no 3 (Supplement), S96-S102.

Mays N. and Dixon, J. (1996) *Purchaser plurality in UK healthcare: Is a consensus emerging and is it the right one?*, London: King's Fund.

Milburn, A. (1997) *£4million to kickstart breakthrough salaried doctors scheme*, London: DoH, Press Release 97/354.

Milner, P. and Meeking, J. (1996) 'Editorial: failings of purchaser-provider split', *Journal of Public Health Medicine*, vol 18, no 4, pp 379-80.

Moran, G. (1996) *Promoting health and local government*, London: Health Education Authority.

MPC (Medical Practices Committee) (1997) *Newsletter issue 3 July*, London: MPC.

NHSE (1993) *Priority and planning guidance for the NHS: 1994/93*, Leeds: NHSE.

NHSE (1994) *Priority and planning guidance for the NHS: 1995/96*, Leeds: NHSE.

NHSE (1995) *Priority and planning guidance for the NHS: 1996/97*, Leeds: NHSE.

NHSE (1996) *Priority and planning guidance for the NHS: 1997/98*, Leeds: NHSE.

NHSE (1997) *1998/99 health authority revenue cash limits exposition book*, Leeds: NHSE.

Nocon, A. (1993) 'Made in heaven?', *Health Service Journal*, vol 23, December, pp 24-6.

O'Donnell, O. and Propper, C. (1991) 'Equity and the distribution of UK National Health Service resources', *Journal of Health Economics*, vol 10, pp 1-19.

Øvretveit, J. (1995) *Purchasing for health*, Buckingham: Open University Press.

Payne, N. and Saul, C. (1997) 'Variations in use of cardiology services in a health authority: comparison of coronary artery revascularisation rates with prevalence of angina and coronary mortality', *British Medical Journal*, vol 314, pp 257-61.

Petticrew, M., McKee, M. and Jones, J. (1993) 'Coronary artery surgery: are women discriminated against?', *British Medical Journal*, vol 306, pp 1164-6.

Reading, R., Jarvis, S. and Openshaw, S. (1993) 'Measurement of social inequalities in health and use of health services among children in Northumberland', *Archives of Disease in Childhood*, vol 68, pp 626-31.

Reading, R., Colver, A., Openshaw, S. and Jarvis, S. (1994) 'Do interventions that improve immunisation uptake also reduce social inequalities in uptake?', *British Medical Journal*, vol 308, pp 1142-4.

Redmayne, S. (1995) *Reshaping the NHS: Strategies, priorities and resource allocation*, Birmingham: NAHAT.

Redmayne, S., Klein, R. and Day, P. (1993) *Sharing out resources: Purchasing and priority setting in the NHS*, Birmigham: NAHAT.

RNIB (Royal National Institute for the Blind) (1997) *Losing sight of blindness*, London: RNIB.

Rudat, K. (1994) *Black and minority ethnic groups in England: Health and lifestyles*, London: Health Education Authority.

Schofield, M. (1996) *The future healthcare workforce: The steering group report*, Manchester: Health Service Management Unit, University of Manchester.

Schorr, L. (1988) *Within our reach: Breaking the cycle of deprivation*, New York, NY: Anchor Books.

Schrijvers, C., Mackenbach, J.P., Lutz, J., Quinn, M. and Coleman, M. (1995) 'Deprivation, stage at diagnosis and cancer survival', *International Journal of Cancer*, vol 63, pp 324-9.

Schrijvers, C., Mackenbach, J.P., Lutz, J., Quinn, M. and Coleman, M. (1997) 'Deprivation and survival from breast cancer', *British Journal of Cancer*, vol 72, pp 738-43.

Sheldon, T. (1997) Editorial, 'Formula fever: allocating resources in the NHS', *British Medical Journal*, vol 315, p 964.

Smaje, C. and Le Grand, J. (1997) 'Ethnicity and the use of health services in the British NHS', *Social Science and Medicine*, vol 45, no 3, pp 485-96.

Smith, P. (1997) 'Examination of witnesses', in Health Committee, *Allocation of resources to health authorities: Minutes of evidence and appendices*, London: House of Commons HC477-II, pp 16-26.

Steele, P. and Willmer, R. (1997) *Modified HES data analysis*, London: DoH (unpublished).

Waller, D., Agass, D., Mant, D., Coulter, A., Fuller, A. and Jones, L. (1990) 'Health checks in general practice: another example of inverse care?', *British Medical Journal*, vol 300, pp 1115-18.

Whitehead, M. (1995) 'Tackling inequalities: a review of policy initiatives', in M. Benzeval, K. Judge and M. Whitehead (eds) *Tackling inequalities in health: An agenda for action*, London: King's Fund, pp 22-52.

Whitehead, M., Evandrou, M., Haglund, B. and Diderichsen, F. (1997) 'As the health divide widens in Sweden and Britain, what's happening to access to care', *British Medical Journal*, vol 315, pp 1006-8.

Worrall, A., Rea, J.N. and Ben-Shlomo, Y. (1997) 'Counting the cost of social disadvantage in primary care: retrospective analysis of patient data', *British Medical Journal*, vol 314, pp 38-42.

Yee, L. (1997) *Breaking barriers: Towards culturally competent general practice*, London: Royal College of General Practice.

8b

Tackling inequalities in health and healthcare – the role of the NHS

Bobbie Jacobson

Introduction

The NHS has two interlinked responsibilities in relation to health inequalities:

- to provide equitable access to effective healthcare in relation to need;
- to work in partnership with other agencies to tackle the broader determinants of health.

This chapter describes the extent to which the NHS has achieved these two objectives, and how further progress might be made.

While equity in access to healthcare in relation to need has been a fundamental founding principle of the NHS (Ross, 1952) and is central to government policy (DoH, 1997, 1998) a clearer, more modern definition of equity is required. This is needed in particular to gain a better understanding of what aspects of equity it is best to tackle at national and local levels.

We welcome the impetus given by government to tackle the determinants of health and reduce health inequalities in its White Paper *The new NHS* (DoH, 1997) and *Our healthier nation* (DoH, 1998) which, if taken together with *Modernising local government* (DETR, 1998a), and the creation of Regional Development Agencies such as the Greater London Authority (DETR, 1998a) re-emphasise the important role of the NHS working with other agencies to tackle inequalities in health and healthcare.

There are five types of equity we could aim for: financial and geographical equality (equality in spending per head of population); equality of health status; equality of service use; equality of treatment outcome; and equality of access to services (Pereira, 1993). Both financial equity and equity of service use imply that all individuals have the same needs. This is clearly not the case and should not be an aim of the NHS. We believe that in terms of equity the objectives of the NHS should be:

- to contribute towards reducing inequalities in health status;
- to achieve equality of access to health services in relation to need;
- to achieve equality of treatment/intervention outcomes.

Underlying these objectives is a clear need to allocate resources equitably.

Reducing inequalities in health status

Because many of the prime determinants of health lie outside the NHS itself we see the NHS as playing a key contributory role that is shared with other partner organisations, including central government, local authorities, the voluntary and business sector and communities. This shared responsibility is central to the "Contract for Health" articulated in the government's Green Paper *Our healthier nation* (DoH, 1998). As we describe elsewhere in this report, major inequalities in health status between different groups and different parts of the country will not be eradicated by *local* action alone, but require actions by central and European government. We see the prime local responsibility as being to

2|

define, reduce and monitor inequalities in health and healthcare *within* a health or local authority area. It remains a national responsibility to define the overall strategic framework for equity within which objectives and targets need to be set at each level.

An effective strategy to reduce inequalities in health whether national or local needs to progress through the following steps:

- equity audit of health and healthcare between and within areas;
- development of objectives/targets for tackling inequalities in partnership with local agencies and communities;
- developing agreed, resourced action plans and monitoring methods;
- regular reports on progress.

There is no requirement nationally, locally or regionally to undertake a systematic review of inequalities in health or healthcare – that is, an equity audit. However, much of the data needed to support such analyses is available from the Census, Public Health Common data set and other health and local authority sources. Initiatives taken round the country have been patchy. A survey of Directors of Public Health in England showed that at least 32 such studies had been undertaken and summarised in Annual Public Health Reports (DoH Variations in Health, 1994).

An assessment of inequalities in health status and its determinants at different levels in the system provides not only a rich source of comparative information, it also offers opportunities for wider collaborative action. The North West Regional Office of the National Health Service Executive (NHSE) has undertaken such an analysis as a stimulus to local action (Flynn and Knight, 1998). Studies within regions across the UK show firm evidence of growing socio-economic inequalities in health status (Phillimore et al, 1991; Bardsley and Morgan, 1996; DETR, 1998b). City level analyses have been undertaken for a number of years within the WHO Healthy Cities initiative (Doyle et al, 1996) and more recently 'Project Megapoles' has allowed comparisons to be made between London and other capital cities across Europe (Agren et al, 1997). Cities such as Birmingham, Liverpool and Sheffield (Birmingham Annual Public Health Report, 1995; Liverpool City

Health Plan, 1996) whose health and local authorities are coterminous, have undertaken detailed analyses of inequalities within their cities.

Equity audit: Liverpool and Birmingham

Liverpool, which was the first city to join the WHO Healthy Cities initiative 10 years ago, has a joint Liverpool City Health Plan (January 1996). An equity audit of health and its social, economic and educational determinants has been published (Liverpool Health Authority, 1996).

More recently, the City's employment economic and regeneration strategies have been more closely aligned to health objectives. While there is little evidence of any reduction in inequalities in most disease areas, there is some evidence of a shift of primary care resources into areas of greatest need with a resultant increase in immunisation uptake (Flynn and Knight, 1998). A new index of quality of life and health has been developed to help monitor progress in implementing the City's Plan. It comprises 21 indicators of social, economic, educational, environmental and health change which can be measured in each of the City's 33 wards. This composite measure can be used to monitor equity in health and healthcare between different parts of the City.

On the basis of a similar equity audit, Birmingham Health Authority has identified the gaps in health and healthcare that need to be addressed (Birmingham Annual Public Health Report, 1995). Similar analyses in London have shown major and growing, socio-economic inequalities in health status and its determinants (Public Health Report for London).

While the national commitment to tackling inequalities in health is evident, there is still little evidence of a comprehensive approach to strategic planning for equity both in health and healthcare (Benzeval and Donald, 1997). The backbone of such a framework is, however, being put into place. Through the White Paper, the government has created five essential new vehicles for improving health and healthcare – some local and some national.

- *A local Health Improvement Programme:* this will need to define health priorities and set out objectives and plans for health improvements over a three-year period.
- *Primary Care Groups (PCGs)/Trusts* which will be cross-sectoral and will work within the local health improvement framework to improve the health of local populations.
- A new system of *clinical governance* backed up by a Legislative Duty of Quality.
- A *Legislative Duty of Partnership* between health and local authorities.
- A new *Performance Assessment Framework* for the NHS which contains six dimensions including health improvement, and aspects of equity together with National Service Frameworks.

However, there is, as yet, no clarity about what the national objectives for reducing inequalities in health are and where the responsibilities for reducing such inequalities lie at each level within the system – including government, health and local authorities and communities. There is therefore a real risk that policy and practice will not be in line with aspirations. This is especially the case at sub-district level where Primary Care Groups (PCGs)/Trust decisions could create new inequities in policy and practice. This might emerge as policy or rationing decisions at PCG level which might reduce access to some services for parts of health authority populations. The potential input of between 600-700 PCGs in England or equity of access to primary and other levels of care is entirely unknown – as is their potential to fragment strategic planning (NHS Confederation, The Development of Primary Care Groups: Policy into Practice, May 1998, Birmingham Research Park, Vincent Drive, Birmingham B15 2SQ).

While the five vehicles for change in the NHS and its partner agencies provide a positive basis for refocusing on health and promoting effective healthcare, none articulate explicitly the equally central importance of tackling inequalities. It is vital, therefore, that the remaining guidance on implementing NHS change should bring these vehicles together to tackle inequity. We welcome the recognition given to the need to target disadvantaged communities in the Health Action Zone initiative and the linkage of Single Regeneration Bidding to health objectives. But

more is needed. An analysis and joint strategy to tackle inequity should be an explicit requirement of every Health Improvement Programme, and should be a required objective of every PCG working with the NHS and other agencies and their communities served. A requirement for the new National Institute of Clinical Excellence and for Clinical Governance mechanisms to address inequities in access to effective care is also needed.

The capacity of health authorities, PCGs and local authorities to tackle such an ambitious public health programme has already been questioned. The Chief Medical Officer's Review of the Public Health Function has concluded that a well-resourced, multidisciplinary public health network is required at each level in the system to tackle the new health strategy (CMO, 1998). There is, as yet, no clear indication of how this is to be achieved. Indeed, there is a real risk of further losses of this public health and health promotion capacity if such resources are shifted to PCGs without any explicit requirement that they should be used to promote the wider interagency health strategy.

Resource allocation in the NHS

Progress has been made in recent years in achieving a more equitable approach to allocating health and related resources. The government's Advisory Committee on Resource Allocation (ACRA), which has succeeded the Resource Allocation Group, is now assessing how resources allocated to primary care (GMS non-cash-limited) can be weighted on a capitation basis in relation to need. This is a step towards a unified needs-based funding stream for the NHS although the ability to reflect real needs is still controversial. We welcome this as it may allow PCGs/Trusts to shift resources more easily to areas of greatest need. There will, however, still be a separate funding stream for social care weighted on a different basis from the NHS, which could exacerbate some aspects of inequalities (Judge and Mays, 1994).

While further work is being undertaken to develop an explicit needs-based weighting for the allocation of GPs to health authority areas by the Medical Practices Committee (MPC), the MPC continues to operate outside system accountability. More importantly, a formulaic approach to the allocating of GPs is unlikely to be sufficient as a policy alone to deal with the growing shortage of GPs in deprived inner-city areas.

The GP deprivation payment system, whereby GPs working in deprived areas receive additional payments, while well-intentioned, has neither been effective in attracting GPs to these areas, nor in increasing access to effective services for disadvantaged populations (Worrall et al, 1997; MPC, 1997). It has methodological shortcomings and has been shown to have failed to compensate GPs adequately for the extra workload of working with deprived communities. Some of this additional work relates to the extra administrative costs of serving highly mobile populations. This is not taken into account at all.

If the 'inverse prevention law' is to be reversed (see below), then a new approach is needed to the way in which other payments such as health promotion and chronic disease management payments are made to GPs which currently serve to reinforce inequity in access to effective preventive care.

If the evaluation of Primary Care Act pilots is shown to provide effective new models of care for disadvantaged groups, then this initiative will merit faster implementation with associated incentives. The impact of other flexibilities such as Section 36 of the Payments (Primary Care Act) should be similarly evaluated.

Resource allocation: Hospital and Community Health Services (HCHS)

Despite the considerable effort made to achieve greater equity in the allocation of HCHS resources (Mays, 1995; Sheldon, 1997), there are a number of major criticisms which still need to be met (Mays, 1995; Sheldon, 1997). First, the methodology for estimating the size of underenumerated, mobile and homeless populations needs to be improved in the Census and inter-Censal years. This is an even greater problem for the allocation of resources to

PCG populations where practice-based estimates can be wildly inaccurate and exclude those who are unregistered. The new formula for allocating resources to PCGs/Trusts will need to address this.

Second, there is no weighting in the HCHS formula for the costs of ethnic diversity (additional to existing disease weightings). These include the direct costs of inputs such as bilingual advocates/interpretation which have been shown to improve health outcome in disadvantaged ethnic groups (Parsons and Day, 1992) and the indirect costs of longer consultations. As many ethnic and cultural needs are not easily quantified (Johnson et al, 1997), weighting the resource allocation formula may not be the most effective solution. The creation of an 'Ethnic Diversity Levy' and allocating it in relation to size, diversity and need identified by health authorities is likely to provide a more effective targeting and accountability mechanism. Combining this resource with Section 11 payments to local authorities to meet communities' additional language needs may offer an effective solution.

While the HCHS formula provides a weighting for mental health needs, it has been widely criticised as being inadequate – especially in recognition of the more recent, rising inflow of mentally disordered offenders from the Criminal Justice System into the NHS, whose costs have been inadequately weighted (DoH, 1997). Experience suggests that the most effective means of targeting resources to meet these needs has been via specifically earmarked Challenge Funds which have ensured that the resource is spent on what is intended.

The means by which HCHS resources are allocated fairly is affected not only by the resource allocation formula itself but by the *pace* by which health authorities move towards their target allocation and the way in which those resources are then spent. Figure 1 shows that in 1998/99 if the top 20% of health authorities in England had been able to move to their target allocation, this would have involved a shift of over £198m from those currently over target. Such shifts of resources are large and would need careful planning, but need to be achieved if HCHS resources are to be distributed equitably.

Figure 1: Distance from resource allocation target – all health authorities in England (1998/99)

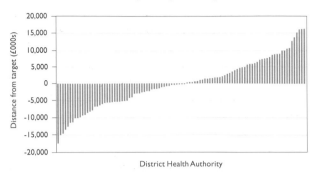

Source: DoH: Resource Allocation Exposition Booklet (1999)

Health promotion

Aside from specific health promotion payments in primary care, and ring-fenced HIV/AIDS and drugs misuse funding, there is no recognition of a capitation, or needs-based allocation to support health promotion. The formulaic, needs-based approach to targeting HIV prevention funds has achieved considerable success in allocating resources where they are most needed (NHSE, 1997) although the use of these resources needs to be targeted and monitored more effectively. This principle of ring-fencing resources with greater accountability for their use could be used both visibly and effectively in local interagency work to support *Our healthier nation*. Areas which are furthest from the *Our healthier nation* targets between and within districts would be expected to benefit. It would be useful to explore whether a body such as the Health Education Authority could fulfil these functions. Health Improvement Programmes could be a powerful vehicle for targeting such a local resource with Annual Public Health Reports reporting back on the impact over time.

Inequities in the NHS

Our consideration of the extent of inequity within the NHS has focused on areas where the evidence base suggests that strong systematic inequity exists. It is important to note that differences in access to care or to treatment do not necessarily indicate inequity on their own – unless they can be adjusted for need. Equally, high levels of intervention are not necessarily a good indication of whether those interventions are inappropriate or ineffective.

We have divided our consideration into those inequities affecting primary care, and those affecting secondary or tertiary (specialist) care and finally mental health services. Our overriding perspective has been that we should be aiming to achieve *equitable access to effective health for those who need it*. In the case of primary care, however, where it is of critical importance that preventive and treatment services are accessible to the *whole* population, it is thus of paramount importance that services are very locally accessible as well as being effective.

For some hospital care – especially tertiary – a different balance needs to be struck between local access and effective 'critical mass' of services and staff to achieve good outcomes. As services become more specialised, good treatment outcomes must be more explicitly balanced against local access. This is most clearly illustrated in government policy on the proper distribution of cancer services as recommended in the Calman/Hine Report (DoH, 1995a). In order to achieve good treatment outcomes for some cancers, not every local district hospital should have either a cancer centre or a cancer unit. We therefore welcome the new discipline that we hope will emerge as a result of the new NHS Service Frameworks – thus avoiding duplication of scarce specialist resources. This will assist in shifting towards a more equitable distribution of NHS resources between regions and between acute and primary healthcare.

A recent systematic review of inequities in access to healthcare has shown that most research on inequities in access to healthcare neither adjusts for need or for socio-economic factors (Goddard and Smith, 1998). We have taken this into account in interpreting our findings.

Inequities in primary care

Access to effective, local primary healthcare is determined by several 'supply' factors:

*   the distribution of GPs, practice staff, dentists, pharmacists, community health staff and other primary care practitioners;
*   the quality of primary care facilities which allow an appropriate range of services to be provided;

- the quality of training and education of primary care staff;
- the ability to recruit and retain GPs and primary care staff;
- resources available to recruit, and train those staff;
- cultural and gender sensitivity of services.

These must be set against demand factors which include knowledge about health and illness and belief systems within the community about entitlement to relevance of services.

There is consistent evidence that higher rates of consultation are associated with greater deprivation (Goddard and Smith, 1998). The evidence suggests that this relationship persists after adjusting for need (Goddard and Smith, 1998). Despite these higher rates, there is also evidence that the quality and length of time of such consultations is poorer for those from lower socio-economic groups than it is for those who are middle class. The data for minority ethnic groups shows that some groups – such as the Chinese, Africans, and young Pakistani women – have low consultation rates relative to need, but that the differences for other ethnic groups are not obvious.

The further away patients live from their GP practice the less likely they are to consult. This is evident in rural areas – although the differences are not as great for serious health problems as for less severe ones (Carr-Hill et al, 1997).

It has been widely reported that women consult more often than men. It is unclear whether this represents a gender inequity for men or whether the differences – mainly ages 15-44 – represent appropriate differences in need during the reproductive and childrearing years (Goddard and Smith, 1998).

The inverse care law is more evident, however, in the inequitable distribution of GPs (Judge and Mays, 1994; Hacking, 1996). Figure 2 shows that the position has been worsening for those living in the most deprived parts of the country while improving in the least deprived.

Figure 2: Trends in the distribution of GPs in relation to deprivation score (UPA)

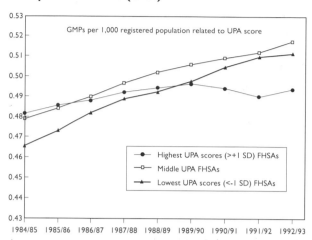

Source: B. Jarman (personal communication)

A number of studies show that deprived areas suffer increasing difficulty in recruiting GPs (MPC, 1997). This situation has been exacerbated – especially in inner London – by the poor quality of primary care premises, large numbers of single-handed GPs, GPs approaching retirement and practices without training status (Johnstone et al, 1996; Boyle and Hamblin, 1997; DoH, 1997).

Evidence from local studies suggests that this inequity extends beyond that of GPs to other primary care staff including practice nurses, health visitors and district nurses (Hirst et al, 1998).

A local analysis of the distribution of practice staff (see Figure 3) shows major inequities in distribution between practices. This has been shown to be associated with the risk of admission to hospital for asthma (Livingstone et al, 1996) and to practices reaching immunisation targets in the GP contract (ELCHA, 1998).

Strong evidence exists to support what might be called the 'Inverse Prevention Law' in primary care in which those communities most at risk of ill-health have least access to a range of effective preventive services including cancer screening programmes, health promotion and immunisation (Goddard and Smith, 1998). While the relationship is strongest for socio-economic factors, it is likely that there are additional inequities in access suffered – especially by Bangladeshi women (Benzeval and Judge, 1996). In addition it has been shown that access to women practitioners has been a deterrent to Asian women

Figure 3: Inequities in the distribution of practice staff* in an inner-city district

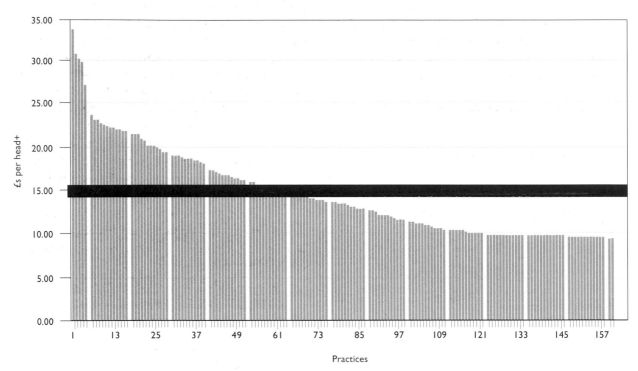

Practices

Notes:

* Funded by General Medical Services.

+ The current staff budgets for all GP practices in ELCHA are shown in the graph above. The £ per head represents the budget claimed by each practice per year per head of the practice population which they serve (the average patient list size per GP in ELCHA in 1996/97 was 2,041). It should be noted that there is no adjustment for list inflation.

Source: ELCHA (1998, Figure 2.2)

taking up an invitation for cervical cancer screening (Naish et al, 1994). Local studies have shown that access to female practitioners is poorest in areas with high concentrations of Asian residents (Birmingham Annual Public Health Report, 1995) and that practices with a female doctor or nurse are more likely to reach the cervical cytology targets set out in the GP contract (ELCHA, 1998).

Sub-regional and small area analyses illustrate this inequity graphically for areas such as Liverpool (Flynn and Knight, 1998) and Birmingham, where the most deprived parts of Birmingham are least well served (Birmingham Annual Public Health Report, 1995). Figure 4 shows that within London health promotion claims by GPs are highest in the least deprived and lowest in the most deprived areas.

Figure 4: Jarman UPA score versus GP health promotion claims, London boroughs (October 1995)

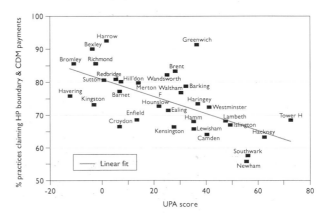

Note: HP = health promotion; CDM = chronic disease management.

Source: After Bardsley et al (1997)

27

Tackling inequalities in health and healthcare

Figure 5 shows the findings of a new analysis we commissioned which groups health authorities into seven deprivation clusters, based on the Jarman UPA score. It shows a clear pattern of inequitable access to immunisation services – with the most deprived clusters having the lowest uptake rates.

Figure 5: Immunisation uptake rates by deprivation cluster

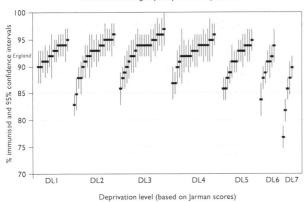

Source: Central Health Outcomes Unit (1998)

It is important to note that Figure 6 shows inequities *between* and also *within* deprivation clusters. This offers potential scope for setting and monitoring targets for PCGs/Trusts and their health authorities to reduce such inequalities within similarly deprived clusters as well as between them.

Figure 6: Regional variations in the effectiveness of the NHS to control high blood pressure

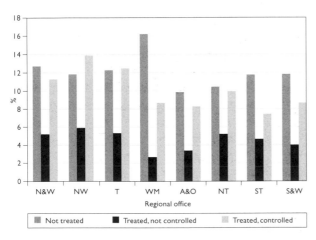

Source: Central Health Outcomes Unit (1998)

Figure 6 provides further evidence of both poor performance and variations in the NHS' performance in treating high blood pressure effectively. This example is important because it is one of the important cost-effective contributions primary care can make to the population prevention of stroke and chronic heart disease (CHD). But it has also been shown that the use of evidence-based guidelines in primary care can reduce socio-economic differences in high blood pressure (NHS Centre for Reviews and Dissemination, 1995). A review of the contribution of the NHS to reducing what was then termed 'Variations in Health' in the five key areas of the *Health of the nation* strategy (DoH, 1995b) showed that while evidence was lacking in many areas, most effective interventions designed to reduce socio-economic or ethnic variations in health had one or more of the following characteristics:

- intensive input
- multifaceted appropriateness
- multidisciplinary
- involved home visiting
- were culturally appropriate with sensitive messages and materials.

The review also showed that most research did not assess cost-effectiveness. This leaves the NHS with difficult choices to make concerning scarce resources.

Policy directed at reducing inequalities in access to primary care will clearly need to address inequities in the allocation of primary care resources – including the Medical Practices Committee (MPC) policy or the distribution of GPs (see resource allocation). But this alone will not be sufficient to address the other factors including recruitment, retention and training of both GPs and other essential primary care staff to areas where they are most needed. Experience within the London Implementation Zone (LIZ) initiative, which was explicitly intended to redress some of these inequities, shows that while some inequities in practice and community staff were reduced, and improvements to premises took place, it has not had a major impact on large parts of London where very high proportions of premises are still well below basic standards (King's Fund London's Mental Health, 1997). Additional education and training support via the LIZ Educational Incentives

Scheme within London has enabled the creation of a new model of inner-city working for GPs, whereby young GPs spend fixed periods of time working in inner-city practices linked to academic departments (North Thames NHSE, the Four Rs). The problems with this model of development are that the resources were only available to London and the funding for these programmes has now come to an end; a medically dominated model of care may not be the most effective long-term solution.

Inequities in hospital care

The interpretation of evidence on variations in the utilisation of hospital care is often difficult. Few studies adjust either for case mix or severity of illness or distinguish between emergency and elective care. Although there is a large body of routine data and a growing number of clinical indicators now available, the data are not adjusted for need and private sector use; ethnic and socio-economic information is almost entirely absent. The failure of the NHS to collect useable information on the use of services by ethnic minorities is wholly unacceptable.

In keeping with our principle that there should be equitable access to *effective* healthcare, we have taken the view that there should be equitable access to local emergency and tertiary services and where the evidence base is strong (NHS Centre for Reviews and Dissemination, 1996) specialist services should be concentrated in fewer, and thus more distant, centres.

At first glance there is little evidence of poor access to overall inpatient care either for people from deprived backgrounds or from most ethnic minorities. The majority of the evidence shows a strong positive relationship between levels of deprivation of an area and hospital admission rates (Chenet and McKee, 1996; Slack et al, 1997). This relationship holds for individuals too (Balarajan et al, 1987) for length of stay (O'Donnell and Propper, 1991) even when adjusted for need (Haynes, 1991). However, these data must be interpreted with caution as higher admission rates may also reflect, in part at least, inequitable access or poor quality primary care – or inappropriate inpatient care – as in the field of diabetes and asthma (Watson et al, 1996).

For outpatients, attendance is either higher in disadvantaged groups or similar to the better-off – after adjusting for need. For most minority groups attendance rates are lower than for whites although it increases with age (Goddard and Smith, 1998). There is some evidence to suggest this may be related to GP referral beliefs and practices (McCormick et al, 1995; Smaje and Le Grand, 1997).

There is, however, a strong body of evidence showing systematic inequities in access to investigation and treatment for specialist cardiac services and socio-economic inequity in survival after cancer treatment (Goddard and Smith, 1998). While claims have been made in other specialist areas, the evidence base is more questionable. In the field of coronary heart disease (CHD) there is strong evidence of inequity in relation to socio-economic factors, ethnic origin, gender, age and geography (Equity of access to health care, March 1998). This needs to be urgently redressed if CHD is really to be at the heart of the national strategy to improve health. Given that mortality from CHD in South Asians is 40% higher than the general population, investigation and intervention rates for CHD in areas with large Asian communities would be expected to be higher than average. The evidence shows the opposite to be the case (Goddard and Smith, 1998) after adjusting for socio-economic and geographical factors. By contrast, the evidence on renal replacement therapy suggests more equitable access, with treatment rates being appropriately higher in Asian groups after adjustment for confounding factors (London Renal Services Group, 1993; Roderick et al, 1994, 1997).

While research has played a vital role in establishing the existence of inequities within the NHS, it is also vital that routine information systems become capable of alerting clinicians and managers to changing patterns of inequity within the system. We therefore welcome the government's intention to produce, and make public, comparative information on clinical outcomes. But it must be used with great caution. The bald publication of 'league tables' of clinical indicators without explanation or any adjustment for need, case severity or activity in the private sector could be counterproductive. We believe that the best way of encouraging effective clinical governance is to ensure that the data provided is presented in a helpful manner and that there is a requirement led by the new National Institute of Clinical Excellence on all responsible within the NHS system to explain apparent variations through the accountability and performance routes soon to be in place. The emergent National Service Frameworks should reinforce this by setting minimum standards.

The recent consultation document on the new Performance Assessment Framework (DoH, 1999) and the subsequent proposals for clinical effectiveness indicators (NHSE, 1998) illustrate the potential advantages and pitfalls. On the one hand, it is very helpful for health authorities and PCGs to be asked to address the significant regional variations in intervention rates shown, and to see the indicators grouped into similar regional clusters for comparative purposes. However, the lack of adjustment for need, private sector use and the lack of information either on ethnic minority rates or on socio-economic differences means that many dimensions of inequity will continue to be invisible or misinterpreted.

Despite this we believe that routine data are important. We therefore commissioned the Central Health Outcomes Unit to conduct an analysis of routine data across a wide range of NHS interventions/services (A. Lakhani, personal communication). In addition to the cluster analyses recently published for consultation (NHSE, 1998), new analyses of variation in NHS interventions by area deprivation score (using the Jarman UPA score) were undertaken. All the caveats we have already discussed apply to this data to which we should add the 'ecological fallacy' which implies that inequities between regions do not necessarily mean inequities between *individuals*. The findings showed, however, that for many areas of intervention there was little variation between clusters or deprivation groups. Below we focus on two key areas of the analysis which highlight effective NHS interventions in two priority areas in *Our healthier nation*: coronary heart disease and cancers. We also use total hip replacement as an example of a highly cost-effective NHS intervention whose rate would not be expected to vary between social groups or areas – thus allowing easier interpretation of the routine data.

Coronary heart disease – access to effective treatment

Figure 7: Differences in intervention rates for coronary artery bypass grafts and coronary angioplasty (persons) – English health authorities grouped by level of deprivation*

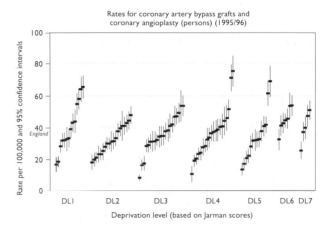

Note: * The deprivation levels DL1 to DL7 are obtained from the distribution of the health authority Jarman UPA scores such that variations are assessed in terms of the Standard Deviation. The least deprived being DL1 and the most DL7. The methodology for handling the skewed form of the distribution is described in Raleigh and Kiri (1997).

Source: Central Health Outcomes Unit (1998)

Figure 7 confirms the published evidence and demonstrates inequity between the most and least deprived groups, with no significant tendency towards higher intervention in the most deprived groups where the need is greatest. There are, however, also major inequities *within* each deprivation grouping. While the addition of private sector information might result in a clearer gradient between groupings, the presentation of information in this way helps inform the debate about equity of access to effective care and about targets that might need to be set locally and nationally to redress the observed inequities.

Cervical cancer – access to effective treatment

Figure 8: Five year relative survival (%) from cervical cancer in women aged 15+ diagnosed in 1989-90 – English health authorities grouped by level of deprivation

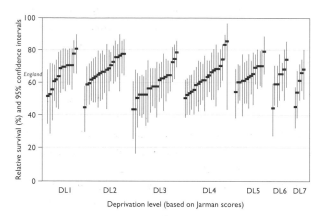

Source: Central Health Outcomes Unit (1998)

Figure 8 shows that once diagnosed, women from the most deprived parts of the country do not appear to fare significantly worse than women from the least deprived parts of the country. This is contrary to earlier evidence that cancer survival is poorer in more disadvantaged groups (Davey Smith et al, 1998). However, the figure shows significant inequity of outcome *within* individual deprivation clusters.

Total hip replacement – access to cost-effective treatment

Figure 9: Primary total hip replacement (persons aged 65+) (1995/96) – English health authorities grouped by level of deprivation

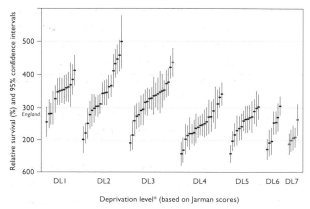

Note: * For details of how the seven-part deprivation categorisation was derived see Raleigh and Kiri (1997)

Source : Central Health Outcomes Unit (1998)

For total hip replacement, Figure 9 clearly shows that the more deprived the health authority the less access its elderly residents have to total hip replacements. The explanations for this inequity may be manifold and include patient and doctor factors as well as the impact of long waiting lists on the threshold for referral in some parts of the country.

The role of the private sector in inequity in access to healthcare

No assessment of inequities in access to healthcare would be complete without a consideration of the role of the private sector. We have focused here on its contribution and impact on inequities in acute, mainly elective, surgical care. The value of privately funded acute healthcare provided both within and independently of the NHS was estimated at £2.35bn in 1996 (Laing, 1997) – representing 7% real growth on the previous year. Independent hospitals and clinics now account for the largest part of this market – estimated at nearly £1.5bn in 1996. Of this surgeons, anaesthetists and physicians earned an estimated £550m in the same year.

Private revenue within the NHS is projected at £252m for 1996/97, and represents what has been a declining proportion of private patient revenue now at 15% of the total compared with 40% during the 1970s. Information on private sector activity or quality is not routinely available for scrutiny. This not only hampers the proper interpretation of clinical indicators, it does not allow detailed analysis of the full extent of inequities in access to elective care – as we have shown in our earlier examples. This is an unacceptable situation if equitable access to effective care is a central objective of the NHS.

It might be argued that there are a number of interrelated ways in which private practice could introduce inequities into the system of healthcare:

- private health insurance – especially that provided by employers – may serve to distort equity in the allocation of NHS resources;
- the ability to pay rather than clinical need may determine access to care;
- high levels of private practice in some parts of the country may lengthen waiting lists for treatment and reduce NHS access to consultant surgeons and anaesthetists;

- movements from private to NHS sector for patients during treatment may represent 'queue-jumping';
- there may be inequities in treatment outcomes between patients receiving private sector and NHS care.

The evidence supporting many of these assertions is unavailable. A number of individual studies, however, have shown that those who are better off, or who live in affluent parts of the country, are more likely to access private care (Marang-van de Mheen et al, 1998) at the expense of the less affluent. More important still is the evidence that for known effective interventions such as coronary artery bypass surgery and angioplasty, over 22% are now privately funded in some parts of the country (Clinical Standards Advisory Group, 1993). Occasional studies of access to cardiac care which have included the private sector activity have shown clear evidence of socio-economic inequalities in access to this type of care (Black et al, 1996). Similar inequities may exist for other elective procedures now very common in the private sector, such as hip replacements and herniorrophy. Generally, it is widely known that for procedures where waiting lists are long, private sector activity is correspondingly high.

In our view, private practice is here to stay, and it is neither helpful to try to outlaw it nor to ignore it. It is essential, however, that a systematic review is undertaken of its impact on equity of access to healthcare. This is especially important in the light of the priority given by this government to reducing long waiting lists. Such a review should focus particularly on elective surgery including orthopaedics and abortions, for which there is strong evidence of unmet NHS need (Newman et al, 1997). We believe that as a minimum, those providing private healthcare should now be required to provide the same routine information on their activity and quality as the NHS. This is already statutorily required in the case of assisted conceptions, abortions and nursing home care and should be compulsory for all forms of private healthcare. This should be implemented within the Performance Assessment Framework.

An independent review of private practice would enable wider public debate on many of the unresolved issues in this area, including the relationship between clinical governance and private practice and resource allocation and private medical insurance.

Mental health services

Mental health services, although specialist in nature, are both community- and hospital-based. They thus belong neither wholly in the primary nor the hospital sector.

We have shown elsewhere in this report a strong positive association between socio-economic factors and all major forms of mental illness and the role of socio-economic and education policy in reducing the risk of mental illness in the community (Goldberg, Chapter 15). Here we focus briefly on what can be concluded about inequalities in mental health service utilisation. There is widespread evidence that use of psychiatric – especially inpatient – services is strongly positively correlated with high levels of deprivation and unemployment (Goddard and Smith, 1998). There is also widespread evidence of very high inpatient admission rates for schizophrenia among young Caribbean men (Goddard and Smith, 1998). This is not the case for women or men from other minority ethnic groups or for consultation patterns among black Caribbeans in primary care. Most research with South Asian populations has shown much lower rates of GP consultation for mental health problems than for whites (Gillam et al, 1989; McCormick et al, 1996).

There is a lack of consensus about the explanation for these different patterns of utilisation. It is not clear, for instance, whether the overrepresentation in the inpatient sector is due to higher levels of need in young male Caribbeans, or whether there is racial bias within both the NHS and Criminal Justice Systems. Equally it is not clear whether the observed underutilisation by Asians represents inequitable access to services or an appropriate response to lower levels of need (University of York, 1995).

However there is strong evidence of much higher rates of mentally disordered offenders being cared for within psychiatric services in urban, deprived areas (see Goldberg, Chapter 15). This is reflected in the striking differences in diagnoses of patients hospitalised urban environments compared with the average.

This also shows a different underlying inequity in access to mental health services in deprived urban areas. In view of the very high levels of severe mental illness in the inner city and the well-documented difficulty mental health services have in coping with demand (King's Fund London's Mental Health, 1997), the data shows that access to specialist mental health services for the whole spectrum of mental ill-health outside of psychotic illness is very limited. The underweighting of resources for the very severely mentally ill in the resource allocation formula exacerbates this inequity (see resource allocation). Further detailed study of the appropriateness of use of inpatient mental health services show that a significant minority of mental health patients remain in hospital due to a chronic shortage of appropriately supported accommodation in the community (King's Fund London's Mental Health, 1997). Evidence from well-resourced multiagency, community mental health teams and assertiveness outreach teams shows that carefully selected patients with severe mental illness can be cared for effectively in the community – in an urban environment (Sainsbury Centre for Mental Health, 1998). An adjustment of mental health resource allocation, together with a mental health strategy that supports further NHS and local authority community and housing developments, will help to redress this inequity.

Recommendations

A new framework for tackling inequalities in health

- We recommend that reducing inequalities in health should be given *overriding* priority as the primary objective of the government's overall health strategy and that this should be articulated at every level of planning, intervention and delivery of services, from the national contract through to Regional, City and Primary Care Group levels. There should be a clear national commitment to reducing inequalities in health and its determinants. This should be reflected across government departments and in Planning and Priorities Guidance.

Specifically we recommend:

- That responsibilities for reducing inequalities in health by government/national organisations be articulated clearly within the national contract. Government should publish a triennial report to Parliament on progress towards the objectives set in the Contract.
- That at regional or city level there should be an equivalent duty of partnership between the NHS, city or regional government to ensure that health inequalities and their causes are monitored and the findings used to target Urban Regeneration and Health Action Zone resources. Regional Offices should be charged with developing a means of clustering similar health areas and facilitate a peer-led methodology for reviewing progress in tackling inequalities. This should be integrated into the new Performance Management process.
- That each health authority's Health Improvement Programme be required to develop local targets for reducing the main inequalities in health based on an assessment of local health inequalities and their determinants, and in the context of *Our healthier nation*.
- That the Duty of Partnership between health and local authorities should be a *two-way* duty with a requirement for local authorities to show evidence of having considered the Health Improvement Programme in their own planning.
- That Directors of Public Health, working in partnership with local authorities, should produce an equity profile of their district. Directors of Public Health should lead a triennial audit of progress towards achieving objectives to reduce inequalities in health and the findings should be published in their Annual Public Health Report. There should be a requirement for both health, local authorities and PCGs to respond to its findings.
- That consideration be given as to how to set minimum standards for an adequate level of health promotion/public health resource in districts to support the local strategy.

Strengthening the NHS framework for tackling inequity

We recommend that the welcome focus of the new clinical governance system on clinical effectiveness should be extended to give equal prominence to *equity of access* to effective healthcare.

Specifically we recommend:

- That the remit of the National Institute for Clinical Excellence be extended to include equity of access to effective health and healthcare.
- That the National Performance Assessment Framework be directed to focus initially on the key areas in *Our healthier nation*, and to concentrate performance management on achieving a more equitable utilisation of services in relation to need in both primary and hospital sectors. Coronary heart disease and cancers should be the top two priorities at the outset.
- That the National Service Framework be used to develop minimum standards of primary care, staffing, premises and outcomes for all to complement the disease-based approach adopted thus far.
- That health authorities, working with PCGs and providers on local clinical governance systems, should agree priorities and objectives for reducing inequities in access to effective care for disadvantaged areas and communities. These should form part of the Health Improvement Programme.

Resource allocation

We recommend that achieving a more equitable allocation of NHS resources should be the top priority for government. To achieve this requires adjustments to the ways in which resources are allocated and the speed with which resource allocation targets are met.

Specifically we recommend:

- That there should be an immediate revision in the 'pace of change' policy so that the 10% health authorities that are furthest from their capitation targets move more quickly to their actual target. This should aim to fit in with the new planning timetable for Health Improvement Programmes.
- That the principle of needs-based weighting needs to be extended to non-cash limited GMS resources.
- That the Advisory Committee on Resource Allocation (ACRA) reviews the size and effectiveness of deprivation payments in targeting the most disadvantaged populations.
- That the ACRA consider introducing an earmarked Health Promotion Fund to health authorities that would combine the allocation of the existing primary care health promotion payments and be allocated to districts on the basis of distance from targets set out in the *Our healthier nation* strategy. This could be achieved collaboratively within the framework of the Health Improvement Programme (Balarajan et al, 1987).
- We further recommend that the allocation of HCHS resources be adjusted to recognise the need:
  - to estimate underenumerated populations more accurately, especially at PCG level;
  - to create an 'Ethnic Diversity Levy' which would be allocated to health and local authorities jointly on the basis of size, diversity and proxy measures of need within these populations;
  - to increase the currently earmarked Challenge Funds to meet the projected needs of the severely mentally ill over time.

Improved information systems

We recommend that the information strategy develops explicit plans for supporting the production of routine comparative information that is adjusted for need, and relates to deprivation levels and ethnic origin. Analysis of performance by similar clusters should be piloted. It should be developed further at PCG and practice level.

Improved cultural sensitivity of services

We recommend that it should be an overriding priority of the NHS to provide comprehensive ethnic monitoring information in secondary and primary care as well as ethnic monitoring of staff. Equal opportunities policies should be in place in all parts of the NHS and Health Improvement Programmes should address how to improve equity of access to services for relevant minority groups in their populations. This should be a top priority with the National Service Frameworks for mental health and CHD.

Review of private practice

We recommend that the government initiate a fundamental review of the relationship of private practice to the NHS sector – including resource allocation. It should review how private practice and its quality may be explicitly regulated. This should include a consideration of making private practice data available for public scrutiny and the impact of private practice on the NHS waiting lists.

Research and development

We recommend that a Research and Development programme be created with an explicit remit to evaluate the changes being implemented in the NHS and other agencies in relation to the government's objective to reduce inequalities in health and healthcare. Specifically it should address:

- The effectiveness of new flexiblities within the Primary Care Act and Health Action Zones in tackling inequalities in health and healthcare.
- The impact of PCGs on inequities in health and healthcare.
- Effective methods of interagency working to reduce inequalities in health.
- Effective methodologies for local and national Health Impact Assessment.
- The impact of National Service Frameworks and the work of the National Institute of Clinical Excellence (NICE) on inequities in healthcare.

References

Agren, G., Essinger, K. and Tode, K. (1997) '*Project Megapoles*', *A public health network for capital cities and regions*, Stockholm: Stockholm County Council.

Balarajan, R., Yuen, P. and Machin, D. (1987) 'Socioeconomic differentials in the uptake of medical care in Great Britain', *Journal of Epidemiology and Community Health*, vol 41, pp 196-9.

Bardsley, M. and Morgan, D. (1996) 'Health', Chapter 4 in P. Edwards and J. Flatley (eds) *The capital divided: Mapping poverty and social exclusion in London*, London: London Research Centre.

Benzeval, M. and Donald, A. (1997) *The role of the NHS in tackling inequalities in health*, December (Input Paper).

Benzeval, M. and Judge, K. (1996) 'Access to health care in England: continuing inequalities in the distribution of GPs', *Journal of Public Health Medicine*, vol 18, pp 33-40.

Birmingham Annual Public Health Report (1995) *Closing the gap – 10 benchmarks for equity and equality in health*, Birmingham: Birmingham Annual Public Health Report.

Black, N., Langham, S., Coshall, C. and Parker, J. (1996) 'Impact of the 1991 NHS reforms on the availability and use of coronary revascularisation in the UK (1987-1995)', *Heart*, Supplement 4, vol 76, no 4.

Boyle, S. and Hamblin, R. (1997) *The health economy of London: A report to the King's Fund London Commission*, London: King's Fund.

Carr-Hill, R., Place, M. and Posnett, J. (1997) 'Access and the utilisation of healthcare services', in B. Ferguson, T. Sheldon and J. Posnett (eds) 'Concentration and choice in healthcare', London: *Financial Times Healthcare*.

Chenet, L. and McKee, M. (1996) 'Challenges of monitoring use of seconday care at local level: a study based in London, UK', *Journal of Epidemiology and Community Health*, vol 50, pp 359-65.

Clinical Standards Advisory Group (1993) *Access to and availability of CABG and coronary angioplasty*, Report of a CSAG Working Group, London: HMSO.

CMO (Chief Medical Officer) (1998) An Interim Report of a project to strengthen the public health function in England, 23 February.

Davey Smith, G., Hart, C., Hole, D., MacKinnon, P., Gillis, C., Watt, G., Lane, D. and Hawthorne, V. (1998) 'Education and occupational social class: which is the more improtant indicator of mortality risk?', *Journal of Epidemiology and Community Health*, March, vol 52, no 3, pp 153-60.

DETR (Department of the Environment, Transport and the Regions) (1998a) *Modernising local government: Local democracy and community leadership*, London: DETR.

DETR (1998b) *A mayor and assembly for London*, London: The Stationery Office.

DoH (Department of Health) Variations in Health (1994) *What can the DoH and NHS do?*, Variations Sub-Group of the Chief Medical Officer's *Health of the nation* Working Group.

DoH, A Policy Framework for Commissioning Cancer Services [EL(95)51] (1995a) *A report by the Expert Advisory Group on Cancer to the CMOs of England and Wales*, April.

DoH Variations in Health (1995b) *What can the DoH and NHS do?*, A Report produced by the Variations Sub-Group of the CMO's *Health of the nation* Working Group, October.

DoH (1997) *The new NHS – modern, dependable*, London: The Stationery Office.

DoH (1998) *Our healthier nation: A contract for health. A consultation paper*, London: The Stationery Office.

DoH (1999) *The NHS Performance Assessment Framework*, London, March.

Doyle, Y., Brunning, D., Cryer, C., Hedley, R. and Hodgson, C. (1996) *Healthy Cities indicators: Analysis of data from cities across Europe*, Copenhagen: WHO Regional Office for Europe.

ELCHA (East London and The City Health Authority) (1998) Annual Public Health Report 1997/98, *Health in the East End*.

Flynn, P. and Knight, D. (1998) *Inequalities in health in the North West*, NHSE North West.

Gillam, S.J., Jarman, B., White, P. and Law, R. (1989) 'Ethnic differences in consultation rates in urban general practice', *British Medical Journal*, vol 299, pp 953-7.

Goddard, M. and Smith, P. (1998) *Equity of access to health care*, York: University of York, Centre for Health Economics, March.

Hacking, J. (1996) 'Weight watchers', *Health Services Journal*, pp 28-30.

Haynes, R. (1991) 'Inequalities in health and health service use; evidence from the general household survey', *Social Science and Medicine*, vol 33, pp 361-8.

Health of Londoners, A Public Health Report for London (1998) *Health of Londoners Project*.

Hirst, Lunt and Aitken (1998) 'Were practice nurses equitably distributed across England and Wales 1988-1995?', *Journal of Health Services Research & Policy*, vol 3, no 1, pp 31-8.

Johnson, M., Clark, M., Owen, D. and Szczepura, (1997) ' "The unavoidable costs of ethnicity": a review for the NHSE: Executive summary', The Centre for Research into Ethnic Relations and The Centre for Health Services Studies.

Johnstone, F., Lucy, J., Scott-Samuel, A. and Whitehead, M. (1996) *Deprivation and health in North Cheshire: An equity audit of health services*, Liverpool Public Health Observatory: EQUAL.

Judge, K. and Mays, N. (1994) 'Allocating resources for health and social care in England', *British Medical Journal*, vol 308, pp 1363-6.

King's Fund London's Mental Health (1997) *The Report to the King's Fund London Commission 1997*.

Laing's Review of private healthcare (1997) Chapter 2, 'Private acute health services', A41–A89.

Liverpool City Health Plan (1996) *Liverpool Healthy City 2000*.

Liverpool Health Authority (1996) *Annual Public Health Report 1996*.

Livingstone, A.E., Shaddick, G., Grundy, C. and Elliott, P. (1996) 'Do people living near inner city main roads have more asthma needing treatment? Case control study', *British Medical Journal*, 16 March, vol 312, no 7032, pp 676-7.

London Renal Services Group (1993) *Report of an independent review of specialist services in London*, London: HMSO.

London Strategic Review Independent Advisory Panel, Chair: Sir Leslie Turnberg (1997) *Health services in London – A strategic review* (Turnberg Report) London: DoH.

McCormick, A., Fleming, D. and Charlton, J. (1995) *Morbidity statistics from general practice: Fourth national study 1991-1992*, London: OPCS.

McCormick, A., Fleming, D. and Charlton, J. (1996) *Morbidity statistics from general practice: Fourth national study 1991-1992*, London: OPCS.

Marang-van de Mheen, P.J., Davey Smith, G., Hart, C.L. and Gunning-Schepers, L.J. (1998) 'Socioeconomic differentials in mortality among men within Great Britain: time trends and contributory causes', *Journal of Epidemiology and Community Health*, April, vol 52, no 4, pp 214-18.

Mays, N. (1995) 'Geographical resource allocation in the English National Health Service, 1971-1994: the tension between normative and empirical approaches', *International Journal of Epidemiology*, vol 24, no 3 (Supplement), S96-S102.

MPC (Medical Practices Committee) (1997) *Newsletter issue 3 July*, London: MPC.

Naish, J., Brown, J. and Denton, B. (1994) 'Intercultural consultations: investigation of factors that deter non-English speaking women from attending their general practitioners for cervical screening', *British Medical Journal*, 29 October, vol 309, no 6962, pp 1126-8.

Newman, M., Bardsley, M., Morgan, D. and Jacobson, B. (1997) *Contraception and abortion services in London: Are we meeting the need?*, London: HOLP.

NHS Centre for Reviews and Dissemination (1995) *Review of research on effectiveness of health service interventions to reduce variations in health*, Report 3, York: University of York (and unpublished update).

NHS Centre for Reviews and Dissemination (1996) *Hospital volume and health care outcomes, costs and patient access effective health care*, December 1996, Volume 2, Number 8, York/Leeds: Nuffield Institute for Health, University of York, University of Leeds.

NHSE (1997) *HIV/AIDS Funding*, EL (97) 18, Leeds: NHSE.

NHSE (1998) *Clinical effectivness indicators: A consultation document*, May.

North Thames NHSE, The Four Rs, Recruitment, Retention, Refreshment and Reflection, *London Initiative Zone, Educational Incentives*, NHSE, Annual Report 1996/97.

O'Donnell, and Propper, C. (1991) 'Equity and the distribution of UK National Health Services resources', *Journal of Health Economics*, vol 10, pp 1-19.

Parsons, L. and Day, S. (1992) 'Improving obstetric outcomes in ethnic minorities: an evaluation of health advocacy in Hackney', *Journal of Public Health Medicine*, June, vol 14, no 2, pp 183-91.

Pereira, J. (1993) 'What does equity in health mean?', *Journal of Social Policy*, vol 22, no 1, pp 19-48.

Phillimore, P., Beattie, A. and Townsend, P. (1991) 'Widening inequality of health in Northern England 1981-1991', *British Medical Journal*, vol 309, pp 1125-8.

Raleigh, V. and Kiri, V. (1997) 'Life expectancy in England: variations and trends by gender, health authority and level of deprivation', *Journal of Epidemiology and Community Health*, vol 51, pp 649-58.

Roderick, P.J., Martin, D. and Diamond, I. (1997) *How do population need, access and supply factors influence acceptance onto renal replacement therapy in England?*, Report to South and West Regional Office.

Roderick, P.J., Jones, I., Raleigh, V.S., McGeown, M. and Mallick, N. (1994) 'Population need for renal replacement therapy in Thames regions: ethnic dimension', *British Medical Journal*, vol 309, pp 1111-14.

Ross, J.S. (1952) *The National Health Service in Great Britain*, Oxford: Oxford University Press.

Sainsbury Centre for Mental Health (1998) *Keys to engagement: Review of care for people with severe mental illness who are hard to engage with services*, London: Sainsbury Centre for Mental Health.

Sheldon, T. (1997) 'Formula fever: allocating resources in the NHS', *British Medical Journal*, vol 315, p 964.

Slack, R., Ferguson, B. and Ryder, S. (1997) 'Analysis of hospitalisation rates by electoral ward: relationship to accessibility and deprivation data', *Health Services Management Research*, vol 10, pp 24-31.

Smaje, C. and Le Grand, J. (1997) 'Ethinicity, equity and the use of health services in the British NHS', *Social Science and Medicine*, vol 45, pp 485-97.

University of York (1995) *Review of the research on the effectiveness of health service interventions to reduce variations in health*, October.

Watson, J.P., Cowen, P. and Lewis, R.A. (1996) 'The relationship between asthma and admission rates, routes of admissiomn, and socioeconomic deprivation', *European Respiratory Journal*, vol 9, pp 2087-93.

Worrall, A., Rea, J.N. and Ben-Shlomo, Y. (1997) 'Counting the cost of social disadvantage in primary care: retrospective analysis of patient data', *British Medical Journal*, vol 314, pp 38-42.

9

Nutrition and health inequalities

Michael Nelson

Executive summary

General

There is good evidence that inequalities in access to and consumption of a healthy diet lead to inequalities in health. The underlying cause of these inequalities are financial, educational, and environmental, but age and gender are also important. The policies of the Treasury and of the Departments of Health, Social Security, Education and Employment, Environment, Trade and Industry, the Ministry of Agriculture Fisheries and Food, the Food Standards Agency, and food suppliers need to be coordinated at the highest level in order to maximise access by all segments of the population to a healthy and affordable food supply and to encourage the adoption of healthy eating habits, with the specific objective to reduce nutrition-related inequalities in health. There is also a need to improve the information base which guides the formulation of appropriate nutrition-related policies and evaluates their impact. If it were necessary to identify the groups most likely to benefit from interventions, women of childbearing age and children from low-income households are those whose short- and long-term health, growth and development are most likely to be impaired by poor nutrition.

Policy **The Minister for Public Health should create an interdepartmental forum to integrate government policy to reduce nutrition-related inequalities in health.**

Benefits
- Creation of policies which coordinate the diverse aims of different sectors of government, industry and the community.

- Rapid reduction in inequalities in nutrition-related ill-health and associated costs of care and health service provision.

- Provide a forum in which the conflicts of interest of different sectors can be discussed and resolved.

- Rational prioritising and continuing policy development through implementation of recommendations contained in this report, the Nutrition Task Force Low Income Project Team, and the submission from the National Food Alliance.

Evidence The rise in inequalities in nutrition-related health is due in part to a failure to integrate the diverse needs of food providers, tax payers and consumers. A coordinated approach with a clear health agenda has been shown to have long-term and sustainable benefits (eg Norway).

Policy **The government should introduce a programme that focuses specifically on women of childbearing age and children in low-income households and which integrates the provision of food (through healthy living centres, schools, nurseries, etc), nutrition education, and the development of cooking and budgeting skills.**

Benefits
- Breaking the vicious cycle of poor maternal nutrition being passed on to the children.
- Alleviation of hunger, especially among mothers on low income who go without food to protect their children's intakes.
- Reintroduction of cooking and budgeting skills currently missing in schools and homes.

Evidence The Women, Infant and Children (WIC) scheme in the United States has shown benefits in terms of reduced neonatal care costs and better socialisation of children, with long-term health and social benefits.

Policy **Provide financial support through local government, health authorities, social services and planning departments to set up, maintain, and evaluate local initiatives which aim to improve nutritional health in the community, schools and the workplace. Mapping food provision on a local level should be carried out to identify areas of greatest need.**

Benefits
- Promote continuity of initiatives shown to be effective in reaching their target audience.
- Improve health-related life-style among individuals who are clustered in high risk groups.

Evidence Targeted interventions which are part of a national strategy are more effective than untargeted population-based interventions. The current scale of intervention is too small to have a major impact on nutrition-related health inequalities. If a local strategy is to be pursued it needs proper support at central and local government level.

Policy **Government should provide guidelines for maintaining food security, and planning the retail provision of food at the local level. Such guidelines should integrate the needs of communities for food provision, transport policy, taxation policy, the need to maintain local services, and the need for retailers to sustain profitability.**

Benefits
- Increased availability of low-cost food for low-income households.
- Revitalisation of local economies, including opportunities for employment.

Evidence Successful partnerships between food retailers, local government and local communities have led to concrete improvements in the provision of food at low cost (eg Easterhouse, Glasgow).

Policy **The government should promote the development and use of Budget Standards.**

Benefits:
- Scientifically-based evidence of the levels of expenditure needed to sustain a healthy life-style.
- Reference points for social security payments and minimum wage levels which sustain health and which can be paid for by reduced costs to the NHS, higher educational attainment, increased employability and productivity, and lower crime.

Evidence Several European countries (Sweden, Denmark, Holland, Finland, Norway) with smaller inequalities in health use Budget Standards as a reference point when setting social security and minimum wage levels. Studies in developing countries show clear benefits of improved employee health in terms of increased productivity.

And more generally, but with the highest priority:

Policy **Reform the tax and benefit systems to increase net (after tax) incomes at the bottom end of the income distribution.**

Benefits • Higher disposable income facilitates the purchase of a healthier diet.

• Improved incentives to work for increased returns from employment.

Evidence The current systems of benefits and taxation provide virtually no financial incentive for people who are unemployed to return to work. People who take full-time employment at low wages, often in menial tasks, need better returns for the additional responsibilities and outgoings which they are being asked to assume.

Inequalities in nutrition lead to inequalities in health

There is substantial evidence to show that nutrition is an important cause of health inequalities, particularly in relation to socio-economic differences (James et al, 1997). This evidence is based mainly on cross-sectional or ecological (rather than longitudinal) studies concerned primarily with variations in health across a range of nutritional exposures. Clustering of nutritional risk factors in poorer sections of society together with higher rates of nutrition-related diseases suggest that these relationships may be causal. Other factors associated with being poor (bad housing, less education, etc) contribute independently to higher disease rates, and are often inextricably bound with nutrition. The associations between these factors and access to healthy diets are discussed in the next section.

Socio-economic differences

Table 1 shows the relationship between disease patterns and diet in lower socio-economic groups in Great Britain. The evidence is based on data from the *Health Survey for England* (Colhoun and Prescott-Clarke, 1996), the *National Food Survey* (MAFF, 1981-97), the *National Diet and Nutrition Surveys* (DHSS, 1989; Gregory et al, 1990, 1995), plus many surveys which have measured diet in relation to disease, even if it is not specifically with respect to socio-economic differences (eg Woodward et al, 1992). The weight of evidence varies with different illnesses or disorders. The sum of evidence, however, tends to reinforce consistent messages about the balance of a healthy diet likely to reduce nutrition-related inequalities.

The diet in low socio-economic groups is characterised by low levels of vegetables and fruit and their associated anti-oxidant vitamins, foods rich in dietary fibre, and lower fat foods. This pattern is repeated in all of the population sub-groups for which data have been reported separately (Table 2). The average differences in food consumption by social class (Figure 1a) are more clearly revealed when analyses are carried out for a specific household type (eg two adults and one or two children) (Figure 1b). (It should be noted that in the British Adult Survey [Gregory et al, 1990], higher intakes of lower fat foods in higher social classes, and higher P:S ratios were not associated with reduced total fat intake in these groups, nor in reduced cholesterol levels.)

38

Table 1: Excess disease rates in lower socio-economic classes and their relation to diet in Great Britain

Excess disease	Risk factors	Dietary contributors
Anaemia of pregnancy low intake of meat; physical	Low iron; folate status	Low intake of vegetables and fruit; inactivity
Premature delivery	Lower folate; lack of n-3 fatty acids	Low intake of vegetables, fruit and appropriate oils and fish
Neural tube defect	Lower folate	Low intake of vegetables and other folate sources
Low birthweight or disproportion	Adolescent pregnancy; lower folate; lack of n-3 fatty acids; low weight gain in pregnancy; smoking	Low intake of vegetables, fruit; and possibly trans-fatty acids
Anaemia in children and adults	Iron; folate; vitamin C and B_{12} deficiency	Possibly premature use of cow's milk; low intake of vegetables and fruit; low intake of meat; diet low in nutrients, with low intake linked to physical inactivity
Dental disease	Low fluoride content of drinking water	Sweet snacks and drinks between meals
Eczema/asthma	Parental smoking; air pollution	Low breastfeeding rates; low intake of fruit
Insulin dependent diabetes mellitus	Viral infections	Low breastfeeding rates
Obesity in children and adults	Poor recreational facilities; intense traffic; excessive	Physical inactivity; energy dense (high fat) diets
Hypertension	Processed foods high in salt; low birthweight; slow weight gain in infancy; adult weight gain	Salty, energy dense foods with high sodium and low potassium, magnesium and calcium content; alcohol; low intake of vegetables and fruit; inactivity
Low IQ, poorer cognitive function	Prematurity; anaemia in childhood and adolescence; teenage pregnancy	Low breastfeeding rates; lower intake of iron rich foods, especially in adolescent girls
Resistance to infection	Poorer vitamin and mineral status	Low intakes of vegetables and fruit; lower zinc intakes (elderly)
High cholesterol	Excess weight gain	Excess dairy fats and (some) hydrogenated vegetable oils; trans-fatty acids
Low high density lipoprotein or high triglycerides	Excess weight gain	Physical inactivity; energy dense diets; low intake of fish
Non-insulin dependent diabetes	Excess weight gain television watching	Physical inactivity; energy dense diets

Table 1: cntd

Excess disease	Risk factors	Dietary contributors
Coronary artery disease	Hypertension; lipid abnormalities; smoking; low folate and anti-oxidants; low birth weight and slow weight gain in infancy; homocysteinaemia	Salty, energy dense foods with high sodium and low potassium, magnesium, calcium; alcohol; low intake of vegetables, fruit and fish; low activity; poor maternal nutrition
Peripheral arterial disease	Smoking; low folate; lipid abnormalities	Low intake of vegetables, fruit and possibly fish
Cerebrovascular disease	Hypertension; low folate; high cholesterol	Salty, energy dense foods with high sodium and low potassium, magnesium, calcium; alcohol; low intake of vegetables and fruit
Cancers; lung, stomach, oropharyngeal, oesophagus	Smoking, especially with excess alcohol intake	Low intakes of vegetables and fruit; low intake of dietary fibre
Cataracts, macular degeneration		Low intake of vegetables, fruit and n-3 fatty acids
Bone disease in elderly people	Vitamin D deficiency; confined living and travel opportunities; poor peak bone mass	Physical inactivity; low intake of calcium in childhood and adulthood; high phosphate intake (soft drinks)

Source: Adapted from James et al (1997)

Table 2: Food consumption and nutrient intake by social class or income group

Data source	Reference	Comparison	Higher in low-income/ socio-economic group	Lower in low-income/ socio-economic group
National Food Survey (1995)	MAFF (1996)	Income Group A (high) versus Income Group D & E2 (low)	*Foods:* White bread Full fat milk Carcase meat and meat products Eggs Total fats Sugar Potatoes Tea	Reduced fat milk Cheese Poultry Fish Fresh green vegetables Other fresh vegetables Fruit Brown and wholemeal bread Breakfast cereals Coffee Soft drinks Alcholic beverages Confectionery
			Nutrients (as % DRV): Retinol equivalents Vitamin D Sodium Thiamin Vitamin B_6	Magnesium Vitamin C
Infants up to 1 year	Martin and White (1988) Mills and Tyler (1992)	Social class I versus IV + V Socio-economic groups ABC1 versus C2DE	*Foods:* Infant formulas Potatoes Biscuits Confectionery Squashes and soft drinks	Breast milk Cow's milk and milk products Fruit
			Nutrients: Saturated fatty acids Dietary cholesterol	Carotene Vitamin C
Toddlers 1½-4½ years	Gregory et al (1995)	Social class I, II, IIIN (non-manual) versus IIIM, IV, V (manual) Not in receipt of benefit versus in receipt of benefit	*Foods:* White bread Non-high fibre breakfast cereal Milk puddings Skimmed milk Margarine (non-PUFA) Coated chicken Burgers and kebabs Meat pies and pastries Chips and crisps Sugar Chocolate and confectionery Soft and alcoholic beverages Tea and coffee	Pizza Wholewheat/soft grain bread Biscuits and fruit pies Sponge puddings Semi-skimmed milk Infant formula Cottage cheese Lamb, chicken, turkey, liver Raw and salad vegetables Fresh vegetables Fruit Fruit juice Commercial infant drinks
			Nutrients: Energy (lone-parent children) Non-milk extrinsic sugar Starch Sodium	Non-starch polysaccharides ß-carotene equivalents Vitamin C Iron Calcium Iodine
School children 10-15 years	Wenlock et al (1986) DHSS (1989)	Social class I versus V Not in receipt of supplementary benefit versus in receipt of benefit Father employed versus unemployed	*Foods:* Total bread White bread Eggs Total potato Chips Baked beans (older children) Sugar	Milk Carcase meat Chicken Citrus fruit Apples and pears
			Nutrients:	Carotene Vitamin C
Adults 16-64 years	Gregory et al (1990) MAFF (1994)	Social classes I + II versus IV + V	*Foods:* White bread Soft margarine Chips Total potatoes Sugar	High fibre breakfast cereal Semi-skimmed milk Salad vegetables Total fruit Apples and pears Chocolate Wine, fortified wine and spirits
			Nutrients:	Calcium Iron ß-carotene Vitamin C Vitamin E

Figure 1(a) Food acquisitions, all households, by income group

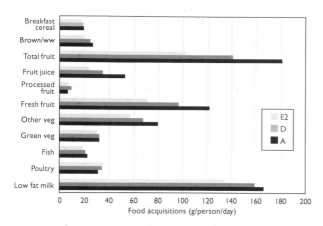

Note: A: £570/week and over

D: <£140/week (earner)

E2:< £140/week (no earner)

Figure 1(b) Food acquisitions, all households, by income group

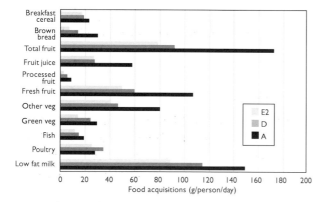

Source: *National Food Survey* (1995)

Figure 2 (a): Dietary adequacy (% RNI), households with two adults and one or two children, by income group

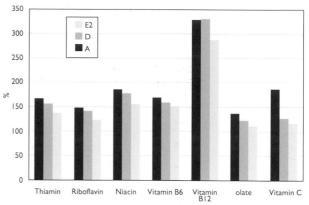

Note: A: £570/week and over

D: <£140/week (earner)

E2:< £140/week (no earner)

Figure 2 (b): Dietary adequacy (% RNI), households with two adults and one or two children, by income group

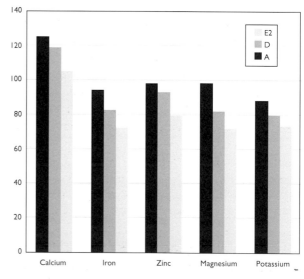

The food consumption patterns are reflected in differences in nutrient intake between the highest income group (A) and the lowest (D and E2) (Table 3). Income group D (low-income households with earners) appear to be worse off nutritionally than those in E2 (low-income primarily on Income Support) possibly because of loss of benefits associated with Income Support (eg free school meals). Analysis by specific household type (eg two adults with one or two children) reveals more consistent patterns showing lower intakes in income group E2 for all vitamins (Figure 2a) and minerals (Figure 2b).

Table 3: Nutritional value of household food (% of Reference Nutrient Intake [DoH, 1991]) by income group, *National Food Survey* **(1995) and the** *Dietary and Nutritional Survey of British Adults* **(1986/87)**

Nutrient	National Food Survey (1995)			Dietary and Nutritional Survey of British Adults (1986/87)			
	Group A (>=£570 /week)	Group D (with earner, <£140/ week)	Group E2 (no earner, <£140/ week)	Men, 16-64 years		Women, 16-64 years	
				I + II	IV + V	I + II	IV + V
Calcium	116	115	118	144	124	113	94
Iron	87	88	93	172	147	87	78
Zinc	93	95	96	124	114	128	109
Magnesium	86	80	82	114	100	97	77
Sodium	162	176	168	210	210	149	141
Potassium	80	79	79	96	85	75	63
Thiamin	154	159	162	250	170	200	175
Riboflavin	136	136	139	208	154	182	145
Niacin	178	178	182	252	225	251	206
Vitamin B_6	149	160	158	214	178	275	158
Vitamin B_{12}	332	319	334	490	480	400	313
Folate	127	126	127	160	147	118	98
Vitamin C	167	118	121	242	134	240	140
Retinol equivalents	152	166	173	248	222	287	203
% in sample	*6.3*	*6.2*	*15.5*	*35*	*17*	*35*	*20*

Source: After Gregory et al (1990); MAFF (1996)

Vitamin intakes, when expressed as a percentage of Reference Nutrient Intake (RNI) (DoH, 1991), are generally above 100% in both the *National Food Survey* and the British Adult Survey. The RNI were determined originally in relation to prevention of deficiency disease. The more recently derived Dietary Reference Values strive to take into account newer knowledge of the relationships between intake and development of chronic disease, but it is important to note that for many nutrients intakes may need to be substantially above 100% RNI to confer protection. The *relative* intake between socio-economic groups is therefore a better measure to relate to health inequalities. Table 3 shows that, especially in the individual survey of adults, intakes in social classes IV+V are often substantially below those in I+II. Moreover, the distribution of intakes in poorer households is likely to include a larger proportion with intakes substantially below the population mean. The intakes of minerals are, with the exception of calcium, consistently below 100% of the RNI, with striking gradients by social class for individual surveys of adults (Table 3) or specific household types (Figure 2(b)). Analysis of food consumption patterns provides useful clues about

dietary profiles likely to be associated with better health (Pryer et al, 1995).

Pregnancy

Folate intakes are 20% lower in women from social classes IV+V than I+II (Gregory et al, 1990) (Table 3). Preconceptual and first trimester diets low in folate are associated with increased risk of neural tube defects, stillbirth, prematurity and lower birthweight. Intakes of n-3 fatty acids are 10%-20% lower in women from social classes IV+V compared with I+II. These are associated with poorer placental function, which may predispose to hypertension, diabetes, abdominal obesity and coronary heart disease in later adulthood. Median red cell folate concentrations and serum vitamin B_{12} concentrations were lower in social classes III manual, IV and V than in I, II and III non-manual. Lower socio-economic groups have higher rates of teenage pregnancy, prematurity, and low birthweight, consistent with these nutritional associations. Some of these associations may be confounded by smoking and other health behaviours.

Breastfeeding

Rates of breastfeeding have remained relatively static over the last 15 years (Table 4). At birth, social class I mothers are almost twice as likely as social class V mothers to breastfeed (90% vs 50%). At four months, they are more than four times more likely to be still breastfeeding. Breastfeeding is associated with lower rates of infection in infancy, better immune development, fewer food intolerances and less eczema and atopic allergy in childhood and adolescence, lower risks of development of insulin dependent diabetes mellitus, higher IQ at age eight (in preterm babies fed breast milk compared with formula), and lower risks of breast cancer in breastfeeding mothers. Again, smoking and other health behaviours may confound some of these associations.

Table 4: Incidence of breastfeeding by socio-economic group (% breastfeeding at each age)

Duration	Social class I			Social class IV + V		
	1980	1985	1995	1980	1985	1995*
Birth	87	87	90	52	54	50
I week	82	83	84	43	44	40
2 weeks	80	79	83	38	40	36
6 weeks	74	71	73	27	27	23
4 months	59	54	56	11	14	13
6 months	50	45	42	8	11	11
9 months	31	23	31	6	4	5

Note: * social class V.
Source: Foster et al (1997); Crown ccopyright is reporduced with the permission of the Controller of Her Majesty's Staionery Office

Anaemia

Diets which are low in iron in relation to requirements, and low in vitamins which are likely to increase levels of iron absorption (especially vitamin C, but riboflavin and retinol may also have a role) will lead to iron deficiency anaemia.

Anaemia in infancy and early childhood results in poorer immune status, retarded growth and development and reduced cognitive function (British Nutrition Foundation, 1995). The findings in the survey of toddlers (Gregory et al, 1995) showed 16% of children under four years of age with iron intakes below the Lower Reference Nutrient Intake [LRNI], and 8% of toddlers with haemoglobin levels below 110 g/l (the WHO cut-off point for anaemia). There was no association with social class, but there

was a trend towards lower mean haemoglobin levels with lower educational status of the mother. Prevalence of anaemia in infancy and early childhood is higher in Asian groups (Duggan et al, 1991).

In adolescence, estimates of iron deficiency anaemia range from 3% to 20%, higher in girls of Asian and Afro-Caribbean origin than white girls. Lower iron status in girls is significantly associated with poorer performance on IQ tests (Pollitt, 1990) and reduced activity levels (Nelson et al, 1994). Girls from lower social classes show poorer iron status but the trends fail to reach statistical significance.

Among adults (Gregory et al, 1990), men and women from social classes IV+V had lower iron intakes than those from social classes I+II (Table 3), but there were no differences by social class in levels of haemoglobin or ferritin. Red cell folate and vitamin B_{12} were lower in the lower social classes.

Among people 65-74 years of age, up to 8% of men and 29% of women have marginal haemoglobin levels and minimal iron stores. Over 75, these values rise to 17% and 39%, respectively. It is often linked with the presence of chronic disease, and the levels are substantially lower in healthy older people (British Nutrition Foundation, 1995). Evidence from the 1972 report on the diets of elderly people (DHSS, 1972) showed higher proportions of elderly subjects with low haemoglobin among those spending less per week on food or whose main sources of income were social security payments or state pensions, the relationships most evident among men living alone.

Obesity

The British Adult Survey shows higher levels of overweight body mass index ([BMI] 25-30) in men (37%) than in women (24%), but obesity (BMI>30) is higher in women (12%) than in men (8%). Prevalence of obesity is strongly inversely associated with lower social class in women, and moderately associated in men (Gregory et al, 1990). These findings are confirmed in the *Health Survey for England* (Colhoun and Prescott-Clarke, 1996) (Table 5) and in the longitudinal data from the Whitehall Study (Davey Smith and Brunner, 1997). The issue of inequality therefore relates to both gender and socio-economic status. Fetal origins of adult obesity are probable, and an early increase in adiposity in the age range two to six may also predispose to adult overweight. The problem is effectively one of imbalance between energy intake and expenditure, and therefore has bearing on issues related to physical education in children and activity levels in adulthood. The problems associated with obesity are manifold: diabetes, hypertension, hyperlipidaemia, some cancers, menstrual and obstetric complications, back pain, arthritis, and varicose veins. Rates of obesity are rising.

Table 5: Percentage of men and women with BMI over 30, by social class

	Social class					
	I	II	IIIN	IIIM	IV	V
Men	10.5	14.0	14.6	16.7	15.0	13.3
Women	11.1	13.9	13.9	19.9	23.6	21.3

Source: Colhoun and Prescott-Clarke (1996); Crown Copyright is reproduced with the permission of the Controller of Her Majesty's Stationery Office

Gender

Women are more likely than men to drink semi-skimmed milk (68% and 62%, respectively), eat wholemeal bread (29%, 22%), eat fruit at least once a day (54%, 44%) and vegetables at least once a day (71%, 64%). More men drink more heavily than women (Colhoun and Prescott-Clarke, 1996) (Table 6). Nutrient intakes (as per cent of RNI) are lower in women than in men in all social classes for iron, calcium, magnesium Vitamin B_{12} and folate (Table 3). The lowest levels of adequacy are reported for women in social classes IV+V. While there is evidence that women are more likely than men to under-report their diet (Pryer et al, 1994), women are also more likely to be dieting, and the low levels of adequacy may reflect low intakes at any one time in a substantial segment of the female adult population. The consequences of anaemia have been discussed above. There is growing evidence that low calcium intakes throughout life may be associated with increased risk of osteoporosis (Murray, 1996; Heaney, 1996). Recent evidence from Suleiman et al suggest that higher calcium intakes in postmenopausal women is associated with higher bone mass (1997), and Cadogan and co-workers

(1997) suggest that milk drinking in childhood may play an important role in promoting higher bone mass, at least in the short term. This may be especially important if activity levels are declining among girls (Armstrong et al, 1990) and women in manual occupations whose levels of activity may hitherto have been protective against bone loss.

Table 6: Drinking habits of men and women in England

	% describing level of drinking (Number of units consumed per week)	
	Heavy drinking	Very heavy drinking
Men	20% (22-50)	7% (>50)
Women	10% (15-35)	2% (>35)

Source: Colhoun and Prescott-Clarke (1996); Crown Copyright is reproduced with the permission of the Controller of Her Majesty's Stationery Office

What are the underlying causes of inequalities in nutrition?

Lack of money at the household level is the primary cause of inequalities in nutrition and the associated ill health. This is compounded by:

- the absence of a coherent strategy to address food poverty;
- structural changes in the food supply system which tend to reduce access to cheap, healthy foods for low-income communities;
- benefit and wage levels which are not linked to an analysis of the cost of a healthy life-style;
- a reduction in cooking skills (especially among the young);
- lack of nutritional standards for institutions (such as schools and workplaces);
- failures in support for local community initiatives which address these issues;
- the effects of inequality per se (Wilkinson, 1996);
- tax and benefit systems where tax is levied on incomes below benefit levels, where non-means tested family income support (Child Benefit and married couple's tax allowance) has fallen sharply in real terms, and where public sector rents have risen faster than earnings, resulting in falling disposable incomes especially in single wage households.

Low income contributes to the poor diet–health relationship in many ways. For example:

Less money spent on health-enhancing foods: cheaper foods of the types most commonly purchased by low-income households (Table 2) tend to be higher in fat, saturated and trans-fatty acids and sugar, and lower in fibre, vitamins and minerals than the more expensive alternatives. Low-income households are more efficient purchasers of nutrients than richer households (Figure 3), and while less money is spent on protective foods such as fruits and vegetables, more is spent as a proportion of their total food budget. Where economy line healthy options exist, unattractive and stigmatising packaging may reduce uptake.

Figure 4: Car ownership by tenths of income

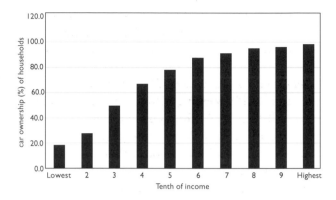

Source: Family Expenditure Survey 1995/96

Figure 3: Spending efficiency (g of food/pence), by income group

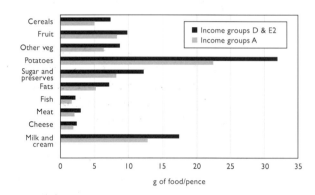

Note: A: £570/week and over

D: <£140/week (earner)

E2:< £140/week (no earner)

Source: *National Food Survey* (1994)

Access to private (and public) transport: this is needed to reach the out-of-town supermarkets which now dominate food retailing and where food is cheaper (Piachaud and Webb, 1996). Car ownership is income-dependent (Figure 4). The problem is concentrated among lone-parent households (only 41% with a car), pensioner households (43%), and those living in local authority or housing association rented accommodation (34%). Public transport is needed especially for households on peripheral housing estates who have no nearby major shopping facilities. In rural areas, 40% of villages have neither a shop nor a bus service.

Poor housing: rented accommodation has poorer food storage and preparation facilities than owner-occupier accommodation. This may restrict food choice. Housing tenure is a key feature of locality, and locality is strongly associated with changes in mortality (Dorling, 1997). In Scotland (Woodward et al, 1992), the odds ratios for housing tenure are the highest of all social factors, being 1.63 and 1.55 for men and women, respectively, comparing those who live in rented accommodation with owner-occupiers. After adjustment for a number of coronary heart disease risk factors (smoking and fibrinogen are the most important confounding variables for men, and BMI, high-density lipoprotein cholesterol, and triglyceride levels, the most important for women), most, if not all, of the significant effect of education and occupation on coronary heart disease is removed, but housing tenure remains highly significant (p<0.001), with odds ratios of 1.48 and 1.45 for men and women, respectively. When relationships among the social factors themselves are investigated, housing tenure is found to remove the significant effects of education and occupation in men, and of education in women. No other social factor removes the significant effect of housing tenure (p<0.001). Housing tenure in Scotland is thus found to be the most discriminatory measure of social status in relation to coronary heart disease, and is closely tied with unemployment and low income. Housing tenure is also likely to dictate access to shopping facilities: many peripheral housing estates are poorly served by supermarkets and by public transport.

Unemployment: unemployment leads to loss of income, and is highly localised across Britain. The diet–health problem is therefore related to locality as well as income and social class. This is reflected in the previous comments relating to housing tenure.

Social class: social class tends to cross generations (Power et al, 1991) taking with it unhealthy dietary patterns which persist for both cultural and physiological reasons. The clearest physiological expression of this phenomenon is the cycle of poor maternal nutrition, worse outcomes of pregnancy, reduced childhood development (physical and cognitive) and less education, leading once again to poor maternal nutrition.

What can be done to reduce inequalities in nutrition?

There is an urgent need to act as soon as possible to avoid prolonging the inequalities which exist. It would be rash to act without deciding which strategies for action are most likely to be of greatest benefit, weighting our judgement to achieve a balance between short-term and long-term goals. But it must be recognised that while we wait for 'the evidence', many more people are being condemned to lifetimes of ill-health and early mortality.

A clear message is emerging regarding the targeting of interventions. Those programmes which are most successful at bringing about change are:

- constructed on sound theoretical bases which characterise the social and psychological mechanisms whereby individuals are likely to change their habits (Benzeval et al, 1995; Roe et al, 1997), and
- targeted at high risk groups (Wilkinson, 1996; Piachaud and Webb, 1996; Brunner et al, 1997).

If it were necessary to identify the groups most likely to benefit from interventions, women of childbearing age and children from low-income households are those whose short- and long-term health, growth and development are most likely to be impaired by poor nutrition. Geographical concentration of effort to maximise benefit may be more effective than broader population-based strategies.

Any programmes which are aimed specifically at low-income households should be in addition to, not in place of, broader programmes which aim to change food culture (changing what foods are available in tuck shops in schools, at work canteens, etc).

The Executive summary at the beginning of this report attempts to prioritise the actions which need to be put in place to have maximum impact on both the short and long term. It is intended to strike a balance between actions which are likely to have more immediate effects and those which provide a broad sustainable base for improvement in the long term.

Policies

The following comments amplify the points raised in the Executive summary.

> **Policy** **The Minister for Public Health should create an interdepartmental forum to integrate government policy to reduce nutrition-related inequalities in health.**

Part of the reason for the rise in nutrition-related inequalities in health over the last 20 years has been the absence of a coherent government strategy on food and nutrition. Creation of policies is urgently required which will coordinate the diverse aims of different sectors of government, industry and the community. The more rapid the reduction in inequalities, the more quickly the quality of life will improve for the most at-risk segments of society, and the more rapidly the associated costs of care and health service provision will decline.

The policies of the Treasury and of the Departments of Health, Social Security, Education and Employment, Environment, Trade and Industry, the Ministry of Agriculture, Fisheries and Food, the Food Standards Agency, and food suppliers need to be coordinated at the highest level in order to maximise access by all segments of the population to a healthy and affordable food supply and to encourage the adoption of healthy eating habits, with the specific objective to reduce nutrition-related inequalities in health. A forum is urgently required in which the conflicts of interest of different sectors can be discussed and resolved. This requires representation at the highest levels in order to facilitate this process. Where the forum is placed (in the Department of Health, in the Food Standards Agency, or the Cabinet Office) is a matter for discussion.

It is clear that the rise in inequalities in nutrition-related health is due in part to a failure to integrate the diverse needs of food providers, consumers and taxpayers. A coordinated approach with a clear health agenda has been shown to have long-term and sustainable benefits (eg Norway).

The forum should:

- prioritise actions recommended in this report, the report of the Low Income Project Team, and the National Food Alliance submission;
- make recommendations to government regarding the most effective ways of reducing nutritional inequalities in health;
- develop a five-year plan to reduce nutritional inequalities in health which identifies the specific actions to be taken by government departments, communities, and retailers, and which sets targets for improvements in risk factors and morbidity and mortality for nutrition-related illnesses.

Policy   **The government should introduce a programme that focuses specifically on mothers and children and which integrates the provision of food, nutrition education, and the development of cooking and budgeting skills.**

It is important to break the vicious cycle of poor maternal nutrition being passed on to the next generation. It is unacceptable that hunger continues to exist in Britain on a wide scale, especially among mothers on low income who go without food to protect their children's intakes. The most effective way of breaking the cycle is to provide food to those most in need, and to reintroduce cooking and budgeting skills which are currently absent from the school curriculum and in many homes.

Evidence from the Nutrition Program for Women, Infants and Children (WIC) in the United States has shown benefits in terms of reduced neonatal care costs and outcomes of pregnancy (Owen and Owen, 1997) and better socialisation of children, with long-term health and social benefits (Committee on Scientific Evaluation of WIC Nutrition Risk Criteria Food and Nutrition Board, 1996).

A programme of this kind must be integrated (i) with a scheme to ringfence social security payments for food, for example, by limiting the demands which can be made on low incomes in the form of rent, debt and utility deductions: current regulations allow household incomes to be driven far below Income Support levels, resulting in reduced expenditure on food and serious dietary inadequacy (Dowler and Calvert, 1995); and (ii) with improved access for low-income households to healthy and affordable food supplies (see the next two policies).

Policy   **Provide financial support through local government, health authorities, social services and planning departments to set up, maintain and evaluate local initiatives which aim to improve nutritional health in the community, schools and the workplace. Mapping food provision on a local level should be carried out to identify areas of greatest need.**

There is a growing number of small projects at the local level whose aim is to improve diet, through direct provision of food (eg coops), better skills (eg cooking skills classes) and other approaches. It is important to allow those initiatives which are shown to be effective in reaching their target audience and changing food habits to continue their work. Many projects are set up with small grants from local authorities but cease when the funding runs out.

The main advantage of these projects is that they are designed to improve health-related life-style among individuals who are clustered in high risk groups. They are low in cost because there exists a network of services through the health authority, local government environmental offices, health promotion teams, and so on to implement and support initiatives.

Targeted interventions which are part of a national strategy are more effective than untargeted population-based interventions. The current scale of intervention is too small to have a major impact on nutrition-related health inequalities, but provides an important focus for development that can be integrated into a wider strategy of improvement. If a local strategy is to be pursued it needs proper support from central and local government.

Mapping the areas of greatest need must be a priority. The identification of 'shopping deserts' and action through coordination with the community and retailers is required. The relative mix of shops, local transport and housing needs to be evaluated for need and appropriate intervention.

Policy   Government should provide guidelines for planning the retail provision of food at the local level to generate food security for low-income communities. Such guidelines should integrate the needs of communities for food provision, transport policy, taxation policy, the need to maintain local services and the need for retailers to sustain profitability.

In just six years the number of greengrocers in Britain declined by 25%. The total number of retail food outlets continues to decline. Many of the smaller shops were accessible to low-income neighbourhoods which are now left without adequate shopping facilities. The result is more expensive food for those least able to afford it (Wilkinson, 1996).

Action is needed to increase food security for communities with a high proportion of low-income households and improve the availability of low-cost food. By engaging food retailers in the development of this provision, there will be a revitalisation of local economies, including opportunities for employment. True food security includes improved local food economies and citizen involvement (Whitehead, 1995). Mere improvements in the local physical environment will not address the problems of

vandalism and staff safety which have led to some supermarkets (eg Kwik Save) withdrawing from areas regarded as unsafe.

The government needs to provide direct incentives to encourage retailers to work closely with local government and local communities in the provision of low-cost and healthy food. Such partnerships have in the past led to concrete improvements in the provision of food at low cost (eg Easterhouse, Glasgow). This may be achieved through tax incentives which encourage the retention of existing shops (eg extend rate relief now provided to village shops to those in inner-city areas) as well as the development of new facilities.

Policy   The government should use Budget Standards when setting benefit levels and minimum wage.

There is strong evidence to show that low income and its sequelae (especially poor diet and housing) are powerful causes of poor health even after smoking has been taken into account. If government is to recommend changes in life-style which relate to improvements in health, then the costs of these improvements to individual householders need to be made explicit. Equally, there is a responsibility of government to show that the tax and benefit systems are constructed so as to allow those on low income to achieve a healthy life-style. This will require Budget Standards as reference points.

Budget Standards are baskets of goods and services which, when priced, represent a particular living standard. There is substantial evidence from physical, health and social sciences to identify the levels of goods and services associated with good health. Several European countries (Sweden, Denmark, Holland) with smaller inequalities in health than Britain already use Budget Standards as a reference point when setting social security and minimum wage levels.

Expenditure on food (after housing costs) represents 30% of total expenditure in the poorest tenth and 18% in the richest tenth of the income distribution, although total expenditure on food per person per week tends to increase with income (Figure 5). Moving off benefit and into work entails additional expenditure that is likely to squeeze the food budget, resulting in a *reduction* in expenditure on food per person. This may explain the fall in expenditure in households in the second tenth of the distribution of income. If inequalities in nutrition-related ill-health are to be reduced, realistic appraisals of food costs are needed to allow for more sensible tapering of Council Tax Benefit, Housing Benefit and Family Credit in relation to increases in income (see the next policy).

Figure 5: Per cent of household spending on food and amount spent per person per week, by tenth of income

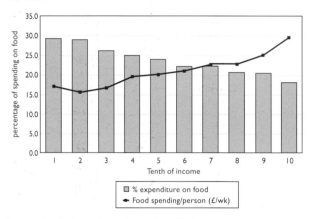

Source: *Family Expenditure Survey* (1995/96)

Policy **Reform the tax and benefit systems to make employment more attractive to people on low incomes by replacement of existing social security benefits, income tax allowances and tax reliefs by a system of transferable tax credits or basic incomes.**

Higher disposable income facilitates the purchase of a healthier diet. Of this there is no question. It is vital to improve the incentives to work for increased returns from employment. A reduction in basic rate tax from 20% to 10% is likely to help rich taxpayers more than poor taxpayers because the poorest may not have enough income to set against the whole of the 10% band. They need to be lifted out of income tax. In advance of wholesale reform of tax and benefit, a reduction from 20% to 10% will be of no value to the low paid if:

- personal allowances are not increased;
- allowances for lone parents are abolished;
- thresholds for payments of Council Tax Benefit, Housing Benefit and Family Credit are not increased to allow a larger proportion of earned income to be retained.

The current tax and benefits systems provide virtually no financial incentive for people who are unemployed to return to work. People who take full-time employment at low wages, often in menial tasks, need better returns for the additional responsibilities and outgoings which they are being asked to assume. Additional costs relating to transport, clothing, childcare, convenience foods and food preparation facilities will all squeeze the food budget when employment does not result in an appreciable increase in net income after tax. As an example, a lone mother with two young children in full-time employment and £60.00 per week childcare costs can double her gross income from £130 to £260 per week, but be only £10 per week better off after housing costs (Table 7). Where is the incentive to return to work and take on the burden of arranging childcare and assume the responsibilities of showing up for work in what may be unmotivating, menial work?

The costs of lifting the lower paid out of direct taxation and of increasing non-means-tested family Income Support (convertible tax credits or basic income) would in part be paid for by reduced costs to the NHS and increased employee productivity. The modelling recommended below (see Further action) should be used to demonstrate how reduced costs related to improved health, fewer working days lost through ill-health, and improved productivity can finance these changes in tax and benefit. Studies in developing countries show clear benefits of improved employee health in terms of increased productivity.

Table 7: Families whose head is a full-time employee

Lone parent with 2 children: 1 under 5, 1 aged 5-10 and childcare costs   **Local authority tenant**

Tax threshold £104.18pw   Rent £43.89pw   Council Tax £8.80pw   No Family Credit 30 hour credit
Net income on Income Support: Before housing costs £158.17pw   Childcare costs £60.00pw   Child Benefit = £26.10pw
After housing costs £105.48pw

£ per week

Gross earnings	Income tax	Not contracted out NICs	Take home pay	Family Credit	Housing Benefit	Council Tax Benefit	Net income Before housing costs	After housing costs	Marginal deduction rate	Replacement ratio
130.00	5.16	8.04	116.80	71.75	27.87	3.87	246.39	133.70	89.5%	78.9%
140.00	7.16	9.04	123.80	71.75	23.32	2.47	247.44	134.75	89.5%	78.3%
150.00	9.16	10.04	130.80	71.75	18.77	1.07	248.49	135.80	89.5%	77.7%
160.00	11.26	11.04	137.70	71.37	14.53	–	249.70	137.01	93.0%	77.0%
170.00	13.56	12.04	144.40	66.68	13.23	–	250.40	137.71	93.0%	76.6%
180.00	15.86	13.04	151.10	61.99	11.92	–	251.10	138.41	93.0%	76.2%
190.00	18.16	14.04	157.80	57.30	10.61	–	251.81	139.12	93.0%	75.8%
200.00	20.46	15.04	164.50	52.61	9.31	–	252.51	139.82	93.0%	75.4%
210.00	22.76	16.04	171.20	47.92	8.00	–	253.21	140.52	93.0%	75.1%
220.00	25.06	17.04	177.90	43.23	6.69	–	253.92	141.23	93.0%	74.7%
230.00	27.36	18.04	184.60	38.54	5.39	–	254.62	141.93	93.0%	74.3%
240.00	29.66	19.04	191.30	33.85	4.08	–	255.33	142.64	93.0%	74.0%
250.00	31.96	20.04	198.00	29.16	2.78	–	256.03	143.34	93.0%	73.6%
260.00	34.26	21.04	204.70	24.47	1.47	–	256.73	144.04	93.0%	73.2%
270.00	36.56	22.04	211.40	19.78	–	–	257.27	144.58	79.9%	73.0%
280.00	38.86	23.04	218.10	15.09	–	–	259.28	146.59	79.9%	72.0%
290.00	41.16	24.04	224.80	10.40	–	–	261.29	148.60	79.9%	71.0%
300.00	43.46	25.04	231.50	5.71	–	–	263.30	150.61	79.9%	70.0%
310.00	45.76	26.04	238.20	1.02	–	–	265.31	152.62	79.9%	69.1%
320.00	48.06	27.04	244.90	–	–	–	271.00	158.31	33.0%	66.6%
330.00	50.36	28.04	251.60	–	–	–	277.70	165.01	33.0%	63.9%
340.00	52.66	29.04	258.30	–	–	–	284.40	171.71	33.0%	61.4%

Source: DSS (1997); Crown Copyright

Lone parent with 2 children: 1 under 5, aged 5-10 and childcare costs, local authority tenant

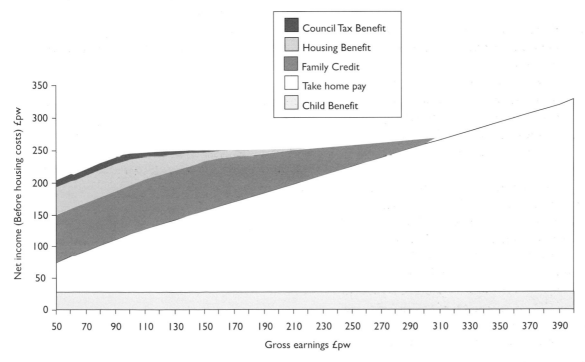

Source: DSS (1997); Crown Copyright

Further action

There are many specific initiatives that can be taken. These include:

- *Reintroduction of school milk:* recent evidence relating milk consumption and calcium intake to bone density in adolescent girls suggests it could be important in relation to long-term bone health and a reduction in osteoporosis (Cadogan et al, 1997).
- *Introduction of school fruit:* universal introduction of school fruit would be likely to have significant impact on fruit consumption nationally, and be of especial benefit in children from low-income households where consumption levels are lowest.
- *Programmes at work:* making salad and fruit widely available in canteens (possibly cross-subsidised from sales of other foods) would have a dramatic impact on consumption nationally and particularly in manual social class workers.
- *Reinstate entitlement to free school meals to those receiving Family Credit:* the loss of free school meals effectively undermines all of the benefit which Family Credit is intended to provide. This would have an immediate and positive benefit for these families.

There are also many research priorities which should be pursued, among which are the following.

The Department of Health should finance the development of computer models of health benefits and harm which are likely to arise from the implementation of specific nutrition policies, with special reference to health inequalities. This would help to evaluate the likely effects of policy recommendations in light of health objectives and knowledge of diet–health interactions, and provide better estimates of the costs, both in financial and human terms, of changes in nutrition policy. At present, the Department of Health Committee on Medical Aspects of Food and Nutrition (COMA) recommendations relate to single foods or nutrients.

The effects of the adoption of such recommendations on the balance of the diet is rarely considered (eg if red meat consumption is reduced to avoid saturated fats, what might be the effect on rates of anaemia and associated consequences, for example, low birth weight). In targeted groups, it could be used to help evaluate the notion of cumulative high-risk exposure.

The development of appropriate indicators of food-related health is needed, including community indices of food availability which are applicable at local level, to identify the pockets of the poor who are at greatest risk.

In the absence of a coordinated government policy on nutrition and health inequalities, there have been no longitudinal UK-based studies which have looked systematically at baseline and follow-up measurements of changes in health related specifically to changes in food choice and nutritional status. While valuable evidence is available from the *National Diet and Nutrition Surveys* (DHSS, 1989; Gregory et al, 1990, 1995) and other studies such as the Whitehall Study (Davey Smith and Brunner, 1997), these are not longitudinal in inception. Such research needs urgent implementation.

Better evidence is needed of the ways in which change in socio-economic patterns of food consumption are related directly to changes in risk factors for ill-health. Appropriate cohort studies need to be initiated. Part of this aim could be achieved through appropriate follow-up of subjects who participate in the *National Diet and Nutrition Surveys*.

Addendum

Following the presentation of my paper on nutrition and health inequalities to the Acheson Committee, it was clear that a number of policy options mentioned in the main body of the paper did not find their way into the Executive summary but which, on reflection, were felt to be worth highlighting.

5.0

The direct provision of food to low-income households

Direct provision of food allows families to improve their diets but would not be considered a part of income. An increase in Child Benefit, for example, would be deducted from Income Support and Family Credit, so any increase in Child Benefit would be of value only to those not receiving benefits. Specific policy recommendations in addition to those already suggested should therefore include:

- reinstatement of entitlement to free school meals to families receiving Family Credit;
- provision of free school milk (see comments below on osteoporosis);
- provision of free school fruit.

A further point was raised concerning milk formula tokens given to mothers of newborn children. A similar incentive needs to be provided to mothers who choose to breastfeed. Food vouchers (the value of which is not deducted from other benefit payments) should be considered.

Reduction of salt intake

Hypertension rates are higher in social classes IV and V, and a reduction in salt intake is likely to be beneficial. Figure 6 shows that National Food Survey estimates of sodium intake from food acquisitions (as a per cent of RNI) is higher in income groups D and E2 than A, and that lower-income households have higher consumption of processed foods rich in sodium (eg white bread, meat products, and processed vegetables other than frozen). Similar gradients are revealed in the survey of toddlers (Gregory et al, 1990) whose sodium intakes from food and whose dietary sodium densities (per 1,000 kcal) are higher in households from manual social classes, who are receiving benefits, where mothers have no educational qualifications, who are unemployed or economically inactive, or where there is a lone parent. (No such gradients were observed in the adult survey, however, but the reason for this inconsistency is not clear.) The government should make specific and binding recommendations to:

- reduce the sodium content of processed foods;
- increase the provision of economy line foods with low sodium content.

Figure 6: Sodium intake (% RNI) and food consumption of proposed foods (g/person/week), by income group

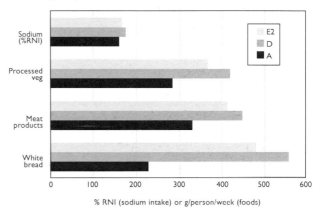

Note: A: £570/week and over
D: <£140/week (earner)
E2: <£140/week (no earner)

Source: *National Food Survey* (1995)

Reduction of hunger

A number of recent surveys (National Children's Homes, 1991; Dobson et al, 1994; Owens, 1997) have reported hunger as a regular event in many low-income households. A total of 20% of parents and 10% of children reported having gone hungry or without food in the previous month due to lack of money (National Children's Homes, 1991). A total of 25% of children had gone hungry because they did not like what was on offer, a special problem in low-income households where alternative, acceptable foods may not be available. Ironically, hunger coexists with higher rates of obesity in this group, although whether hunger and obesity coexist within the same households or individuals is not known. The government should:

- undertake surveys to identify the demographic and socio-economic characteristics of individuals and households where hunger occurs, and examine its association with measures of nutritional status;
- identify and implement the steps necessary to reduce hunger.

Osteoporosis

There is a steep gradient in osteoporosis rates between genders, being three times more common in women. Some of this difference is attributable to factors such as lower body mass and the decline in oestrogen levels at the menopause. Part of the difference may also be due to low intakes of calcium and low activity levels. Recent evidence in the UK suggest that adolescent girls who are supplemented with milk over 18 months have higher bone mass (Cadogan et al, 1997), and higher calcium intakes and physical activity levels are associated independently of other risk factors with higher bone mass in white postmenopausal women (Suleiman et al, 1997). The lack of a social class gradient may be an historical artefact relating to patterns of work and physical activity, women from manual social classes having had lower calcium intakes but whose bone mass has been protected by higher levels of physical activity. This pattern of diet and activity explains the low rates of osteoporosis in developing countries. In the UK, declining levels of domestic and manual labour, unemployment (especially among lone mothers), and continuing levels of calcium intake in women from low-income households may presage a rapid rise in osteoporosis among poorer women. Government should:

- promote increases in dietary calcium intake among women, especially those from low-income households, through increased promotion and availability of calcium rich foods at affordable prices;
- promote higher intakes of dietary calcium in school children at all ages through the provision of free school milk.

Evidence which relates calcium intake in pre-school children to adolescent and adult bone mass is lacking. Follow-up studies of pre-school and primary school children from the *National Diet and Nutrition Surveys* should relate measures of bone mass in adolescence to calcium intakes at earlier ages.

References

Armstrong, N., Balding, J., Gentle, P. and Kirby, B. (1990) 'Pattern of physical activity among 11 to 16 year old British children', *British Medical Journal*, vol 301, pp 203-5.

Benzeval, M., Judge, K. and Whitehead, M. (eds) (1995) *Tackling inequalities in health*, London: King's Fund.

British Nutrition Foundation (1995) *Iron: Nutritional and physiological significance*, London: Chapman and Hall.

Brunner, E., White, I., Thorogood, M., Bristow, A., Curle, D. and Marmot, M. (1997) 'Can dietary interventions change diet and cardiovascular risk factors? A meta-analysis of randomized controlled trials', *American Journal of Public Health*, vol 87, pp 1415-22.

Cadogan, J., Eastell, R., Jones, N. and Barker, M.E. (1997) 'Milk intake and bone mineral acquisition in adolescent girls: randomised, controlled intervention trial', *British Medical Journal*, vol 315, pp 1255-60.

Colhoun, H. and Prescott-Clarke, P. (1996) *Health Survey for England 1994*, London: HMSO.

Committee on Scientific Evaluation of WIC Nutrition Risk Criteria Food and Nutrition Board (1996) 'Summary of WIC nutrition risk criteria: a scientific assessment', Institute of Medicine, National Academy of Sciences, *Journal of the American Dietetic Association*, vol 96, pp 925-30.

Davey Smith, G. and Brunner, E. (1997) 'Socio-economic differentials in health: the role of nutrition', *Proceedings of the Nutrition Society*, vol 56, pp 75-90.

DHSS (Department of Health and Social Security) (1972) *A nutrition survey of the elderly*, Reports on Health and Social Subjects No 3, London: HMSO.

DHSS (1989) *The diets of British schoolchildren*, London: HMSO.

Dobson, B., Beardsworth, A., Keil, T. and Walker, R. (1994) *Diet, choice and poverty: Social, cultural and nutritional aspects of food consumption among low income families*, Loughborough: Centre for Research in Social Policy, Loughborough University of Technology.

DoH (Department of Health) (1989) *The diets of British schoolchildren*, Report on Health and Social Subjects, No 36, London: HMSO.

DoH (1991) *Dietary reference values for food energy and nutrients for the United Kingdom*, Report on Health and Social Subjects, No 41, London: HMSO.

Dorling, D. (1997) *Death in Britain. How local mortality rates have changed: 1950s-1990s*, York: Joseph Rowntree Foundation.

Dowler, E. and Calvert, C. (1995) *Nutrition and diet in lone-parent families in London*, London: Family Policy Studies Centre.

DSS (Department of Social Security (1997) *Tax/benefit model tables*, April, London: Government Statistical Service.

Duggan, M.B., Steel, G., Elwys, G., Harbottle, L. and Noble, C. (1991) 'Iron status, energy intake, and nutritional status of healthy young Asian children', *Archives of Disease in Childhood*, vol 66, no 12, pp 1386-9.

Foster, K., Lader, D. and Cheesbrough, S. (1997) *Infant feeding 1995: A survey of infant feeding practices in the United Kingdom carried out by the Social Survey Division of ONS on behalf of the Department of Health, the Scottish Office Department of Health, the Welsh Office and the Department of Health and Social Services in Northern Ireland*, London: The Stationery Office.

Gregory, J., Foster, K., Tyler, H. and Wiseman, M. (1990) *The dietary and nutritional survey of British adults*, London: HMSO.

Gregory, J., Collins, D.L., Davies, P.S.W., Hughes, J. and Clarke, P.C. (1995) *National diet and nutrition survey: Children aged 1½ to 4½ years*, London: HMSO.

Heaney, R.P. (1996) 'Bone mass, nutrition, and other lifestyle factors', *Nutrition Reviews*, vol 54, pp S3-10.

James, W.P.T., Nelson, M., Ralph, A. and Leather, S. (1997) 'The contribution of nutrition to inequalities in health', *British Medical Journal*, vol 314, pp 1545-9.

MAFF (Ministry of Agriculture, Fisheries and Food) (1981-97) *National Food Survey 1980-1996*, London: HMSO.

Martin, J. and White, A. (1988) *Infant feeding 1985*, London: HMSO.

Mills, A. and Tyler, H. (1992) *Food and nutrient intakes of British infants aged 6-12 months*, London: HMSO.

Murray, T.M. (1996) 'Prevention and management of osteoporosis: consensus statements from the Scientific Advisory Board of the Osteoporosis Society of Canada. 4. Calcium nutrition and osteoporosis', *Canadian Medical Association Journal*, vol 155, pp 935-9.

National Children's Homes (1991) *NCH poverty and nutrition survey*, London: NCH.

Nelson, M., Bakaliou, F. and Tivedi, A. (1994) 'Iron deficiency anaemia and physical performance in adolescent girls from different ethnic backgrounds', *British Journal of Nutrition*, vol 72, pp 427-33.

Owen, A.L. and Owen, G.M. (1997) 'Twenty years of WIC: a review of some effects of the program', *Journal of the American Dietetics Association*, vol 97, pp 777-82.

Owens, B. (1997) *Out of the frying pan*, London: Save the Children Foundation.

Piachaud, D. and Webb, J. (1996) *The price of food: Missing out on mass consumption*, London: STICERD.

Pollitt, E. (1990) *Malnutrition and infection in the classroom*, Geneva: UNESCO.

Power, C., Manor, O. and Fox, J. (1991) *Health and class: The early years*, London: Chapman and Hall.

Pryer, J.A., Vrijheid, M., Nichols, R. and Elliott, P. (1994) 'Who are the "low energy reporters" in the Dietary and Nutritional Survey of British Adults', *Proceedings of the Nutrition Society*, vol 53, p 235A.

Pryer, J., Brunner, E., Elliott, P., Nichols, R., Dimond, H. and Marmot, M. (1995) 'Who complied with COMA 1984 dietary fat recommendations among a nationally representative sample of British adults in 1986-7 and what did they eat?', *European Journal of Clinical Nutrition*, vol 49, no 10, pp 718-28.

Roe, L., Hunt, P., Bradshaw, H. and Rayner, M. (1997) *Health promotion interventions to promote healthy eating in the general population: A review*, London: Health Education Authority.

Suleiman, S., Nelson, M., Li, F., Buxton-Thomas, M. and Moniz, C. (1997) 'Effect of calcium intake and physical activity level on bone mass and turnover in healthy, white, postmenopausal women', *American Journal of Clinical Nutrition*, vol 66, pp 937-43.

Wenlock, R.W., Disselduff, M.M. and Skinner, R.K. (1986) *The diets of British schoolchildren: Preliminary report*, London: HMSO.

Whitehead, M. (1995) 'Tackling inequalities: a review of policy initiatives', in M. Benzeval, K. Judge and M. Whitehead (eds) *Tackling inequalities in health*, London: King's Fund, pp 22-52.

Wilkinson, R. (1996) *Unhealthy societies: The afflications of inequality*, London: Routledge.

Woodward, M., Shewry, M.C., Smith, W.C. and Tunstall-Pedoe, H. (1992) 'Social status and coronary heart disease: results from the Scottish Heart Health Study', *Preventive Medicine*, vol 21, pp 136-48.

10

Education and health inequalities[1]

Geoff Whitty, Peter Aggleton, Eva Gamarnikow and Paul Tyrer

Inequalities in education and health

British data appear to show a clear correlation between social inequality, levels of educational attainment and the state of the nation's health (see, for example, Morris et al, 1996)[2]. The present paper explores recent evidence, drawn from Britain and elsewhere, about one particular aspect of this relationship – the extent to which education impacts upon health[3]. After discussing the importance of 'social capital' in this context, it then seeks to identify educational interventions that might contribute to a reduction in health inequalities.

According to recently published data from the 1970 birth cohort study, those without educational qualifications are, at age 26, four times more likely to report poor general health (23%) than those with highest educational qualifications (6%). There is a similar inverse relationship between educational qualifications and depression, measured by the Malaise Inventory, where very high levels of depression are evident, particularly among women without educational qualifications (Montgomery and Schoon, 1997). There are strikingly similar findings in research on those with poor basic skills in the 1958 cohort: 36% of women and 18% of men with very low literacy skills suffered from depression, compared with around 6% of those with good literacy skills (Bynner and Parsons, 1997). Another conclusion to be drawn from cohort studies is that "children who do well in education tend strongly to make healthier choices in adult life in health related habits of diet, alcohol consumption, smoking and exercise" (Wadsworth, 1997a, p 200).

However, in many studies, level of education acts as a marker for the effects of other influences, such as class, occupational level or life-style, as Marmot et al (1997) have recently described. Because so few studies have controlled adequately for relevant variables, the extent to which there is a separate and distinct educational influence on health remains unclear. Nevertheless, some studies do seem to demonstrate a clear independent effect of education on, for example, levels of risky behaviour and associated morbidity. Indeed, a number suggest that qualification level is a better predictor of non-smoking than social class (Shewry et al, 1992; Winkleby et al, 1992; King's Fund, 1996; Whitehead and Drever, 1997).

Notwithstanding this uncertainty about the relationship between educational, health and other forms of disadvantage, many studies have drawn attention to the cumulative effects of low social class of origin, poor educational achievement, reduced employment prospects, low levels of psychosocial well-being and poor physical and mental health (Benzeval et al, 1995; Wilkinson, 1994, 1996). A life-course perspective on human development hypothesises a chain of causality which links critical periods of biological development, sensitive periods of psychosocial development and adult health risks (Wadsworth, 1996, 1997a, 1997b; Kuh, 1997). At each stage risks can accumulate, adding to disadvantage. Education is thus linked to health through the differential opportunities for income, employment and security associated with different levels of educational attainment. The 'pathway' perspective advocated by Power and Hertzman (1997) points to the importance of early experience but also to the possibility of changing trajectories through experiences in later life.

In short, although the extent to which education has an independent effect on medium to longer-term health status remains unclear, it does appear to have such an influence. How it achieves this, both directly and indirectly, requires further exploration. Nevertheless, it may plausibly be hypothesised that education has both a potentiating and a protective role – potentiating in relation to the triggering of healthier life-styles and behaviour, protective in that higher levels of education provide access to the kinds of employment opportunities and life chances that can protect individuals from disadvantage in later life.

The importance of social capital

Unfortunately, many children live in such disadvantaged circumstances that their opportunities to benefit from education, and its potentiating and protective role, are severely limited. Robinson (1997, p 17) rightly argues that "a serious programme to alleviate child poverty might do far more for boosting attainment ... than any modest intervention in schooling", and much the same could be said in relation to health. However, even though substantial increases in material resources for disadvantaged groups may seem the most obvious way of tackling inequalities, interventions that increase 'social capital' may also be useful in reducing risk, leading to consequent improvements in health, education and, indeed, economic prosperity.

Social capital has been defined by Putnam (1993, p 167) as the "features of social organization, such as trust, norms, and networks, that can improve the efficiency of society by facilitating coordinated actions". He suggests that communities with high and long-established levels of social capital are significantly more successful than those which lack them. Some of the earliest American research on social capital demonstrated its particular relevance to education (Coleman, 1988) and these findings have been supported by more recent research. Teachman et al (1996), for example, found that children who change schools regularly – and therefore have less access to lasting school-related social relationships and networks – are more likely to drop out of school early. Similarly, Furstenberg and Hughes (1995, p

589) have suggested that social capital is a factor determining school staying-on rates among disadvantaged African-American young people. They further found that those with a higher level of social capital are less likely to be depressed, more likely to be in work, less likely to be teenage parents and more likely to have "avoided serious trouble". Fuchs and Reklis (1994) have concluded that the strength of parental relationships and the influence of other social networks is crucial in affecting children's 'readiness to learn' in pre-school contexts.

Data from British birth cohort studies similarly suggest the importance of social capital in maximising educational potential, thus bringing likely health benefits. For example, Wadsworth's analyses (1996, 1997a, 1997b) indicate that parental interest in children's education impacts positively on educational outcomes, and on achievements and opportunities in adulthood, irrespective of social class. Willms (1999) cites studies in Catholic schools, suggesting that the success of these institutions may be in part dependent upon strong levels of social capital within the communities that the schools serve. School effectiveness and improvement research similarly provides evidence that high levels of trust between head teacher and staff, between staff and pupils, and between home and school, are associated with beneficial outcomes (Mortimore and Whitty, 1997). Moreover, although participation in community and voluntary organisations is strongly differentiated by social class and education, women with low literacy and numeracy skills appear more likely to be involved in schools' PTA activities (6% and 12% respectively) than in any other local networks (Bynner and Parsons, 1997).

One of the challenges facing efforts to generate and reinforce social capital with a view to reducing inequalities, however, is that disadvantaged communities are institutionally constructed over long periods of time. As Putnam points out, "where norms and networks of civic engagement are lacking, the outlook for collective action appears bleak" (1993, p 183). In other words, there may be levels of poverty or disadvantage which make it difficult for people to engage in the social activities and civic duties thought to be crucial to the production of social capital. Nevertheless, Gillies and Spray (1997) have cited a number of health promotion projects based in disadvantaged communities, suggesting that building local networks and institutions with the direct involvement of local people can have major and relatively speedy health benefits. Gillies (1997, p 2) singles out volunteer activities, peer programmes and civic activities as potentially effective social capital building initiatives, particularly those working alongside "durable structures which facilitate planning and decision-making".

Priorities for intervention

Taken together, this evidence suggests that interventions that seek to enhance educational attainment for disadvantaged groups, while working to develop social capital within their communities, could make some contribution directly and indirectly to the reduction of health inequalities. Early interventions seem likely to be particularly effective in this respect. Indeed, Wadsworth argues that the "chances of reduction of inequalities for any given generation will be greater the earlier attempts at reduction are begun. It is unlikely that health inequalities can be easily or rapidly reduced, increasingly so as the individuals carry an accumulation of health potential which is hard to change" (1997b, p 867). On the other hand, Power and Hertzman's (1997) work should counsel against neglecting the potential of later interventions in, for example, school settings.

However, the experience of past interventions is not altogether hopeful. Mortimore and Whitty (1997) cite findings from a longitudinal study of primary schools which show that even the most effective schools tend not to reverse the 'within school' pattern whereby advantaged children outperform those from disadvantaged backgrounds. Furthermore, the finding that in effective schools disadvantaged children made more progress than advantaged children in less effective schools is double-edged. If all schools improved to the level of the most effective, the effect would merely be to increase the gap in achievement between advantaged and disadvantaged children. This increase in educational inequality might in turn lead to increased and starker social inequalities and hence to increased health inequalities. Health gains come, Wilkinson (1994, 1996) argues, not from the further raising of a rich nation's overall standard of living, but

from policies that seek to narrow the gap between the richest and the poorest in that society.

All this suggests that strategies that seek to reduce inequalities, rather than merely raise standards overall, will need to be more effectively targeted towards disadvantaged groups than has previously been the case (Mortimore and Whitty, 1997). Various suggestions have been made about the possible form of such interventions. Some are general strategies to enhance achievement among disadvantaged groups which, on the basis of the evidence cited here, may impact indirectly on health outcomes by raising qualification levels and employment prospects. Some aim to influence health knowledge and behaviours more directly through work in educational settings. Others focus on ways of building social capital in disadvantaged communities. Still others entail coordinated strategies that seek to do all these things at the same time. The evidence would seem to point to the importance of this last approach and here we focus on three areas of policy in which work of this nature is being developed and might be carried forward.

Pre-school provision

A large number of studies conducted in the US and elsewhere highlight the significant benefits of pre-school interventions, some of which have a direct effect on health outcomes, while others produce educational and other benefits which may affect later health status. A range of health benefits have been attributed to early education interventions, ranging from improved neurological and social functioning (Begley, 1996) to a possible delay in the onset of dementia (Hertzman and Wiens, 1996).

Although still controversial, findings from two of the longest established US initiatives, High/Scope and Project Headstart, do seem to demonstrate impressive gains in health and social outcomes, particularly when pupils are compared with those staying at home or experiencing other forms of intervention (Schweinhart et al, 1993; Case et al, 1999; Schweinhart and Weikart, 1997a). For example, only 6% of those attending High/Scope – a programme based on a constructivist theory of child development – are reported as having received treatment for emotional difficulties during their primary or secondary education compared with 47%

of a group that had undergone an intervention involving direct instruction. Similarly, Headstart students have been reported as staying on at secondary school for an average of two years longer than those who did not attend a pre-school programme. They also seem to have experienced fewer teenage pregnancies, less delinquency, "higher feelings of empowerment and a more positive attitude towards the education of their children" than the control group (Case et al, 1999, p 10). These direct and indirect social benefits suggest that every dollar invested in High/Scope-style pre-school education nets $7 in long-term savings on crime, health, and other social expenditure (Schweinhart and Weikart, 1997b).

As Law (Chapter 1 of this report), among others, has pointed out, we cannot assume that findings from the US are necessarily applicable here. However, there is some evidence – from a range of initiatives piloted in the last 20 years – to suggest that good quality pre-school interventions can have positive effects in the UK too (see, for example, Jowett and Sylva, 1986; Athey, 1990; Shorrocks et al, 1992; Sylva and Wilshire, 1993). Interventions that focus on developing what has sometimes been called a 'readiness to learn' seem likely to bring particular benefits to disadvantaged children (Sylva and Wilshire, 1993; Ball, 1994; Sylva, 1997). Support for parents can also be of vital importance in this context (Smith and Pugh, 1996). Although, over the years, many UK-based programmes have either been marginalised or abandoned before their outcomes could be properly evaluated (Mortimore and Whitty, 1997), there is now a broad consensus among UK educationalists, developmental psychologists, child and adolescent psychiatrists and researchers that high-quality interventions in the early years are one of the more effective ways of improving educational performance, self-esteem and emotional well-being, with accompanying benefits for health in general. There is also a growing awareness of the role that building social capital through parental involvement can play in the success of such initiatives.

With this in mind, the announcement by the Minister for School Standards that all local education authorities (LEAs) are to prepare Early Years Development Plans to address issues of inequality in pre-school childhood is a welcome one. However, as some disadvantaged LEAs already have relatively high

levels of public provision, careful attention will need to be given to the style and focus of any pre-school interventions undertaken. The current Department for Education and Employment study, by Sylva and others, of the effects of different kinds of pre-school provision on children's attainment and behaviour should provide important evidence about what works and why.

Making schools healthier

The Ottawa Charter for Health Promotion recognised that power and control were central issues in health promotion, and pointed to the importance of community empowerment as a key process in the promotion of health (Kickbusch, 1990). Thereafter, health promotion came to be widely understood as the process of enabling people to increase control over and to improve their health. Schools, one of the few contexts in which interventions can reach the majority of children and young people, have increasingly been moving beyond a narrow concern with health education in the curriculum towards a broader health-promoting approach.

Although evaluations of specific programmes of health education in schools are notoriously difficult to interpret, there is some evidence of the effectiveness of school-based work on nutrition (King, 1988), substance use (Hansen, 1992), accident prevention (Clayton et al, 1995) and sexual health (UNAIDS, 1997). This suggests that schools can and do play a positive role in promoting health among young people. However, if it is not to reinforce existing health inequalities, health education needs to connect sensitively with young people's experiences which are differentiated by class, region, ethnicity and gender.

The notion of 'health promoting schools' represents a more broadly-based approach, in which health promotion is a whole-school undertaking encompassing its ethos and environment, and links between the school, parents and community, as well as health education itself (Tones, 1996). A recent evaluation of the English schools in the European Network of Health Promoting Schools (Hamilton and Saunders, 1997) suggests that such approaches to health promotion can lead to pupil gains in knowledge, attitudes, self-esteem and health behaviours. These improvements are particularly apparent in primary schools, adding further weight to Wadsworth's call to make health interventions at an early age. The evaluation also recommends that "pupils need to be effectively involved and consulted in the most appropriate way for their age" (Hamilton and Saunders, 1997, p 35).

The newer concept of 'healthier schools' suggests that health-related activities in schools can also impact on levels of educational achievement which, in turn, will have an additional indirect effect on health (Healthier Schools Partnership Project, 1997). This facilitates closer links between health-related activities and broader strategies of school improvement. Advocates of the approach also imply that partnership between schools, businesses and community-based agencies can be an important conduit for building social capital. Such schemes will, however, need rigorous evaluation before we know how far a healthier school approach can have an impact on school effectiveness, particularly for disadvantaged pupils, at the same time as impacting more directly upon pupils' health knowledge and behaviours.

Developing and evaluating the various ways in which school-based interventions can impact both directly and indirectly upon health outcomes within local communities, and particularly the reduction of health inequalities, should therefore be made a priority.

Interagency working

The Ottawa Charter also states that health requires coordinated healthy public policies resulting from links between different policy sectors; effective empowerment of communities to set up and implement their own priorities; and improved, more accessible, less hierarchical, community-centred health services.

It is well established that such coordinated multiagency work, when directed towards tackling multiple disadvantage, is most effective in reducing both health and education inequalities. In a broad-based and multi-sited initiative in Karelia, Finland, for example, smoking prevalence among young people was reduced for at least eight years (Vartiainen, 1994). Similarly, in a Minnesota programme on heart health, significant and long-lasting benefits in nutritional

knowledge and behaviour among young people were noted (Perry et al, 1988). The WHO Healthy Cities Initiative, formally launched in 1986, aimed to consolidate and build social networks and facilitate community empowerment as part of a broader process of health promotion. Preliminary, if somewhat impressionistic, evaluation suggests that this approach can be associated with positive health gains (Davies and Kelly, 1993).

In England, an historical lack of coordination between housing, education and social services has been shown to exacerbate disadvantage, and recent policies have sometimes added to the problem (Power et al, 1995). However, there has of late been renewed interest in the Hillfields project, initiated in Coventry in the 1970s. Recently chosen to become one of the seven model Early Learning Centres, Hillfields aims to combine learning with childcare and integrated services (including education and mental health services) for parents and other community members (Lepkowska, 1997). Similar projects elsewhere have already been identified by the OECD (1996) as examples of best practice. The Huhtasuo Social Welfare and Health Centre in Jyvaskyla, Finland, built next door to a comprehensive and a special school, provides a range of health and emotional support systems for the local disadvantaged community. In Woodstock in New Brunswick, Canada, impressive links developed between education, social services and health providers have led to the more effective targeting of resources, case-planning and intervention. Such initiatives can help to foster the "horizontal diverse networks among individuals and groups of equal status" constitutive of high levels of social capital, which are likely to be associated with high levels of health and well-being (Gillies and Higgins, 1995) and hopefully, we would add, enhanced educational outcomes.

Better coordination between different agencies in areas where their interests coincide, and better liaison where they do not, is clearly essential if the cumulative effects of disadvantage are to be addressed effectively and efficiently.

Summary and recommendations

Although there is a growing body of literature on health and educational inequalities, further research is needed to develop our understanding of the causal pathways which link educational and health inequalities in the lives of individuals, families, and social groups. This is particularly the case with respect to research on gender and ethnicity. However, education may be hypothesised as having both direct and indirect effects on health outcomes. This should be borne in mind when developing programmes and interventions.

Existing research on health and educational inequalities suggests that disadvantage is cumulative and that educational and health opportunities are heavily skewed towards the advantaged. In the longer term, programmes and interventions that shift opportunities towards disadvantaged individuals, families and communities are more likely to reduce educational and health inequalities, than are more broadly-based initiatives catering for all. Existing and proposed government policy initiatives – such as the Welfare to Work Programme, the statutory minimum wage and the work of the Social Exclusion Unit – may make a useful contribution here.

In addition, educational initiatives may, if carefully planned and targeted, be able to make an impact on inequalities when located within appropriate policy and legislative frameworks. Virtually all the evidence points to the positive effects of good pre-school provision on both educational and health outcomes. We therefore strongly encourage the continuing development and evaluation of coordinated, good quality pre-school provision. However, pre-school interventions must be sensitive to different childhoods and work to build social capital within local communities in order to move towards meeting their needs and aspirations.

Health education in schools should be further developed, preferably within a wider institutional structure of health promoting/healthier schools and, where possible, related to broader initiatives to improve schools and enhance performance. Efforts to persuade young people to adopt healthier behaviours and life-styles should take place within a supportive and enabling context for the promotion of health and educational achievement.

In the first instance, such interventions should be concentrated in areas of greatest disadvantage. In addition to enhanced levels of resourcing, attention will need to be given to developing social networks in and around schools. Given the apparent connectedness of education and health inequalities, and the evidence in support of interagency working, there is a strong case for achieving some form of linkage between the proposed Education Action Zones and Health Action Zones. However, in the light of the experience of earlier intervention programmes, it will also be important to address the needs of disadvantaged groups beyond these zones.

Acknowledgements

We would like to thank the following individuals for their help and advice in preparing this overview. Michaela Benzeval (King's Fund), Professor John Bynner (City University), Dr Cathy Campbell (London School of Economics), Frances Drever (Office of National Statistics), Professor Philip Graham (National Children's Bureau), Professor Sally MacIntyre (Glasgow University), Professor Michael Marmot (University College London), Dr Barbara Maughan (Institute of Psychiatry), Professor Peter Moss (Thomas Coram Research Unit, Institute of Education), Dr Chris Power (Institute of Child Health), Professor Sir Michael Rutter (Institute of Psychiatry), Dr Marjorie Smith (Thomas Coram Research Unit, Institute of Education), Professor Mike Wadsworth (University College London Medical School), Hilary Whent (Health Education Authority) and Dr Margaret Whitehead (King's Fund). We are also grateful for comments on the paper by Professor Kathy Sylva (Oxford University) and Professor Sally Tomlinson (Goldsmiths College).

Notes

[1] This chapter has been previously published in the *Journal of Education Policy* (1998), vol 13, no 5, pp 641-52.

[2] The relationship is clearer in terms of class and regional differences than it is in relation to gender and differences of ethnicity. A note on this is included in the Appendix to this chapter.

[3] Studies that focus purely on the ways in which health impacts upon education are not therefore a central concern of this particular paper.

Appendix: Class, region, ethnicity and gender

There are striking and well-documented similarities in large-scale patterns of social class inequality in health and education in the UK (Kumar, 1993; Benzeval et al, 1995; Smith and Noble, 1995; Bynner and Parsons, 1997; ONS, 1997a, 1997b; Smith et al, 1997). There are similar large-scale regional contrasts in health and education inequalities, particularly between the North West and South East of England, but with marked differences between affluent and disadvantaged communities within regions (Eames et al, 1993; Smith and Noble, 1995). However, patterns of educational and health inequality in relation to ethnicity and gender are somewhat more complex.

In most respects, Pakistani, Bangladeshi and African-Caribbean groups appear to experience greater disadvantage than Indian/African Asians, Chinese and white groups. Overall health differences between minority ethnic groups and whites become less marked after controlling for standard of living, suggesting that much, but not all, of the variation can be attributed to social class (Nazroo, 1997). However, participation in post-16 education is higher for all major minority ethnic groups than for the white population (Gillborn and Gipps, 1996), although this partly reflects greater difficulties in gaining access to the labour market. There are also likely to be important differences in the health and education status of recently arrived refugee groups.

Gender-based evidence on health inequalities is mixed. More men than women report having a limiting long-standing illness, but consultation and hospitalisation rates are higher for women and women are more likely than men to be diagnosed with significant neurotic psychopathology. A higher proportion of men drink and smoke heavily, but young women are more likely to smoke. Overall, women are more likely to eat healthier foods than men (ONS, 1997b). Gender-based educational evidence is similarly mixed. Girls are now achieving at a higher level than boys at all stages of compulsory education and the gender gap in favour of young men at A-level and entry to higher education has been progressively eroded (Arnot et al, 1996). However, young men remain more likely than women to study for vocational qualifications, and men have retained their advantages in employment and earning power, even in relation to women with similar qualifications (Power et al, 1998).

It might appear that the higher participation rates among minority ethnic groups and women, reported above, hold the potential to interrupt current patterns of health inequality. However, in investigating this, it will be important to utilise appropriate measures. Indicators for education which attempt to profile the whole population may be inappropriate for investigating more subtle differences. For example, an undifferentiated category of post-compulsory education will obscure variations in a population with high staying on rates into differentiated forms of post-compulsory provision. In this context, as in others, the nature of the education and its occupational consequences may be crucial to actual health outcomes.

References

Arnot, M., David, M. and Weiner, G. (1996) *Educational reforms and gender equality in schools*, Research Discussion Series 17, Manchester: Equal Opportunities Commission.

Athey, C. (1990) *Extending thought in young children: A parent-teacher partnership*, London: Paul Chapman.

Ball, C. (1994) *Start right: The importance of early learning*, London: RSA.

Begley, S. (1996) 'Your child's brain', *Newsweek*, 19 February.

Benzeval, M. (1997) 'Health', in A. Walker and C. Walker (eds) *Britain divided: The growth of social exclusion in the 1980s and 1990s*, London: Child Poverty Action Group, pp 153-69.

Benzeval, M., Judge, K. and Whitehead, M. (eds) (1995) *Tackling inequalities in health*, London: King's Fund.

Bynner, J. and Parsons, S. (1997) *It doesn't get any better: The impact of poor basic skills on the lives of 37 year olds*, London: Basic Skills Agency.

Case, R., Griffin, S. and Kelly, W.M. (1999) 'Socioeconomic gradients in mathematical ability and their responsiveness to intervention during early childhood', in D.P. Keating and C. Hertzman (eds) *Developmental health and the wealth of nations: Social, biological and educational dynamics*, New York, NY: Guilford, pp 125-49.

Clayton, A.B., Platt, C.V., Colgan, M.A. and Butler, G. (1995) *A child based approach to road safety education for 8-11 year-olds*, Basingstoke: AA Foundation for Road Safety Research.

Coleman, J.S. (1988) 'Social capital in the creation of human capital', *American Journal of Sociology*, vol 94, Supplement 95, pp S95-S120.

Davies, J.K. and Kelly, M.P. (1993) *Healthy cities: Research and practice*, London: Routledge.

Eames, M., Ben-Shlomo, Y. and Marmot, M.G. (1993) 'Social deprivation and premature mortality: regional comparison across England', *British Medical Journal*, vol 307, no 6912, pp 1097-102.

Fuchs, V.R. and Reklis, D.M. (1994) 'Mathematical achievement in eighth grade: interstate and racial differences', NBER Working Paper 4784, Stanford, CA: NBER.

Furstenberg, F.F. Jr and Hughes, M.E. (1995) 'Social capital and successful development among at-risk youth', *Journal of Marriage and the Family*, vol 57, pp 580-92.

Gillborn, D. and Gipps, C. (1996) *Recent research on the achievement of ethnic minority pupils*, OFSTED Review of Research, London: HMSO.

Gillies, P. (1997) 'Social capital: recognising the value of society', *Healthlines*, vol 45, pp 15-17.

Gillies, P. and Higgins, D. (1995) 'Measuring outcomes from co-ordinated community interventions to prevent and control HIV transmission', Notes from ACT/HIV meeting, University of Nottingham, 31 January.

Gillies, P. and Spray, J. (1997) *Addressing health inequalities: The practical potential of social capital*, London: Health Education Authority.

Hamilton, K. and Saunders, L. (1997) *The health promoting school: A summary of the ENHPS Evaluation Project in England*, London/Windsor: Health Education Authority/National Foundation for Educational Research.

Hansen, W. (1992) 'School-based substance abuse prevention: a review of the state of the art in curriculum, 1980-90', *Health Education Research*, vol 7, no 3, pp 403-30.

Healthier Schools Partnership Project (1997) *Project handbook*, London: Lewisham Education.

Hertzman, C. and Wiens, M. (1996) 'Child development and long-term outcomes: a population health perspective and summary of successful interventions', *Social Science and Medicine*, vol 43, no 7, pp 1083-95.

Jowett, S. and Sylva, K. (1986) 'Does kind of pre-school matter?', *Educational Research*, vol 25, no 1, pp 21-31.

Kickbusch, I. (1990) *A strategy for health promotion*, Copenhagen: WHO Regional Office for Europe.

King, A. (1988) 'Promoting dietary change in adolescents: a school-based approach for modifying and maintaining healthful behaviour', *American Journal of Preventive Medicine*, vol 4, pp 68-74.

King's Fund (1996) *Society and health*, vol 3, Summer.

Kuh, D. (1997) 'The life course and social inequalities in health', Evidence to the Independent Inquiry into Health Inequalities.

Kumar, V. (1993) *Poverty and inequality in the UK: The effects on children*, London: National Children's Bureau.

Lepkowska, D. (1997) 'Inner city nursery is named as pioneer', *Times Educational Supplement*, vol 4251, p 8.

Montgomery, S.M. and Schoon, I. (1997) 'Health and health behaviour', in J. Bynner, E. Ferri and P. Shepherd (eds) *Twentysomething in the 1990s: Getting on, getting by, getting nowhere*, Aldershot: Ashgate, pp 77-96.

Marmot, M., Ryff, C.D., Bumpass, L.L., Shipley, M. and Marks, N.F. (1997) 'Social inequalities in health: next questions and converging evidence', *Social Science and Medicine*, vol 44, no 6, pp 901-10.

Morris, J.N., Blane, D.B. and White, I.R. (1996) 'Levels of mortality, education, and social conditions in the 107 local education authority areas in England', *Journal of Epidemiology and Community Health*, vol 50, pp 15-17.

Mortimore, P. and Whitty, G. (1997) *Can school improvement overcome the effects of disadvantage?*, London: Institute of Education, University of London.

Nazroo, J.Y. (1997) *The health of Britain's ethnic minorities*, London: Policy Studies Institute.

OECD (Organisation for Economic Cooperation and Development) (1996) *Successful services for our children and families at risk*, Paris: OECD.

ONS (Office for National Statistics) (1997a) *Summary of socio-economic differences*, London: ONS.

ONS (1997b) *Summary of gender differences*, London: ONS.

Perry, C.L., Luepker, R.V., Murray, D.M., Kurth, C., Mullis, R., Crockett, S. and Jacobs, D.R. (1988) 'Parental involvement with children's health promotion: the Minnesota Home Team', *American Journal of Public Health*, vol 78, pp 1156-60.

Power, C. and Hertzman, C. (1997) 'Social and biological pathways linking early life and adult disease', *British Medical Bulletin*, vol 53, no 1, pp 210-21.

Power, S., Whitty, G. and Youdell, D. (1995) *No place to learn: Homelessness and education*, London: Shelter.

Power, S., Whitty, G., Edwards, T. and Wigfall, V. (1998) 'Schoolboys and schoolwork: gender identification and academic achievement', *International Journal of Inclusive Education*, vol 2, no 2, pp 135-53.

Putnam, R.D. with Leonardi, R. and Nanetti, R.Y. (1993) *Making democracy work: Civic traditions in modern Italy*, Princeton, NJ: Princeton University Press.

Robinson, P. (1997) *Literacy, numeracy and economic performance*, London: CEP, London School of Economics and Political Science.

Schweinhart, L.J., Barnes, H.V. and Weikart, D.P. (1993) 'Significant benefits: the High/Scope Perry pre-school study through age 27', *Monographs of the High/Scope Educational Research Foundation*, vol 10.

Schweinhart, L.J. and Weikart, D.P. (1997a) 'Lasting differences: the High/Scope pre-school curriculum comparison study through age 23', *Monographs of the High/Scope Educational Research Foundation*, vol 12.

Schweinhart, L.J. and Weikart, D.P. (1997b) 'The High/Scope pre-school curriculum comparison study through age 23', *Early Childhood Research Quarterly*, vol 12, pp 117-43.

Shewry, M.C., Smith, W.C.S., Woodward, M. and Tunstall-Pedoe, H. (1992) 'Variation in coronary risk factors by social status: results from the Scottish Heart Health Study', *British Journal of General Practice*, vol 42, pp 406-10.

Shorrocks, D., Daniels, S., Frobisher, L., Nebon, N. Waterson, A. and Bell, S. (1992) *Enca 1 Project: The evaluation of national curriculum assessment at Key Stage 1*, Leeds: School of Education, University of Leeds.

Smith, C. and Pugh, G. (1996) *Learning to be a parent: A survey of group-based parenting programmes*, London: Family Policies Studies Centre.

Smith, G., Smith, T. and Wright, G. (1997) 'Poverty and schooling: choice, diversity or division', in A. Walker and C. Walker (eds) *Britain divided: The growth of social exclusion in the 1980s and 1990s*, London: Child Poverty Action Group, pp 123-39.

Smith, T. and Noble, M. (1995) *Poverty and schooling in the 1990s*, London: Child Poverty Action Group.

Sylva, K. (1997) 'The early years curriculum: evidence-based proposals', in SCAA, *Developing the primary school curriculum*, London: School Curriculum and Assessment Authority (SCAA).

Sylva, K. and Wilshire, J. (1993) 'The impact of early learning on children's later development: a review prepared for the RSA Inquiry "Start Right"', *European Early Childhood Education Research Journal*, vol 1, no 1, pp 17-40.

Teachman, J.D., Paasch, K. and Carver, K. (1996) 'Social capital and dropping out of school early', *Journal of Marriage and the Family*, vol 58, pp 773-83.

Tones, K. (1996) 'The health promoting school: some reflections on evaluation', *Health Education Research*, vol 11, no 4, pp R1-R8.

UNAIDS (1997) *Impact of HIV and sexual health education on the sexual behaviour of young people: A review update*, Joint United Nations Programme on HIV/AIDS, Geneva.

Vartiainen, E. (1994) 'The North Karelia Youth Project: fifteen year follow-up of an adolescent smoking prevention programme', Paper presented at the IXth World Conference on Tobacco and Health, Paris.

Wadsworth, M.E.J. (1996) 'Family and education as determinants of health', in D. Blane, E. Brunner and R. Wilkinson (eds) *Health and social organisation: Towards a health policy for the 21st century*, London: Routledge, pp 152-70.

Wadsworth, M.E.J. (1997a) 'Changing social factors and their long-term implications for health', *British Medical Bulletin*, vol 53, no 1, pp 198-209.

Wadsworth, M.E.J. (1997b) 'Health inequalities in the life course perspective', *Social Science and Medicine*, vol 44, no 6, pp 859-69.

Whitehead, M. and Drever, F. (1997) *Health inequalities: Decennial supplement*, London: HMSO.

Wilkinson, R.G. (1994) 'Health, redistribution and growth', in A. Glyn and D. Miliband (eds) *Paying for inequality: The economic cost of social justice*, London: IPPR/Rivers Oram, pp 24-43.

Wilkinson, R.G. (1996) *Unhealthy societies: The afflictions of inequality*, London: Routledge.

Willms, J.D. (1999) 'Quality and inequality in children's literacy: the effects of families, schools and communities', in D.P. Keating and C. Hertzman (eds) *Developmental health and the wealth of nations: Social, biological and educational dynamics*, New York, NY: Guilford, pp 72-93.

Winkleby, M.A., Jatulis, D.E., Frank, E. and Fortman, S.P. (1992) 'Socioeconomic status and health: how education, income and occupation contribute to risk factors for cardiovascular disease', *American Journal of Public Health*, vol 82, p 816.

Geographical inequalities in mortality, morbidity and health-related behaviour in England

Sally Macintyre

Evidence of inequalities

Inequalities in mortality by social stratum and geographical location have been observed in Britain since comprehensive record keeping started in the mid-19th century. Table 1, from Edwin Chadwick's monumental report to the Poor Law Commission (Chadwick, 1842), shows differences between different types of towns and cities in the average age of death of three 'social orders': gentry and professionals; farmers and tradesmen; and labourers and artisans. The rank order by place of age at death was not the same for the different groups; the top group did best in Bath, the bottom did best in Rutland, and while the top and bottom groups did worse in Liverpool, the middle group did worst in Manchester. This suggested that both place and socio-economic position may influence health, and that they may interact to produce distinctive patterns.

Table 1: Age at death among different social orders, by district

District	Gentry and professional	Farmers and tradesman	Labourers and artisans
Rutland	52	41	38
Bath	55	37	25
Leeds	44	27	19
Bethnal Green	45	26	16
Manchester	38	20	17
Liverpool	35	22	15

Source: Chadwick (1842)

There is considerable historical continuity in the patterning of death by area in the UK. For the last 150 years death rates have been highest (Britton, 1990):

- in the North and West, compared to the South and East;
- in highly urbanised areas, compared to rural areas;
- in areas with high concentrations of households characterised as materially and socially deprived, compared to areas with high concentrations of affluent households.

Further general observations are that:

- area differences seem to have been increasing over the last few decades, particularly between 1981 and 1991;
- male mortality seems to be slightly more sensitive to geographical variation than female mortality;
- there are spatial differences in the association between socio-economic status and health at both the individual and small area levels.

For example, in his study of mortality from the 1950s to the 1990s (using county boroughs, and urban and rural remainders of counties existing in 1951), Dorling (1997) found relatively low death rates in 1990-92 in both the South East of England (eg Essex, Kent, and Surrey) and in the South West (eg Gloucestershire, Wiltshire and Somerset), and relatively high death rates in the North West and North East of England (eg Liverpool, Manchester, Durham, Newcastle) and in Scotland, especially the West (Glasgow, Lanark). In the early 1990s a resident of Glasgow was 31% more likely to die than someone of the same age and sex living in Bristol, and 66% more likely to die than a resident of rural Dorset. Some inner-city London areas bucked the

North West/South East trend; Lambeth, for example, had relatively high death rates for young adults, and Islington had relatively high rates for female infant mortality, despite the generally low rates in the London area. Differences between areas widened over the period studied: the three areas with the highest death rates in the 1990s (Oldham, Salford, and Greenock) had mortality rates nearly a third higher than the national average in the 1990s compared with only a fifth higher in the 1950s (Dorling, 1997).

A similar picture was provided by a study of life expectancy in district health authority (DHA) areas in England between 1984 and 1994. Men and women in DHAs with the longest life expectancy live on average 6.7 and 4.7 years longer than same sex counterparts in Manchester, which had the lowest life expectancy in both 1984-86 and 1994-96. Liverpool, Sunderland, South of Tyne and St Helen and Knowsley also had low life expectancy. There was a clear North/South gradient in life expectancy, but with low life expectancy for men in the inner London DHAs of South East London, East London and the City, and Camden and Islington. Improvements over the decade were lowest in places with low life expectancy in the early 1980s (for example, by only 0.10% for males and 0.22% for females in Manchester, compared with Eastern Surrey which showed increases of 0.45% for men and 0.22% for women), so that over the decade studied, differences in life expectancy between the highest and lowest ranking DHAs had widened by 29% (1.5 years) among males and by 9% (0.5 years) for females. There was a correlation (of -0.77 for males and -0.56 for females) between level of deprivation in DHAs (measured by Jarman scores) and life expectancy, and the difference in life expectancy between deprived and affluent areas increased over the decade (Raleigh and Kiri, 1997).

In general the geographical patterning of morbidity and other health indicators such as birthweight is similar to that of mortality (Shouls et al, 1996a, 1996b; Sloggett and Joshi, 1998).

An important question is whether these observed geographical inequalities are simply a reflection of the composition of the population in different areas (poor people die earlier, so areas with lots of poor people will have high death rates; and poor people

will have the same death rates wherever they live), or additionally reflect something to do with the physical and social context (most poor people may have no choice but to live in areas which have health damaging characteristics; and the death rates of poor or affluent individuals will vary depending on what sort of area they live in). A mainly compositional explanation for geographical differences might tend to direct research and policy more towards individuals, while an explanation which added a contextual explanation might also direct attention towards health damaging and health promoting features of areas.

The relative importance of compositional and contextual explanations has been studied fairly extensively in the UK recently, aided in some cases by developments in multilevel modelling. Some studies suggest few effects of aggregate levels of deprivation in the area of residence, once individual levels of deprivation are taken into account, on mortality and morbidity (Sloggett and Joshi, 1994), health-related behaviours (Duncan et al, 1993), psychiatric morbidity (Duncan et al, 1995), and adverse fertility events (stillbirth, underweight birth, birth to a teenage mother and sole registered birth) (Sloggett and Joshi, 1998). However, these studies do observe a North–South difference within England, even after controlling for population characteristics (Sloggett and Joshi, 1994).

Others have observed contextual effects over and above, or in interaction with, individual socio-economic status, on mortality (Britton, 1990; Congdon, 1995; Congdon et al, 1997), long-standing illness (Congdon, 1995; Gould and Jones, 1996; Shouls et al, 1996a), health-related behaviour (Forsyth et al, 1994; Duncan et al, 1996), and cardiovascular risk factors (Jones and Duncan, 1995; Ellaway et al, 1997; Hart et al, 1997; Davey Smith et al, 1998). Although cautioning that the finding of contextual effects may be due to unmeasured individual effects, these authors have tended to conclude that where you live matters for health, although probably not as much as who you are.

Recent observations from multilevel studies additionally show: a North-West/South-East gradient in morbidity (controlling for socio-economic position) (Sloggett and Joshi, 1994; Congdon et al, 1997); particularly steep health gradients between more deprived and affluent individuals or small areas, in more affluent places; generally higher rates of illness among all residents in more deprived areas; and a non-linear relationship between rurality and health (health being poorest in very urban areas, but higher in remote rural areas than in semi-rural areas) (Shouls et al, 1996a; Congdon et al, 1997). Thus, the relationship between socio-economic status and health at both an individual and small-area level seems to vary by latitude, by type of ward, district or region, and by rurality.

Policy implications

Examining geographical differences in health tends to direct attention to features of the social and physical environment which might be health promoting or health damaging, and thus to offer a complementary perspective to that which focuses on the characteristics of individuals. It also reminds us of the importance of the historical dimension, and of local, and macro-economic forces. The distinction made between people and places implicit in much multilevel modelling studies could create a false dichotomy. The social class composition of an area is not independent of characteristics of the area: for example, the proportion of the population living in families headed by men in skilled manual occupations has declined in Sheffield and Glasgow since the demise of the steel and shipbuilding industries respectively, even if it is the same families who live in these places. Further, a key feature of personal wealth or poverty is the opportunities that these provide or preclude for living in salubrious places.

Aspects of the local environment which are probably important for the generation of social inequalities in health include:

- employment opportunities
- educational provision
- transport
- housing
- retail provision
- recreation facilities
- the prevalence of 'incivilities' such as graffiti, litter, vandalism, drug dealing, crime (Smith, 1989; Herbert, 1993)

- policing
- land use
- health services
- environmental hazards (air pollution, noise, hazardous waste, industrial effluents)
- social networks and social cohesion
- cultural norms and values
- geology
- climate.

I say 'probably' since, despite the intuitive plausibility of a model in which features of the local area help to explain inequalities in health, there has been very little systematic research examining which aspects of the area of residence influence which facets of health, in which population groups, over what time period, and how they combine to generate social inequalities in health. There is even less research systematically evaluating the effects on health or health inequalities of interventions at the area level. This is because:

- many features of the local physical or social environment which might influence health and inequalities in health are governed by agencies and policies with goals other than health (eg policing, retail distribution, road building, education, economic regeneration);
- even in the case of something as obviously potentially relevant to health as housing policies and standards, there is (surprisingly) little research which shows unequivocally causal associations with health;
- there is even less research examining the effects of interventions on health or inequalities in health, either in the short or long term (Bunton et al, 1994; Arblaster et al, 1996);
- many community-based initiatives (such as the Healthy Cities Programme) have multiple and diffuse goals, the achievement of which is therefore difficult to measure; such initiatives also tend to engage in process rather than outcome evaluations (Bruce et al, 1995);
- methods for health impact assessment, or for health inequalities impact assessment, for non-healthcare interventions are not well developed (Harding and Greer, 1993; Ratner et al, 1997), and those in the health field are usually applied to disasters rather than policies (see, for example, Narayan, 1990; Evans, 1993).

However, what is clear from descriptive studies of local areas is that an 'inverse care law' tends to apply, across the whole range of potential environmental influences on health, to localities in which poorer people are concentrated. Environmental deprivation then tends to amplify individual deprivation. For example, in neighbourhoods we have studied in Glasgow, 'healthy' foods are less available, and more costly, in areas inhabited by poorer people; despite fewer people in such areas having gardens or cars, there are fewer safe play areas, and public transport is worse; and having an address in such areas may increase the cost of insurance and reduce the chances of being given credit (Macintyre et al, 1993; Sooman et al, 1993; Sooman and Macintyre, 1995; Ellaway and Macintyre, 1998). (Sometimes these deprivation amplification effects are explicit in supply policies; for instance, in deciding where to site supermarkets, the big chains use data on local levels of car ownership, and try to site outlets in areas of high car ownership.)

Since health services (and issues such as resource allocation to health services) are being covered in another input paper, I will not cover them here. Neither am I competent to cover larger macro-economic issues relating to inward industrial investment, urban or regional regeneration policies, or housing finance.

Policy recommendations

1   **In considering how best to reduce inequalities in health, policies should not focus exclusively on either places or people, but should be directed towards both.**

An exclusive targeting of deprived areas would fail to help materially and socially deprived persons or households living in less deprived areas (where the gap between rich and poor may be particularly marked); an exclusively individually targeted set of policies (for example, income redistribution or health education) would fail to address geographical and social variations in opportunity structures (employment, education, land use etc).

2   **Central and local government, and the private and voluntary sectors, should be encouraged to undertake health impact**

assessments, and health inequalities impact assessments, of all policies which might have an impact on the health, and ability to lead healthy lives, of the local population.

This requires a broad view to be taken of determinants of population health: for example, a reduction in beat policemen patrolling public parks in urban areas could lead to an increase of 'incivilities' and fear of crime, and deter young working-class mothers from taking their babies or toddlers to the park; this in turn might deprive both mothers and children of social contact and shared recreation with other families, and access to fresh air and exercise. Policies on the siting (and rating) of supermarkets can influence the price and availability of food meeting current dietary guidelines, and policies on public transport can influence access to a range of health promoting goods and service (food, recreation, healthcare, education, employment).

This also requires assessment of the validity and reliability of how the impact on health or health inequalities of a range of policies is measured: health impact methodologies are less developed than environmental impact assessments (we can probably assess the potential impact of a road-building scheme on the local flora and fauna more accurately than we can assess its impact on human health). Further refinement and development are needed to assess the impact, and the balance of costs and benefits, of interventions and policies on health inequalities. Community health gain might be accompanied by an increase in inequalities (if, for example, more socially and materially advantaged residents are better able to benefit from improvements in local services), and impact assessments need to be able to measure both gain and inequalities.

The cost/utility of using health, and health inequalities impact assessments should itself be monitored and evaluated: the use of these impact assessments is intuitively attractive but as with other intuitively attractive policies, it might be ineffective, harmful, costly, or end up as an excuse for inaction.

Many other more specific policy recommendations have already been covered in other input papers, and/or are not (and cannot be) supported by rigorous evidence. The ones listed (rather than being fully justified by supporting evidence) below consist of 'best guesses' from current social and epidemiological research, and all focus on the environment (ie improving the 'supply' side rather than the 'demand' side for health promoting goods and services).

3   Consideration should be given to the following:

- Supplementation of bread with folic acid (*aim: to reduce rates of neural tube defects, stillbirth, prematurity, etc, in women from lower social classes*).
- Fluoridation of the water supply (*aim: to reduce class gradients in dental health*).
- Rates rebates and other incentives for food suppliers in socially deprived and remote rural areas (*aim: to improve diet, in particular fruit and vegetable consumption, in such places*).
- The reintroduction of nutritional guidelines for school meals (*aim: reduce social class gradients in diet, in particular in fruit and vegetable consumption, and vitamin and iron intake*).
- Reintroduction of free school milk and the introduction of free school fruit (*aim: to reduce social class gradients in diet, in particular in calcium intake and fruit and vegetable consumption*).
- Improved separation of motor vehicle, bicycle and pedestrian use (*aim: to flatten the class gradient in deaths and injuries from road traffic accidents, and in physical exercise*).
- Improved public transport, and subsidies to, or imaginative use of, other transport (car- or taxi-sharing pools, mail delivery services), in remote rural areas or areas with low car ownership (*aim: to reduce class and geographical inequalities in diet, exercise and social contacts by improving access to healthy food, recreation facilities and community activities*).
- Zero-tolerance crime prevention and community policing in poorer areas (*aim: to improve mental health and physical health by facilitating safe use of local external spaces and thereby enhancing social contacts, outdoor recreation, and physical exercise among all age groups, including children, and reducing social isolation, drug abuse, injuries and obesity*).
- Tax credits for environmental improvement of landfill and gap sites (*aim: to create more opportunities for healthy sociability, recreation and physical exercise in poorer areas*).
- Greater use of local schools for after-school and holiday period childcare, and for community activities for children and adults (*aim: to reduce the deterrent effect of lack of childcare on employment among parents, and to enhance social contacts and opportunities for physical exercise and skills learning among all age groups, and thereby reduce social class gradients in social isolation, drug abuse, injuries [from unsupervised play in dangerous environments], and obesity, and improve self-esteem, employability and social cohesion*).
- Improving insulation, heating systems, smoke-detector/fire-alarm systems and security systems in public- and private-sector housing (*aim: to reduce social class gradients in respiratory disease, deaths and injuries from fires and exposure to crime and vandalism*).
- Increase tenure diversification (*aim: to reduce social exclusion and the concentration of incivilities, crime and low morale in highly spatially segregated council housing areas*).

All such initiatives or demonstration projects should be subject to systematic evaluation of their costs and benefits, since it is possible that they may be ineffective or harmful as well as beneficial (for example, traffic-calming schemes may simply displace traffic, and accidents, to other areas; locating supermarkets in poor areas may attract car-owning people from more affluent areas, who then raise the road traffic accident rate among children in the poor area; it might lead to the closure of small local shops serving the needs of non-car owners; and it could also operate to reduce inequalities more by creating local employment than by promoting fruit and vegetable consumption). Such initiatives also need to be sensitive to local conditions and local variations (for example in Wester Hailes, a council housing estate near Edinburgh, it was local working-class residents who were doing the 'rat run' through the area, while in Drumchapel, a similar estate in Glasgow, it was residents of a nearby middle-class suburb who were doing this).

This input paper has been unable to provide a list of policy recommendations supported by reliable evidence. Its aim has therefore been to focus attention on the role of the local and regional environment in the creation and maintenance of socio-economic and geographical inequalities in health, and to argue for the application of health impact assessments.

Acknowledgements

I am grateful to Sarah Curtis, Danny Dorling, Anne Ellaway, Heather Joshi and Graham Moon for their inputs to this paper. The views expressed here are my own.

References

Arblaster, L., Lambert, M., Entwistle, V., Forster, M., Fullerton, D., Sheldon, T. et al (1996) 'A systematic review of the effectiveness of health service interventions aimed at reducing inequalities in health', *Journal of Health Services Research and Policy*, vol 1, no 2, pp 93-103.

Britton, M. (ed) (1990) *Mortality and geography*, Series DS 9, London: OPCS/HMSO.

Bruce, N., Springett, J., Hotchkiss, J. and Scott-Samuel, A. (eds) (1995) *Research and change in urban community health*, Aldershot: Avebury.

Bunton, R., Burrows, R., Gillen, K. and Muncer, S. (1994) *Interventions to promote health in economically deprived areas: A critical review of the literature*, Report to the Northern Regional Health Authority, Newcastle: Northern Regional Health Authority.

Chadwick, E. (1842) *Report of an enquiry into the sanitary conditions of the labouring population of Great Britain*, London: Poor Law Commission.

Congdon, P. (1995) 'The impact of area context on long-term illness and premature mortality: an illustration of multilevel analysis', *Regional Studies*, vol 29, no 4, pp 327-44.

Congdon, P., Shouls, S. and Curtis, S. (1997) 'A multi-level perspective on small-area health and mortality: a case study of England and Wales', *International Journal of Population Geography*, vol 3, pp 243-63.

Davey Smith, G., Hart, G., Watt, G., Hole, D. and Hawthorne, V. (1998) 'Individual social class, area-based deprivation, cardiac disease risk factors and mortality: the Renfrew and Paisley study', *Journal of Epidemiology and Community Health*, vol 52, no 6, pp 399-405.

Dorling, D. (1997) *Death in Britain. How local mortality rates have changed: 1950s-1990s*, York: Joseph Rowntree Foundation.

Duncan, C., Jones, K. and Moon, G. (1993) 'Do places matter: a multilevel analysis of regional variations in health related behaviour in Britain', *Social Science and Medicine*, vol 37, no 6, pp 725-33.

Duncan, C., Jones, K. and Moon, G. (1995) 'Psychiatric morbidity: a multi level approach to regional variations in the UK', *Journal of Epidemiology and Community Health*, vol 49, no 3, pp 290-5.

Duncan, C., Jones, K. and Moon, G. (1996) 'Health related behaviour in context – a multi level modeling approach', *Social Science and Medicine*, vol 42, no 6, pp 817-30.

Ellaway, A. and Macintyre, S. (1998) 'Does housing tenure predict health in the UK because it exposes people to different levels of housing related hazards in the home or its surroundings?', *Health and Place*, vol 4, no 2, pp 141-50.

Ellaway, A., Anderson, A. and Macintyre, S. (1997) 'Does area of residence affect body size and shape?', *International Journal of Obesity*, vol 21, no 4, pp 304-8.

Evans, C. (1993) 'Public health impact of the 1992 Los Angeles civil unrest', *Public Health Reports*, vol 108, no 3, pp 265-72.

Forsyth, A., Macintyre, S. and Anderson, A. (1994) 'Diets for disease? Intraurban variation in reported food consumption in Glasgow', *Appetite*, vol 22, pp 259-74.

Gould, M.I. and Jones, K. (1996) 'Analyzing perceived limiting long-term illness using UK Census microdata', *Social Science and Medicine*, vol 42, no 6, pp 857-69.

Harding, A. and Greer, M. (1993) 'The health impact of hazardous waste sites on minority communities: implications for public and environmental health professionals', *Journal of Environmental Health*, vol 55, no 7, pp 6-10.

Hart, C., Ecob, R. and Davey Smith, G. (1997) 'People, places and coronary heart disease risk factor: a multilevel analysis of the Scottish Heart Health Study archive', *Social Science and Medicine*, vol 45, no 6, pp 893-902.

Herbert, D. (1993) 'Neighbourhood incivilities and the study of crime in place', *Area*, vol 25, pp 45-54.

Jones, K. and Duncan, C. (1995) 'Individuals and their ecologies: analysing the geography of chronic illness within a multilevel modelling framework', *Health and Place*, vol 1, no 1, pp 27-40.

Macintyre, S., Maciver, S. and Sooman, A. (1993) 'Area, class and health: should we be focusing on places or people?', *Journal of Social Policy*, vol 22, pp 213-34.

Narayan, T. (1990) 'Health impact of Bhopal disaster: an epidemiologic perspective', *Economic and Political Weekly*, vol 25, no 34, pp 1905-14.

Raleigh, S. and Kiri, V. (1997) 'Life expectancy in England: variaton and trends by gender, health authority, and level of deprivation', *Journal of Epidemiology and Community Health*, vol 51, no 6, pp 649-58.

Ratner, P., Green, L., Frankish, C., Chomik, T. and Larsen, C. (1997) 'Setting the stage for health impact assessment', *Journal of Public Health Policy*, vol 18, no 1, pp 67-79.

Shouls, S., Congdon, P. and Curtis, S. (1996a) 'Geographic variation in illness and mortality: the development of a relevant area typology for SAR districts', *Health and Place*, vol 2, no 3, pp 139-55.

Shouls, S., Congdon, P. and Curtis, S. (1996b) 'Modelling inequality in reported long term illness in the UK: combining individual and area characteristics', *Journal of Epidemiology and Community Health*, vol 50, no 3, pp 366-76.

Sloggett, A. and Joshi, H. (1994) 'Higher mortality in deprived areas: community or personal disadvantage?', *British Medical Journal*, vol 309, pp 1470-4.

Sloggett, A. and Joshi, H. (1998) 'Deprivation indicators as predictors of life events 1981-1992', *Journal of Epidemiology and Community Health*, vol 52, no 4, pp 228-33.

Smith, S. (1989) 'Social relations, neighbourhood structure, and the fear of crime in Britain', in D. Evans and D. Herbert (eds) *The geography of crime*, London: Routledge, pp 193-227.

Ethnic inequalities in health

James Nazroo

Introduction

This paper will provide summary descriptions of the demographics and social position of ethnic minority groups in the UK; the relationship between ethnicity and health; explanations for ethnic inequalities in health; and possible interventions to reduce ethnic inequalities in health. The following important limitations to the evidence presented here should be borne in mind.

- The data that are available on these issues are crude. As will be described later, the categorisation of ethnicity in almost all data sources fails to account for the contextual nature of ethnic identity, many data sources combine obviously different groups, and white minority groups are almost never included. Nevertheless, using crude groupings does allow us to establish whether ethnic inequalities exist, even if we cannot describe their full range, and does allow us to begin to explore reasons for differences.
- The data on ethnic inequalities in health used here will be restricted to the UK and, to support the conclusions drawn, will mainly take examples from national surveys (Rudat, 1994; Nazroo, 1997a) and analyses of mortality rates by country of birth (Marmot et al, 1984; Balarajan and Bulusu, 1990; Harding and Maxwell, 1997). Regional studies and work from the US contain important lessons, but space restricts their inclusion here.
- I will not attempt a comprehensive coverage of all possible ethnic groups or all diseases, for example, I will not include sexually-transmitted diseases (see DeCock and Low, 1997) nor mental health (see Nazroo, 1997b). Rather, I will use certain examples to develop principles that will aid understanding and policy development.
- A focus on ethnic inequalities carries two dangers. First, it suggests that the health problems faced by ethnic minority groups are somehow different, have different causes, and require different solutions. This is manifestly not the case, as others have commented the similarities between minority and majority groups are greater than the differences (Bhopal, 1997; Bhopal and Donaldson, 1998), although solutions do have to be sensitive to the particular needs of ethnic minority groups. Second, a focus on inequalities can miss important health promotion opportunities (Bhopal and Donaldson, 1998). For example, all South Asian women have very low rates of smoking (Rudat, 1994; Nazroo, 1997a) and respiratory disease (unpublished data from the Fourth National Survey of Ethnic Minorities), but ignoring health promotion in this area could lead to an increase in rates of smoking and a consequent deterioration in health for this group.

Ethnic minority groups in Britain

This section will provide a brief description of the ethnic minority population of Britain, predominantly covering demographics. Most of what we know about the ethnic minority population comes from the 1991 Census (Coleman and Salt, 1996; Peach, 1996; Ratcliffe, 1996; Karn, 1997) and the Fourth National Survey of Ethnic Minorities (FNS) (Modood et al, 1997). The FNS was a large, representative survey covering whites and the main ethnic minority groups living in Britain. It was conducted by the Policy Studies Institute and Social and Community Planning Research in 1993/94.

Ethnic composition of the population of Britain

The 1991 Census included questions on country of birth and, for the first time, ethnic group. Respondents were asked to indicate which ethnic group they belonged to from a fixed range of choices that encompassed both skin colour and country of origin. Responses to this question are shown in Table 1, along with the percentage in each group who were born in the UK. The table shows that 5.5% of the population (just over 3 million people) identified themselves as belonging to one of the ethnic minority groups. Almost half of these people were born in the UK.

Table 1: Ethnic composition of UK population

Ethnic group	Number (000s)	%	% born in UK
White	51,844	94.5	95.8
All ethnic minorities	3,007	5.5	46.8
All black	885	1.6	55.7
Black-Caribbean	499	0.9	53.7
Black-African	208	0.4	36.4
Black-other*	179	0.3	84.4
All South Asian	1,477	2.7	44.1
Indian	841	1.5	42.0
Pakistani	476	0.9	50.5
Bangladeshi	160	0.3	36.7
Chinese and others	644	1.2	40.6
Chinese	158	0.3	28.4
Other-Asian	197	0.4	21.9
Other-other†	290	0.5	59.8

Note: * The 'Black-other' group contains people recorded as 'Black' with no further details, those identifying themselves as 'Black British', and people with ethnic origins classified as mixed black/white and black/other ethnic group. It seems that most of the 'Black-other' group had Caribbean family origins, but were born in Britain; † The 'Other-other' group contains North Africans, Arabs, Iranians, together with people of mixed Asian/white, mixed black/white and 'other' mixed categories.

Source: Owen (1992), reproduced with permission from the University of Warwick

Geographical locations of ethnic minority people

Analysis of the 1991 Census has shown that the ethnic minority population is largely concentrated in England, mainly in the most populous areas. Key findings from this analysis are (Owen, 1992, 1994):

- more than half of the ethnic minority population lives in South East England, where less than one third of the white population lives;
- Greater London contains 44.8% of the ethnic minority population and only 10.3% of the white population;
- elsewhere the West Midlands, West Yorkshire and Greater Manchester display the highest relative concentrations of people from ethnic minorities;
- almost 70% of ethnic minority people live in Greater London, the West Midlands, West Yorkshire and Greater Manchester, compared with just over 25% of white people;
- there are even greater differences when smaller areas are considered: more than half of ethnic minority people live in areas where the total ethnic minority population exceeds 44%, compared with the 5.5% national average.

There are also important differences between the geographical locations of ethnic minority groups. For example, among South Asians: Indians are more concentrated in London and the West Midlands; Pakistanis are more concentrated in West Yorkshire, Greater Manchester and the West Midlands; Bangladeshis are strongly concentrated in London, Birmingham and Greater Manchester.

Table 2 uses an Office for Population Censuses and Surveys (OPCS) classification to characterise local authorities and shows the percentage of different ethnic groups living in each type. It clearly shows the higher concentration of white people in rural and suburban areas and the higher concentration of ethnic minority people in industrial areas and London.

Age and gender

Differences in gender profiles for different ethnic groups probably reflect differences in the recency and patterns of migration, with men typically migrating first and women and children joining them later. So, analysis of the 1991 Census showed that among the South Asian and Black-African groups, males outnumbered females. For the other groups, including whites, there were more women than men (Owen, 1993).

Table 2: Types of areas ethnic minorities and whites live in (%)

OPCS classification	Whites	Ethnic minorities	Blacks	South Asians
Established high status	14.0	17.1	14.1	16.6
Higher status growth	9.4	3.1	2.8	2.3
More rural areas	13.1	1.6	1.4	0.6
Resort and retirement	5.4	1.1	0.8	0.6
Mixed town and country, some industry	23.3	8.3	5.7	9.3
Traditional manufacturing	8.4	27.8	20.0	39.2
Service centres and cities	13.7	11.3	12.1	9.5
Areas with much local authority housing	8.4	4.2	2.5	5.2
Parts of inner London	3.2	21.8	35.8	14.9
Central London	1.0	3.8	5.2	1.8

Source. Owen (1992), reproduced with permission from the University of Warwick

The 1991 Census also showed the relative youth of ethnic minority groups. Children formed one third of the ethnic minority population, compared with under one fifth of the white population. In contrast, while 16% of the population as a whole was aged over 65, only just over 3% of the ethnic minority population fell within this age group (Owen, 1993). Differences in age profiles are summarised in Figure 1, which also suggests differences in the age structures of particular ethnic minority groups (for example the South Asian group has a high proportion of people in the 5 to 15 age range). In summary, Black-Caribbeans, Chinese, Indians and Other Asians tended to be older, while Bangladeshis, Pakistanis and, not surprisingly, Black-others, were younger.

Figure 1: Age distribution for ethnic groups

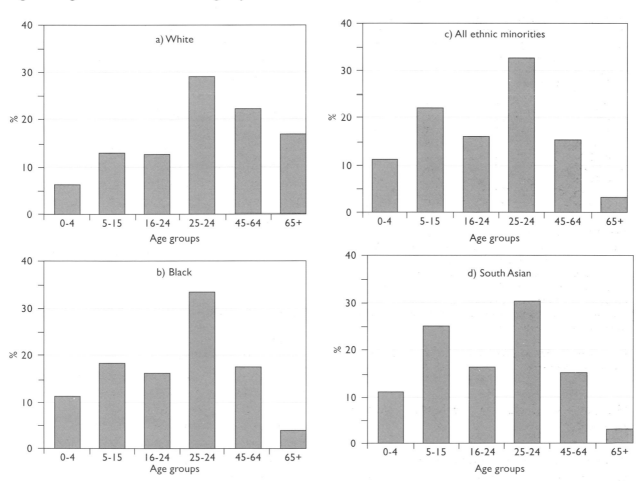

Source: Owen (1993), reproduced with permission from the University of Warwick

Household size and structure

Analysis of the 1991 Census (Coleman and Salt, 1996) and the FNS (Modood et al, 1997) showed that white, Caribbean, Indian and Chinese families had similar numbers of children, while Pakistani and Bangladeshi families had many more children. An analysis of the FNS (Modood et al, 1997) that took into account life-stage suggested that most white families would have one or two children and more than 90% of them would have no more than three children. In contrast, most Pakistani and Bangladeshi families would have four or more children and 85% of them would have three or more children. South Asian households were also larger because of the number of adults they contained (Modood et al, 1997). Half of Pakistani and Bangladeshi households had three or more adults in them, compared with two fifths of Indian and Chinese households, and less than one fifth of white and Caribbean households. Caribbean households were more likely than others to contain one adult with children (ie, were 'lone parent' households), about one in six Caribbean households had this structure, compared with less than one in twenty of other households (Modood et al, 1997).

Economic activity, occupational class and socio-economic status

The FNS provided detailed information on the socio-economic profiles of different ethnic minority groups. The following is a summary of key points.

In terms of economic activity, the most striking findings concerned women. A total of 80% of Bangladeshi and 70% of Pakistani women described themselves as looking after the home or family, compared with about 30% of white and Indian women, and only 13% of Caribbean women (Modood et al, 1997).

In contrast, most men in all of the ethnic groups were in the labour market, differences here were largely due to different rates of unemployment. These are summarised in Table 3, which shows the very high rates of unemployment among Pakistanis and Bangladeshis (almost four times the rate for white men) and the high rate among Caribbeans (more than twice the rate for white men) (Nazroo, 1997a). More detailed analyses showed that these

higher rates of unemployment for Caribbeans, Pakistanis and Bangladeshis persisted regardless of geographical location or qualifications, although the size of the differences varied (Madood et al, 1997).

Table 3: Socio-economic status and ethnicity (%)

	White	Carib-bean	Indian or African Asian	Paki-stani	Bangla-deshi	Chi-nese
% of economically -active unemployed	11	24	15	38	42	7
Registrar General's class						
I/II	35	22	32	20	11	40
IIINM	15	18	21	15	18	26
IIIM	31	30	22	32	32	20
IV/V	20	30	26	33	40	13

Source: Nazroo (1997a)

Table 3 also shows social class differences across ethnic groups, based on the Registrar General's classification of the occupation of the head of household. As for the rates of unemployment, Indians and Chinese compared favourably with whites. Caribbeans and Pakistanis were worse off than these groups and Bangladeshis had a particularly poor profile with 11% in social classes I and II and 40% in social classes IV and V (Nazroo, 1997a).

The FNS included several other indicators of socio-economic status. In terms of housing tenure, about four fifths of Indian and Pakistani households were owner-occupied, compared with about two thirds of white households and half of Caribbean, Bangladeshi and Chinese households. However, Chinese households were far more likely than Caribbean and Bangladeshi households to be privately rented (Modood et al, 1997). Assessments of overcrowding used in the FNS indicated that only one in 50 white households were overcrowded, compared with roughly one in 10 Caribbean and Indian households and more than one third of Pakistani and Bangladeshi households (Modood et al, 1997). About one third of Pakistani and Bangladeshi respondents lived in households that lacked a basic amenity (ie, central heating, hot water from a tap, or exclusive use of bath or shower, bathroom, inside toilet, or kitchen), compared with about one in six of the other respondents (Nazroo, 1997a).

Finally, in terms of income, Table 4 shows the distribution of households according to average incomes. It shows the great extent of poverty among Pakistanis and Bangladeshis – more than four fifths of them lived in households with below half the average income. Two fifths of Caribbean and Indian households were also in this position, compared with one third of Chinese and less than one third of white households (Modood et al, 1997).

Table 4: Household incomes and ethnicity (%)

	White	Carib-bean	Indian	Paki-stani	Bangla-deshi	Chi-nese
More than 1½ times average	23	12	14	1	2	22
½ to 1½ times average	49	47	45	17	14	44
Below ½ of the average	28	41	42	82	84	34

Source: Modood et al (1997)

Racism and racial harassment and violence

No description of the lives of ethnic minority people in Britain would be complete without coverage of racism. Responses to the FNS suggested that more than one in eight ethnic minority people had experienced some form of racial harassment in the past year (Modood et al, 1997). Although most of these incidents involved racial insults, many of the respondents reported repeated victimisation and one quarter of the ethnic minority respondents reported being fearful of racial harassment. White respondents were asked about their own racial prejudice and 26% admitted to being prejudiced against Asians, 20% to being prejudiced against Caribbeans and 8% to being prejudiced against Chinese people. Work carried out for the Commission for Racial Equality has also show that white minority groups, such as the Irish, also face extensive racial harassment (Hickman and Walters, 1997).

Limitations of data on ethnic minority groups

As suggested in the introduction, there are a number of important limitations regarding the data we have available to analyse and understand ethnic inequalities in health. These are summarised here.

Most researchers consider ethnicity to reflect self-identification with cultural traditions that both provide a meaningful social identity and boundaries between groups (Barot, 1996). Ethnicity can act as a marker for a boundary of exclusion, imposed on a minority group, and as a marker for inclusion, providing a sense of identity and access to social resources. And it may be of significance to health for both reasons. In terms of assessing ethnic background, ethnic identity cannot be considered as fixed, because culture is not an autonomous and static feature in an individual's life. Cultural traditions are historically located, they occur within particular contexts and change over time, place and person. The implication is that there are a range of identities that come into play in different contexts and that ethnic identity should be regarded as neither secure not coherent (Hall, 1992). This means that the markers of ethnicity used in the Census and the FNS reflect only one static dimension of ethnicity. The ways in which individuals' and groups' identities change over context, or vary within the broad classifications used, cannot be assessed in such data.

Most epidemiological research on health and ethnicity has taken an even cruder approach than the Census and the FNS to the allocation of individuals into ethnic groups. As might be expected, because country of birth is recorded on death certificates and in the Census, much of the published data in this area has allocated ethnicity according to country of birth (Marmot et al, 1984; Balarajan and Bulusu, 1990; Harding and Maxwell, 1997). This is obviously inadequate for the large number of ethnic minority people born in Britain, as shown in Table 1. It also remains unclear what country of birth really is a marker for – are we measuring genetics, childhood environment, culture, the consequences of racialisation, socio-economic position, etc?

Many studies also use 'ethnic' groupings with quite inappropriate boundaries, such as Black or South Asian. The data are then interpreted as though the individuals within them are ethnically (ie, biologically and culturally) homogeneous, even though such categories are heterogeneous, containing ethnic groups with different cultures, religions, migration histories, and geographical and socio-economic locations (as described in the preceding section). In addition, almost all of the research that is undertaken ignores white minority groups.

The assessment of socio-economic status for comparisons across ethnic groups has two important problems. First, occupational status is frequently inflated on death certificates (where occupation is recorded as the 'skilled' job held for most of the individual's life, rather than the 'unskilled' job held in the last few years of life, or, in the case of the Census, the occupation engaged in during the previous week) (Townsend and Davidson, 1982). This will be particularly significant for immigrant mortality data if migration to Britain was associated with downward social mobility for members of ethnic minority groups, a process that has been clearly documented (Smith, 1977; Heath and Ridge, 1983). So, the occupation recorded on the death certificates of migrants may well be an inaccurate reflection of their experience in Britain prior to death. In addition, given the socio-economic profile of ethnic minority groups in Britain, this inflation of occupational status would only need to happen in relatively few cases for the figures representing the small population in higher classes to be distorted upwards.

There has been an increasing recognition of the limitations of traditional class groupings, which are far from internally homogeneous. A number of studies have drawn attention to variations in income levels and death rates among occupations that comprise particular occupational classes (Davey Smith et al, 1990). And within an occupational group, ethnic minorities may be more likely to be found in lower or less prestigious occupational grades, to have poorer job security, to endure more stressful working conditions and to be more likely to work unsocial hours. Evidence from the FNS illustrates this point clearly. Table 5 shows that ethnic minority people had a lower income than white people in the same class, that unemployed ethnic minority people had been unemployed for longer than equivalent white people and that some ethnic minority groups had poorer quality housing than whites regardless of tenure (Nazroo, 1997a). These differences were particularly marked for the Pakistani and Bangladeshi group, who, as shown in the introduction, are particularly poorly off.

Table 5: Variations within socio-economic bands by ethnic group

	Whites	Carib-beans	Indians	Paki-stanis and Bangla-deshis
Mean weekly income by Registrar General's class (£s)*				
I/II	250	210	210	125
IIIN	185	145	135	95
IIIM	160	145	120	70
IV/V	130	120	110	65
Median duration of unemployment (months)	7	21	12	24
% lacking one or more basic housing amenities†				
Owner-occupiers	11	12	14	38
Renters	27	23	28	37

Notes: * Based on bands of equivalised household income; † ie, exclusive use of bath or shower; bathroom; inside toilet; kitchen; hot water from a tap; and central heating.
Source: Nazroo (1997a)

So, standard indicators of socio-economic status are problematic when making comparisons within ethnic groups, and are of little use for 'controlling out' the impact of socio-economic differences when attempting to compare across ethnic groups. It is vital that this is borne in mind when considering the data shown later or published elsewhere.

Ethnic variations in health – a description

This section will provide a brief description of ethnic variations in health, primarily relying on data from the FNS (Nazroo, 1997a) and the analyses of migrant mortality data conducted by ONS for the period 1991-93 (Harding and Maxwell, 1997; Maxwell and Harding, 1997). Table 6 shows Standardised Mortality Ratios (SMRs) by country of birth for all causes and four specific causes of death (chosen for illustrative purposes). Table 7 shows relative risk for ethnic minority people compared with whites to report fair or poor health and indicators of four specific conditions (a combination of responses to questions on previously diagnosed conditions and symptoms).

Table 6: SMR by country of birth for those aged 20-64 years, England and Wales (1991-93)

	All causes		CHD		Stroke		Respiratory disease[†]		Lung cancer	
	M	W	M	W	M	W	M	W	M	W
Caribbean	89*	104	60*	100	169*	178*	80*	75	59*	32*
Indian subcontinent	107*	99	150*	175*	163*	132*	90	94	48*	34*
India	106*	–	140*	–	140*	–	93	–	43*	–
Pakistan	102	–	163*	–	148*	–	82	–	45*	–
Bangladesh	137*	–	184*	–	324*	–	104	–	92	–
East Africa	123*	127*	160*	130	113	110	154*	195*	35*	110
West/ South Africa	126*	142*	83	69	315*	215*	138	101	71	69
Ireland	135*	115*	121*	129*	130*	118*	162*	134*	157*	143*

Notes: * p < 0.05; † Some causes of death may have been misclassified for this category.
Source: Harding and Maxwell (1997); Maxwell and Harding (1997); Crown Copyright is reproduced with the permission of the Controller of Her Majesty's Stationery Office

Table 7: Age and gender standardised relative risk, all ages, England and Wales (1993-94)

	Fair or poor health	Diagnosed CHD	CHD or severe chest pain	Hypertension	Diabetes	Respiratory symptoms
Caribbeans	1.29*	0.88	0.96	1.47*	3.12*	0.87
All South Asians	1.19*	1.00	1.24*	0.75*	3.65*	0.59*
Indians	1.03	0.79	0.93	0.66*	2.77*	0.55*
Pakistani/ Bangladeshis	1.48*	1.43*	1.83*	0.91	5.24*	0.67*
Chinese	0.96	0.71	0.56	0.42*	1.77	0.43*

Note: * p < 0.05
Source: Nazroo (1997a)

Some general interpretations can be taken from these tables. First ethnic minority groups are not uniformly at greater risk of mortality or poor health. For example, both data sources suggest that Indians have reasonably good overall health. Second, for some outcomes ethnic minority groups appear to be significantly better off than the ethnic majority (eg respiratory symptoms/disease and lung cancer). Third, particular ethnic groups appear to be particularly disadvantaged by different diseases. For example, Caribbeans have high rates of stroke/ hypertension and South Asians have high rates of coronary heart disease (CHD)/severe chest pain.

Although there are similarities in the data presented in the two tables, there are also some inconsistencies. For example, Caribbeans have a low all-cause SMR, but high relative risk of reporting fair or poor general health (though, interestingly, women born in the Caribbean have been shown to have a higher all-cause mortality than men in all three analyses of immigrant mortality data [Marmot et al, 1984; Balarajan and Bulusu, 1990; Harding and Maxwell, 1997]); Indians compared with other South Asians have a lower SMR from CHD and a lower relative risk of reporting a diagnosis or symptoms of CHD, but compared with whites their SMR is elevated, while their relative risk for a diagnosis or reporting symptoms is lower; South Asians have a high SMR from stroke but a lower relative risk of reporting hypertension.

These inconsistencies could be a consequence of a number of factors, including: the data cover different groups (one is restricted to those born outside the UK, the other covers all ethnic minority people); the morbidity data measure prevalence while the mortality data measure a combination of incidence and survival (in the UK); there may be important cohort effects present; there may be data inaccuracies both in the reporting of symptoms or diagnosis (perhaps because of cultural differences in the experience and reporting of symptoms or differences in opportunities for diagnosis) and in the recording of cause of death.

Socio-economic inequalities and ethnic variations in health

Analyses of immigrant mortality data from the 1970s showed no socio-economic gradient for those born in the Indian subcontinent, a reversed gradient for those born in the Caribbean, and that socio-economic effects made no difference to ethnic variations in health (Marmot et al, 1984). Analysis of the more recent data on migrant mortality rates, however, has suggested a relationship between socio-economic status and health for all migrant groups (Harding and Maxwell, 1997). Considering deaths from all causes, men in manual classes had markedly higher SMRs than those in non-manual classes in each migrant group, except those born in West/ South Africa where the difference, although present, was smaller. This pattern was repeated, with only a few exceptions, for each migrant group for the specific causes of death. A similar pattern of findings was present in the FNS data (Nazroo, 1997a). These showed a clear class gradient for reporting fair or poor health in each ethnic group and, again with only very few exceptions, this pattern was clearly repeated for specific diseases. These data have clearly established the presence of socio-economic gradients in health within ethnic minority groups.

However, like the earlier analysis of immigrant mortality data, the most recent analysis has suggested that socio-economic differentials make no contribution to ethnic variations in health (Harding and Maxwell, 1997). Table 8 shows SMRs for migrant groups both unadjusted and adjusted for class. Cells with a large and statistically significant greater unadjusted SMR for the migrant group are shaded, as it is here that a socio-economic effect should be most apparent. The table shows that the only country of birth group for which adjustment gives a clear reduction in SMRs are those born in Ireland, although there is also a reduction for stroke among those born in the Caribbean. For the others, adjustments, if anything, increase the SMRs. So, statistical adjustments for differences in class distribution explained some (but not all) of the raised SMR for those men born in Ireland and the Caribbean, but none of the raised SMR for men in other migrant groups.

It is possible that this is a consequence of the difficulties in adjusted-for social class across ethnic groups, discussed above and illustrated in Table 5. Table 9 uses FNS data to show changes in the relative risk of reporting ill-health upon adjustment for two measures of socio-economic status (Nazroo, 1997a). One is occupational class, the other is an index of standard of living (which took into account housing problems, number of consumer durables owned, and number of cars owned) that was designed to more sensitively reflect ethnic inequalities in socio-economic status. Once again cells that had a large and statistically significant greater unadjusted relative risk for the ethnic minority group are shaded. The table confirms that adjusting for traditional measures of occupational class makes no real difference to the relative risks, but adjusting for the more sensitive standard of living index gives a large reduction in relative risk for all of the ethnic minority groups and for all of the outcomes, except Caribbeans and diagnosed heart disease. It is worth noting that although reductions are present for diabetes, the differences remain large.

Table 8: SMR by country of birth, men aged 20-64, adjusted and unadjusted for class (1991-93)

		All causes	CHD	Stroke	Respiratory diseases	Lung cancer
Caribbean	Unadjusted	89	60	169	80	59
	Adjusted for class	82	55	146	70	49
Indian	Unadjusted	107	150	163	90	48
subcontinent	Adjusted for class	117	165	175	98	52
East Africa	Unadjusted	123	160	113	154	–
	Adjusted for class	137	188	128	162	–
West/	Unadjusted	126	83	315	–	–
South Africa	Adjusted for class	135	79	372	–	–
Ireland	Unadjusted	135	121	130	162	157
	Adjusted for class	129	115	124	143	145

Source: Harding and Maxwell (1997); Crown Copyright is reproduced with the permission of the Controller of Her Majesty's Stationery Office

Table 9: Age and gender standardised relative risk, all ages, adjusted and unadjusted for socio-economic status

		Fair or poor health	Diagnosed CHD	CHD or severe chest pain	Hypertension	Diabetes	Respiratory symptoms
Caribbeans	Unadjusted	1.25	0.95	0.96	1.49	2.6	0.89
	Adjusted for social class	1.15	1.05	0.85	1.56	2.8	0.86
	Adjusted for standard of living	1.15	1.02	0.89	1.33	2.2	0.83
Indians	Unadjusted	0.99	0.77	0.95	0.64	2.6	0.53
	Adjusted for social class	1.00	0.92	0.93	0.70	3.1	0.53
	Adjusted for standard of living	0.94	0.67	0.78	0.60	2.4	0.50
Pakistanis and Bangladeshis	Unadjusted	1.45	1.50	1.88	0.94	4.9	0.65
	Adjusted for social class	1.36	1.49	1.59	0.88	5.2	0.55
	Adjusted for standard of living	1.24	1.24	1.37	0.86	4.1	0.50

Source: Nazroo (1997a)

It should be recognised that although the standard of living index is an improvement over other indicators of social class, it is still far from perfect (Nazroo, 1997a). Nevertheless, the reductions in relative risk achieved with the use of this index suggest that not only are there important socio-economic inequalities in health within ethnic groups, socio-economic inequalities also make a major contribution to ethnic variations in health.

Inequalities in access to health services

A number of studies have shown that members of ethnic minority groups are just as likely as whites to consult with a GP (Balarajan et al, 1989; Rudat, 1994; Car-Hill et al, 1996, Nazroo, 1997a), even after differences in reported health have been taken into account (Nazroo, 1997a). However, they tell us little about whether there are inequalities in access beyond this. Recent indirect evidence has suggested that referral to secondary care is less frequent for ethnic minority people. Ethnic minority people are also less likely than whites to leave the surgery with a follow-up appointment (Gilliam et al, 1989) or to

receive follow-up services such as a district nurse (Badger et al, 1989). South Asians with CHD wait longer for referral to specialist care than whites (Shaukat et al, 1993), despite being more likely to seek immediate care (Ben-Shlomo et al, 1997). One study showed that they were less than half as likely to receive grafts for triple vessel disease, despite having further progressed disease (Shaukat et al, 1997).

None of these studies have been able to explore reasons for these possible differences in quality of care. But it has been shown that ethnic minority people are more likely than whites to find physical access to their GP difficult; have longer waiting times in the surgery; feel that the time their GP had spent with them was inadequate; and to be unhappy with the outcome of the consultation (Rudat, 1994). Part of this might be related to communication problems. In terms of language, a significant number of South Asian (particularly Bangladeshi women) and Chinese people find it difficult to communicate with their GP (Rudat, 1994; Nazroo, 1997a). There may be cultural differences in the expression of symptoms, making the use of western diagnostic approaches inappropriate for some groups, especially as far as mental illness is concerned (Nazroo, 1997b). And many ethnic minority women prefer to consult with female doctors and, to overcome communication difficulties, female doctors with the same ethnic minority background as themselves (Nazroo, 1997a).

Other explanations for ethnic variations in health

The preceding discussion has shown the importance of socio-economic inequalities and has presented evidence suggesting that inequalities in access to health services might also be important to ethnic inequalities in health. However, it is certain that a number of other factors are also important, and that a satisfactory explanation must be multi-factorial and consider interactive effects. Other potentially important factors will be discussed next.

- It is always important to consider the possibility that differences are the result of a statistical artefact. There are numerous problems with data on ethnic variations in health, touched upon above, which may have altered the magnitude of ethnic differences and the significance of socio-economic effects.

- Differences between ethnic groups, particularly those shown in the immigrant mortality data, could be a consequence of migration effects. Those who were more healthy may have been more likely to migrate, particularly if they had to travel some distance (Marmot et al, 1984). Environmental conditions in the country of birth, or the mother's country of birth, may adversely affect the health of an individual. The stress surrounding the process of migration may also be important. Given these possibilities, it is somewhat surprising that the FNS showed little difference between the health of migrants and those born in Britain, and that, where there were differences, migrants were healthier (Nazroo, 1997a). Work in Scotland has also suggested that the health of migrants from the Punjab deteriorates with time spent in the UK, regardless of age (Williams, 1993).

- Cultural differences might contribute to ethnic variations in health in a number of ways, but most importantly through influencing health-related behaviours. Patterns of smoking and drinking have been shown to vary across ethnic groups (Rudat, 1994; Nazroo, 1997a), and the

differences in patterns of smoking have been shown to make a major contribution to ethnic differences in the reporting of respiratory symptoms (Nazroo, 1997a). There are also important cultural differences in diet and there may be differences in the extent to which physical exercise is conducted (Rudat, 1994), although there is no evidence directly relating either of these to differences in health. It is important to remember that culture is not static, and that health behaviours are also influenced by other factors, such as gender and class.

- Genetic differences between ethnic groups may also be important. Some diseases, such as haemoglobinopathies, are clearly related to genetic factors that vary across, but are not exclusive to, particular ethnic groups. There are also research programmes investigating whether more common diseases, such as diabetes, CHD and hypertension, are influenced by genetic factors that vary across ethnic groups (Wild and McKeigue, 1997). Although biological markers have been found, such as insulin resistance syndrome and waist-to-hip ratios, it is not clear whether these are a consequence of genetic differences or environmental effects. The issue is further confused by the possibility that these biological differences may not only be a consequence of current environmental effects, which are hard enough to assess, they could also be a consequence of lifetime-cumulative environmental effects, childhood and prenatal environmental conditions, and the individual's mother's environment (Barker, 1991).

- Class and consumption-based indicators of socio-economic status only partially account for the social disadvantage faced by ethnic minority groups. Other forms of social disadvantage might also effect their health. As described above, racism is a common feature of the lives of ethnic minority people. As well as having an indirect effect on health by influencing socio-economic position, racism could affect health in two further ways. First, ethnic minority people will have a clear recognition of the relative disadvantage they face as a result of the discrimination and racism they experience. This sense of relative disadvantage might have a significant impact on health (Wilkinson, 1996). Second,

experiencing racism and harassment might have a
direct effect on health (Benzeval et al, 1992).
There is almost no evidence on any of these
possibilities.

• The specific geographical locations of ethnic
minority people, described above, might also be
an important source of relative social disadvantage
and contribute to ethnic inequalities in health.
There is a growing body of evidence showing the
importance of geographical effects and how they
might operate (Macintyre et al, 1993; Sloggett
and Joshi, 1994), and it is also clear that ethnic
minority people are more likely to be found in
the most 'unhealthy' areas (Owen, 1992, 1994).
However, the concentration of ethnic minority
people in particular areas might also be protective
of health, by improving levels of social support
and a sense of community (Halpern, 1993; Smaje,
1995). Again there is only very limited evidence
on these possibilities.

Policy recommendations

There are clear ethnic variations in health, and a
growing body of evidence suggesting that these are
probably a consequence of socio-economic
inequalities. There is also a growing body of
evidence suggesting that, although ethnic minority
people make good use of primary care, the quality of
the care received is not as good as that of the ethnic
majority. There are differences in health behaviours
across different ethnic groups, although these have
only been accurately assessed for smoking, which
many ethnic minority groups are less likely to
engage in, and drinking alcohol, which all ethnic
minorities are less likely to do. There is only limited
evidence on the other possible explanations for
ethnic variations or inequalities in health that were
discussed above.

It is important to recognise that a comprehensive
explanation for ethnic inequalities in health will be
multi-factorial. Smoking behaviour, for example,
might explain some of the differences in health, but
it is related to ethnicity, class and gender. And, while
socio-economic status might make a significant
contribution to ethnic inequalities in health, it is
hard to explain how socio-economic effects can lead
to different ethnic groups being disadvantaged by
different diseases. The higher rate of CHD among

South Asians and the higher rate of stroke for
Caribbeans are examples of this. Although both are
related to socio-economic effects, the specific nature
of these differences make it likely that they are not
simple reflections of socio-economic status; other
causal factors that vary across ethnic minority groups
are almost certainly also involved. So, ethnic
inequalities in health are probably a consequence of
multi-factorial and interactive effects. Given the
likely multi-factorial and interactive nature of ethnic
inequalities in health, it is important to identify
where the most effective and efficient points of
intervention lie.

The following policy recommendations are based on
current knowledge of the causes of ethnic
inequalities in health. However, as has been
suggested, the level of knowledge we have is limited.
In order to more adequately inform a policy agenda,
it is crucial that ethnic inequalities in health become
a stronger focus of research and that those
undertaking research consider and evaluate the range
of possible explanations for ethnic inequalities in
health, rather than simply describing variations or
focusing on only one possible explanation. It is also
important that attempts are made to address
concerns about possible artefacts, particularly as far as
cross-cultural assessments of health and assessments of
socio-economic status are concerned.

Recommendations to address socio-economic inequalities

The most recent evidence suggests that there are
socio-economic gradients in health within ethnic
minority groups and that socio-economic
inequalities make an important contribution to
ethnic inequalities in health. The economically
disadvantaged position of some ethnic minority
groups, which is most extreme in the case of
Pakistanis and Bangladeshis, was outlined earlier.
Policies aimed at reducing socio-economic
inequalities and eliminating poverty and
unemployment have value in their own right, but
will also have a major impact on ethnic inequalities
in health. The poorer housing of some ethnic
minority groups was also outlined earlier and policies
aimed at improving housing stock will be of benefit.
Similarly, it seems likely that the specific geographical
locations of ethnic minority groups might be
important, and policies aimed at area regeneration

and reducing geographically-based disadvantages will be important.

So, given the disadvantaged position of some ethnic minority groups across these dimensions, recommendations arising from other input papers to address the economic dimensions of inequalities in health, housing problems, geographical disadvantage and the social environment, will all be of relevance to ethnic inequalities in health. However, relevant policies need to drawn up with the specific problems faced by ethnic minorities in mind. For example, anti-poverty measures and those aimed at improving housing stock need to take into account the greater number of children and larger household size of some ethnic minority groups, the greater rates of lone parenthood in other ethnic minority groups, and that women in some groups are unlikely to participate in formal paid work (Modood et al, 1997). Similarly, the disadvantaged occupational profile of ethnic minority groups is not simply a result of geographical location or poorer training. Note, for example, that during the early 1990s the unemployment rates for ethnic minority groups rose faster than those for whites (Jones, 1993). It is likely that effective anti-discrimination policies will improve the occupational chances of ethnic minority people. Given the younger age profile of ethnic minority groups, some consideration should also be given to the possibilities of preventing those currently living in poor circumstances going on to live in extreme poverty post retirement age.

Recommendations to address inequalities in access to services and information

The provision of health promotion and primary healthcare for ethnic minorities faces a number of difficulties, although, as with socio-economic disadvantage, some of these problems are similar to those faced by their white neighbours. As described above, ethnic minority people are more likely to live in inner-city areas and, consequently, to have to cope with the poorer primary care services faced by all of those living in these areas – for example, one study found that 46% of inner-London GP premises were below standard compared with 7% of those in England as a whole (Jarman and Bosanquet, 1992). Supporting primary care in disadvantaged settings will undoubtedly improve the quality of care available to ethnic minority people and the

establishment of Health Action Zones might be a first step towards this.

However, as with measures to address socio-economic disadvantage, the specific primary healthcare needs of ethnic minority people also need to be addressed. These include:

- **Dealing with language and advocacy needs:** Ethnic minority people may be more likely to be unaware of the services and options open to them in healthcare settings and, as described above, some need language and reading and writing support. Health promotion activities need to be aware of this and provide appropriately translated material and use media such as radio, audiotapes and video in addition to leaflets (Chan, 1997). It is important to recognise that translation services provide only one dimension of a solution – effective advocacy services can be more empowering by providing knowledge and enabling discussion and negotiation (Mason, 1990; Parsons and Day, 1992). However, this is costly and time-consuming; training all health workers to become advocates would be more effective (Bhopal and White, 1993).
- **Dealing with cultural differences in the presentation of illness and the expectations people have for service provision:** Cultural competency training should be a core part of health workers' training curricula (Chan, 1997). This does not mean knowing the detail of the range of cultures that a worker may come into contact with (an impossible task), but learning the principles and skills that enable the health worker to discover the relevant cultural dimensions of the populations they serve (Bhopal and White, 1993).
- **Supporting ethnic minority doctors:** Because of their language needs many ethnic minority patients are attracted to ethnic minority doctors (Rudat, 1994; Nazroo, 1997a); these are often single-handed or small practices in the most deprived areas which have heavy caseloads.
- **Recruiting ethnic minority workers into primary care:** Reducing the need for translation services and cultural competency training (Chan, 1997).

These are models of good practice to help guide a strategy to tackle these issues. In some areas Healthy Living Centres have been established. These provide one-stop facilities covering fitness, leisure, health services, legal and welfare advice, meeting places for community organisations, crèche facilities, and so on, all within a comfortable and convenient location (for example, the West End Health Resource Centre in inner-city Newcastle) (Chan, 1997). Such facilities are dependent on joint commissioning, and there is a clear concern that the health needs of ethnic minority people might fall between the disputed boundaries of social service and healthcare provision. Similarly, the healthcare needs of ethnic minority groups who are not concentrated in particular geographical locations (such as the Chinese) or in areas that do not have large numbers of ethnic minority people, can only be adequately provided by cross-boundary commissioning.

Other models of good practice can undoubtedly be found across the NHS and in the ethnic minority voluntary sector. However, taking advantage of innovations that have been developed within the NHS and by ethnic minority groups, needs proper evaluation of their advantages and disadvantages, adequate dissemination of this information and mainstreaming the funding of those that are successful. Short-term project funding should carry with it a clear commitment to evaluation and long-term funding if shown to be beneficial. However, when mainstreaming it is important to recognise the specific geographical locations of ethnic minority people and that local problems need local solutions.

Central to all of this is adequate needs assessment. This means more than providing Census-type information on the ethnic make-up of providers' populations, for example, through ethnic monitoring. Advocacy needs, level of illness, housing problems, preferences for types and providers of services, and so on, all need to be fed into the planning and provision of health services, and this can only be done through research and full consultation with the communities involved. Community participation in needs assessment and service development is crucial to any assessment of the range of needs particular groups have, the kinds of services people feel they need, and culturally appropriate and sensitive provision of these services (Chan, 1997). This can be developed by encouraging partnership with primary health and

social services, but the inclusion of minority groups that are often excluded from such processes requires careful groundwork. Incorporated in this must be the recruitment of ethnic minority people into decision-making positions and accountability to the communities for which services are provided.

Acknowledgement

This paper draws on information and advice I have received from a great many people. I am particularly grateful to Seeromanie Harding (Office for National Statistics), Raj Bhopal (University of Newcastle), Michael Chan (University of Liverpool), Sunjai Gupta (Department of Health), Gaynor Legall (Director, Afiya Trust), Hamid Rehman (Health Education Authority) and participants in the 'Health' seminar group held during the Policy Studies Institute's 'Ethnic Minorities in Britain' conference, 8 October 1997.

References

Badger, F., Atkin, K. and Griffiths, R. (1989) 'Why don't general practitioners refer their disabled Asian patients to district nurses', *Health Trends*, vol 21, pp 31-2.

Balarajan, R. and Bulusu, L. (1990) 'Mortality among immigrants in England and Wales, 1979-83', in M. Britton (ed) *Mortality and geography: A review in the mid-1980s, England and Wales*, London: OPCS.

Balarajan, R., Yuen, P. and Raleigh, V. (1989) 'Ethnic differences in general practitioner consultations', *British Medical Journal*, no 289, pp 958-60.

Barker, D. (1991) 'The foetal and infant origins of inequalities in health in Britain', *Journal of Public Health Medicine*, vol 13, pp 64-8.

Barot, R. (ed) (1996) *The racism problematic: Contemporary sociological debates on race and ethnicity*, Lewiston: The Edwin Mellen Press.

Benzeval, M., Judge, K. and Solomon, M. (1992) *The health status of Londoners*, London: King's Fund Institute.

Bhopal, R.S. (1997) 'Is research into ethnicity and health racist, unsound, or important science', *British Medical Journal*, no 314, pp 1751-6.

Bhopal, R.S. and Donaldson, L.J. (1998) 'Health education for ethnic minorities – current provision and future directions', *Health Education Journal*, vol 47, pp 137-40.

Bhopal, R.S. and White, M. (1993) 'Health promotion for ethnic minorities: past, present and future', in W.I.U. Ahmad (ed) *'Race' and health in contemporary Britain*, Buckingham: Open University Press, pp 137-66.

Carr-Hill, R.A., Rice, N. and Roland, M. (1996) 'Socio-economic determinants of rates of consultation in general practice based on fourth national morbidity survey of general practices', *British Medical Journal*, no 312, pp 1008-13.

Chan, M. (1997) 'Primary and community healthcare services and ethnic minorities in England', Joint Conference on 'Inequalities in health: Making a difference for black and minority ethnic groups', King's Fund, December.

Chaturvedi, N., Rai, H. and Ben-Shlomo, Y. (1997) 'Lay diagnosis and health care seeking behaviour for chest pain in South Asians and Europeans in London', *Lancet*, vol 350, p 1578-83.

Coleman, D. and Salt, J. (1996) *Ethnicity in the 1991 Census: Volume 1, Demographic characteristics of the ethnic minority populations*, London: HMSO.

Davey Smith, G., Shipley, M.J. and Rose, G. (1990) 'Magnitude and causes of socio-economic differentials in mortality: further evidence from the Whitehall study', *Journal of Epidemiology and Community Health*, vol 44, p 265.

DeCock, K.M. and Low, N. (1997) 'HIV and AIDS, other sexually transmitted diseases, and tuberculosis in ethnic minorities in United Kingdom: is surveillance serving its purpose?', *British Medical Journal*, no 314, pp 1747-51.

Gilliam, S.J., Jarman, B., White, P. and Law, R. (1989) 'Ethnic differences in consultation rates in urban general practice', *British Medical Journal*, no 299, pp 953-7.

Hall, S. (1992) 'The question of cultural identity', in S. Hall, D. Held and T. McGrew (eds) *Modernity and its futures*, Cambridge: Polity Press, pp 274-325.

Halpern, D. (1993) 'Minorities and mental health', *Social Science and Medicine*, vol 36, no 5, pp 597-607.

Harding, S. and Maxwell, R. (1997) 'Differences in the mortality of migrants', in F. Drever and M. Whitehead (eds) *Health inequalities: Decennial supplement*, DS Series No 15, London: The Stationery Office, pp 108-21.

Heath, A. and Ridge, J. (1983) 'Social mobility of ethnic minorities', *Journal of Biosocial Science*, vol 8, supplement, pp 169-84.

Hickman, M. and Walters, B. (1997) *Disability and the Irish community in Britain: Report of research undertaken for the CRE*, London: Commission for Racial Equality.

Jarman, B. and Bosanquet, N. (1992) 'Primary health care in London – changes since the Acheson report', *British Medical Journal*, no 305, pp 1130-3.

Jones, T. (1993) *Britain's ethnic minorities*, London: Policy Studies Institute.

Karn, V. (ed) (1997) *Ethnicity in the 1991 Census: Volume 4: Employment, education and housing among the ethnic minority populations of Britain*, London: HMSO.

Macintyre, S., Maciver, S. and Soomans, A. (1993) 'Area, class and health: should we be focusing on places or people?', *Journal of Social Policy*, vol 22, no 2, pp 213-34.

Marmot, M.G., Adelstein, A.M. and Bulusu, L. (1984) *OPCS immigrant mortality in England and Wales 1970-78: Causes of death by country of birth*, London: HMSO.

Mason, E.S. (1990) 'The Asian mother and baby campaign (the Leicestershire experience)', *Journal of the Royal Society of Health*, vol 55, pp 658-67.

Maxwell, R. and Harding, S. (1997) 'The variation in mortality of migrants living in England and Wales by marital status', Manuscript submitted to *Population Trends*.

Modood, T., Berthoud, R., Lakey, J., Nazroo, J., Smith, P., Virdee, S. and Beishon, S. (1997) *Ethnic minorities in Britain: Diversity and disadvantage*, London: Policy Studies Institute.

Nazroo, J.Y. (1997a) *The health of Britain's ethnic minorities: Findings from a national survey*, London: Policy Studies Institute.

Nazroo, J.Y. (1997b) *Ethnicity and mental health: Findings from a national community survey*, London: Policy Studies Institute.

Owen, D. (1992) *Ethnic minorities in Great Britain: Settlement patterns*, National Ethnic Minority Data Archive 1991 Census Statistical Paper No 1, Warwick: Centre for Research in Ethnic Relations, University of Warwick.

Owen, D. (1993) *Ethnic minorities in Britain: Age and gender structure*, National Ethnic Minority Data Archive 1991 Census Statistical Paper No 2, Warwick: Centre for Research in Ethnic Relations, University of Warwick.

Owen, D. (1994) 'Spatial variations in ethnic minority groups populations in Great Britain', *Population Trends*, vol 78, pp 23-33.

Parsons, L. and Day, S. (1992) 'Improving obstetric outcomes in ethnic minorities', *Journal of Public Health Medicine*, vol 14, pp 183-92.

Peach, C. (1996) *Ethnicity in the 1991 Census: Volume 2: The ethnic minority populations of Great Britain*, London: HMSO.

Ratcliffe, P. (1996) *Ethnicity in the 1991 Census: Volume 3: Social geography and ethnicity in Britain: Geographical spread, spatial concentration and internal migration*, London: HMSO.

Rudat, K. (1994) *Black and minority ethnic groups in England: Health and lifestyles*, London: Health Education Authority.

Shaukat, N., de Bono, D.P., and Cruickshank, J.K. (1993) 'Clinical features, risk factors and referral delay in British patients of Indian and European origin with angina', *British Medical Journal*, no 307, pp 717-8.

Shaukat, N., Lear, J., Fletcher, S., de Bono, D.P. and Woods, K.L. (1997) 'First myocardial infarction in patients of Indian subcontinent and European origin: comparison of risk factors, management, and long term outcome', *British Medical Journal*, no 314, pp 639-42.

Sloggett, A. and Joshi, H. (1994) 'Higher mortality in deprived areas: community or personal disadvantage', *British Medical Journal*, no 309, pp 1470-4.

Smaje, C. (1995) 'Ethnic residential concentration and health: evidence for a positive effect?', *Policy & Politics*, vol 23, no 3, pp 251-69.

Smith, D. (1977) *Racial disadvantage in Britain*, Harmondsworth: Penguin.

Townsend, P. and Davidson, N. (1982) *Inequalities in health*, The Black Report, Harmondsworth: Penguin.

Wild, S. and McKeigue, P. (1997) 'Cross sectional analysis of mortality by country of birth in England and Wales', *British Medical Journal*, no 314, pp 705-10.

Wilkinson, R.G. (1996) *Unhealthy societies: The afflictions of inequality*, London: Routledge.

Williams, R. (1993) 'Health and length of residence among South Asians in Glasgow: a study controlling for age', *Journal of Public Health Medicine*, vol 15, no 1, pp 52-60.

13a

Inequalities of health: road transport and pollution[1]

Adrian Davis

Introduction

Transport is a derived demand. Its primary function is in enabling *access* to people, goods and services. The act of travelling allows the activities for which people travel to happen. These have been described as exchange opportunities and it is argued that people are entitled to the protection of their right to a just and equitable share of exchange opportunities (Engwicht, 1992). Yet road transport currently provides a selective distribution of access. Health benefits are mainly experienced by people travelling, although the most health-promoting and equitable modes of transport (walking and cycling) are vulnerable to the disbenefits imposed by motorised transport. As with health inequalities generally (Benzeval et al, 1995; BMA, 1995; Townsend and Davidson, 1998), the disbenefits of travel fall disproportionately on the lower socio-economic groups, women, ethnic minorities, children and older people. For this reason, in addition to a focus on socio-economic groups, genders, ethnic groups, and geographic areas, issues relating to children and older people are also specifically addressed. Such groups have the greatest travel problems, and together form a majority of the population, not a minority (Goodwin, 1990). Restrictions on independent mobility among members of this majority group amounts to social exclusion because of the restricted access they have compared to those with ready access to a car. In 1994 there were 375 cars per thousand people in Great Britain (ONS, 1997a).

The post-war decline in walking, cycling and public transport use is linked directly with the concomitant increase in the ownership and use of private cars. The decline in walking and cycling has come partly

as perceived and actual danger has risen with car use. Walking is still the most popular physical activity, and surveys continue to show high levels of suppressed demand for cycling (Automobile Association, 1993; Nottinghamshire County Council, 1995) and cycle sales continue to outstrip those of cars (Bicycle Association, 1997). A National Cycling Strategy was launched in 1996 and a National Walking Strategy was launched in 1998. The Cycling Strategy set a target for quadrupling the number of trips made by bicycle by 2012 (from a 1996 baseline). In terms of average trip distance, significant increases in the use of these modes are feasible as 72% of all journeys are under five miles in length and 46% under two miles (DoT, 1995a). In terms of bus use, with every additional car purchased, 300 bus trips are lost each year (Oldfield, 1979)[2]. Bus deregulation in 1986 accelerated the decline in bus patronage. For journeys of over one mile, cars are by far the most frequently used means of travelling for leisure and other personal purposes: to and from work, business, shopping and education. Education trips comprise up to 20% of peak hour travel (DoT, 1995a).

The three health impacts of transport most commonly identified are traffic casualties, air pollution and noise pollution, and are relatively easy to quantify. These are briefly discussed first.

Accidents and pollution

Accidents

Both the number of road deaths and reported serious injuries occurring on Britain's roads are declining. In 1996, 3,598 people were reported killed and

44,473 were seriously injured. Slight injuries, however, have shown a 4% increase to 272,231 people in 1996 compared to the 1995 figure. These are mostly car occupants, although safety for car occupants has increased considerably in recent years. Bus travel is one of the safest forms of travel. For example, each day in London 3,500,000 passengers are carried on buses and in 1996/97 the chances of someone being slightly injured was 1 in 338,983 passengers carried, while the chance of serious injury was 1 in 25,641,025. There has been some concern about Routemaster buses as the number of boarding and alighting accidents reported is higher than for doored vehicles, however, the number of passenger injuries which occur once inside a Routemaster are lower than the number recorded for other vehicle types (Ian Brownhill, Network Monitoring and Safety Manager, London Transport Buses, personal communication, 5 March 1998).

In Britain, vulnerable road users are disproportionately involved in accidents, making up 45% of all road deaths. Pedestrians make up 25% of all killed or seriously injured (KSI) casualties (DETR, 1997a). The British record for child pedestrian casualties is one of the worst in Europe (Jarvis et al, 1995). It is likely that casualties would be higher but for the fact that parents perceive the danger, consequently increasing restrictions on their children's independent mobility (Hillman et al, 1990; Gaster, 1991). The casualty rate (ie, the number of casualties per distance travelled) for all pedestrians fell by 22% between 1981/85 and 1996 as did the KSI rate for cyclists (although the casualty rate for this group increased overall) (DETR, 1997a). Such reductions may be explained, in part at least, by falling exposure rates – people are walking and cycling less.

Cycling has probably declined by about 26% in the 10 years to 1995, accounting for much of the 50% decrease in casualties. It is harder to assess walking, but National Travel Survey data suggests that average distances walked fell 18% between 1985 and 1994, with a drop of 27% for 5- to 15-year-olds (DETR, 1997b). It is important to note that an increase in these modes does not need to lead to an increase in casualties. Where traffic restraint measures are implemented, increases have been achieved while accident rates have declined, as illustrated in York

(Table 1(a) and 1(b)) where a road user hierarchy underpins transport planning.

Table 1(a): Changes to road casualties in York and the UK (% change)*

Casualties	York	UK
All casualties	-40.0	-1.5
Pedestrians	-36.0	-15.0
Cyclists	-29.5	-12.0
Powered two-wheelers	-65.0	-54.0
Car passengers	-16.0	+16.0
Car drivers	+2.5	+41.5

Note: * Average percentage change 1990-94 from 1981-85 average.

Table 1(b): City of York hierarchy of road users, ranked in terms of sustainability

1. Pedestrians
2. People with mobility problems
3. Cyclists
4. Public transport users
5. Commercial/business transport users
6. Car-borne shoppers
7. Coach-borne visitors
8. Car-borne visitors and commuters

Source: House of Commons (1996)

The social class gradient for deaths from road traffic accidents is highest in childhood (at over four times greater for children in social class V as opposed to social class I) but persists into adult life though the gradient is less marked (a ratio of 2:7, class V, to class I, males). In 1991-93 the estimated number of lives that could have been saved in men aged 20-64 (if death rates were equalised), from motor vehicle traffic accidents was 600, with more than half of the saving for those aged under 35. Research has found that accident rates for all casualties – drivers involved in single-vehicle accidents, drivers who failed breath tests, and casualties who did not use seat-belts – were all higher for those from deprived areas relative to those from affluent areas (Abdalla et al, 1997).

A critical issue is speeding by motorists. Speeding generally exacerbates risks for all road users, but especially for pedestrians and cyclists. Of those pedestrians struck by a car, at 40 mph 85% are killed, at 30 mph 45% are killed and many seriously injured. Only 5% of pedestrians struck at 20 mph are killed and most injuries are slight. One thousand deaths per year are directly attributable to speeding and it is the main contributory factor in one third of all road accidents (DETR, 1997b). Speeding is not an activity of a deviant minority: the results of the 1996 speed survey was largely a catalogue of the flouting of all speed limits by most motorists in urban and rural areas, using all types of vehicle, whatever time of day, day of the week, or month of the year (DETR, 1997c).

Pollution

Air

There is a large and growing body of scientific evidence as to the effects of the key emissions from road transport. While a potential hazard to the population generally, a variety of pollutants pose particular risks to vulnerable groups such as pregnant women, older people, people suffering from respiratory and coronary illnesses (Poloniecki et al, 1997) and children (Wjst et al, 1993). In large part, these groups are the same groups who have least access to cars. Moreover, the health costs from pollution due to motor transport are not reflected in the costs of vehicle use. Motor vehicle users only pay a third of the costs that they impose on society (British Lung Foundation, 1998). Key pollutants from road transport are listed in Table 2.

Table 2: Key pollutants emitted by road transport in the UK by end user (1995)

	% share of total emissions
Carbon monoxide	76
Nitrogen oxides	49
Volatile organic compounds	38
Particulates (PM_{10}s)	26*

Note: * by source.

Source: DETR (1997d); Crown Copyright material is produced with the permission of the Controller of Her Majesty's Stationery Office

The Department of Health's Committee on the Medical Effects of Air Pollution (COMEAP) has estimated that up to 24,100 deaths each year in Great Britain may be hastened by a few days or weeks by periods of high air pollution, mainly among older people and the sick. A further 23,900 hospital admissions are brought forward as well as additional admissions. This does not include chronic effects. It is likely that long-term exposure to air pollutants also damages health although this is currently not quantifiable. The estimations made were based on data on PM_{10}s, sulphur dioxide and ozone (DoH, 1998). Correlations between neighbourhood traffic volumes and child respiratory symptoms have been reported (Duhme et al, 1996; Oosterlee et al, 1996) including hospital admissions for asthma (Edwards et al, 1994; Weiland et al, 1994). In general, urban streets with high traffic density are more typical of areas marked by deprivation.

Noise

Traffic noise is the most widespread form of noise disturbance, affecting sleep and mental health. Sleep interference is probably the most important effect in terms of its potential impact on human health and well-being after long-term exposure (World Health Organisation, 1995). Up to 63% of British dwellings are exposed to a level of night-time noise high enough to interfere with sleep (Sergent and Fothergill, 1993). This is likely to include a disproportionately high number of people in low-income groups who live in areas with high levels of traffic. The main effect of exposure is a reduction in the total amount of REM sleep and an increased duration of intermittent waking during hours of exposure (Eberhardt, 1988).

Noise may also have important psycho-social effects with evidence for depression among people exposed to high levels of traffic noise (Ohrstrom, 1991). Overall, traffic noise can reduce perceived environmental quality, increase sleeping problems and health worries which may lead to recourse to health services (Lercher and Kofler, 1996).

Socio-economic groups

Car ownership has been noted to be "probably the best surrogate for current income" (Townsend et al, 1988, p 37) although less so for rural areas (see later under 'Areas: Rural'). Household car ownership is highly dependent on household income, as reflected in Table 3. There is a clear relationship between car access and mortality. Mortality had been found to be lowest among those with access to two cars (but also one car as opposed to no car) (ONS, 1997b). Residents from areas with high percentages of economically inactive adults also have higher traffic casualty rates (Scottish Office, 1996).

Table 3: Households with no car (%)

Professional	5
Managerial	4
Intermediate non-manual	15
Junior non-manual	28
Skilled manual	14
Semi-skilled manual	33
Unskilled manual	45
Economically inactive	55

Source: General Household Survey (1996); Crown Copyright

An important factor influencing household choice in mode of transport used is also multiple car ownership. The growth in multiple car ownership households is greater than ownership take-up among those previously in 'households without a car'. Data has suggested that households without a car make three trips per day, households with one car six trips, and eight for households with two or more cars (Goodwin, 1990). In addition, there is also the issue of company-owned cars. Between 1990 and 1994 52% of all cars registered were company owned. There is a subsidy to these motorists of over £1 billion per year, excluding external costs such as accidents of which company car users are disproportionately involved in (IEEP, 1995).

Cost has an important role in travel in terms of choice between public transport and car use. Low-income households are more reliant on public transport. People in the lowest income quintile make 2.5 times as many bus trips as those in the highest quintile (DoT, 1995a). Bus deregulation in 1986 (outside London) has meant that fare prices are determined by the operator. The level of subsidy provided by local authorities has declined, especially in the English metropolitan areas where fares have risen most steeply (Bradshaw, 1996). Rail and local bus fares have increased by nearly one third in real terms since 1980 while motoring costs have decreased by 5% (Oldfield, 1979). Table 4 shows changes in bus passenger journeys by area pre- and post-bus deregulation.

An example of the value of affordable, accessible and reliable bus transport is South Yorkshire. Prior to bus deregulation in April 1986, South Yorkshire had one of the most comprehensive and cheap public transport systems in the UK, having frozen fares in 1975. There was a large decrease in fare prices in real terms over a 10-year period, and increases in bus patronage relative to other metropolitan counties

during the early 1980s, resulting in an actual increase in distance travelled by bus. The public transport subsidy benefited the health of the local population by providing the social amenity of additional travel at the least additional health cost (Nicholl et al, 1987). After deregulation when bus fares rose by 250% in South Yorkshire, the unemployed and the retired reduced their bus journeys by over 62% and 60% respectively compared with 37% reductions for those in work and 48% reductions for school children. Additionally, social support networks suffered as travel to undertake informal caring roles were more difficult to make. This resulted in increased requests for statutory support services including home helps (Sheffield City Council, 1986).

Table 4: Local bus services: passenger journeys by area 1993-1994 compared to 1983

	1983 (million)	1993-94 (million)	Change (%)
English metropolitan areas	2,011	1,334	-33.7
English shire counties	1,629	1,268	-22.2
England	4,727	1,268	-21.3
Scotland	680	526	-22.6
Wales	180	130	-27.8
All areas outside London	4,500	3,258	-27.6
London	1,087	1,117	+2.7
Great Britain	5,587	4,375	-21.7

Source: DoT (1994, Table 2.1); Crown Copyright

Areas

Urban

People in deprived areas are likely to be exposed to higher traffic volumes than those living in wealthier areas and also exposed to greater risk of injury and higher levels of pollution. Accident rates are generally higher for those living in terrace properties and purpose-built flats (Scottish Office, 1996). There is an inverse relationship between motor traffic volume and street-level non-traffic activity (Appleyard, 1981). Neighbourhoods dominated by high traffic volumes are indicative of communities stripped of their 'social capital' (Gillies, 1997). Cyclists and pedestrians find it harder to get around, and both older people and families with young children report that high road traffic volumes result in feelings of insecurity (Klæboe, 1992). The severance effect of motor traffic reduces access to health-promoting facilities for those on foot or travelling by bicycle, including shops, health facilities, parks and friends. The latter is important because of the health protective function of social support networks (Fox, 1988) and there is evidence that lack of social support can increase mortality from coronary heart disease by up to four times (Greenwood et al, 1996).

People in the lowest income groups are over-represented in council housing. Most council housing is built in large, separate, single-purpose estates with poor transport links, which has a major effect on access to work and training opportunities (Power, 1996; Ong and Blumenberg, 1998). The poor quality of the information on public transport scheduling, routing and costs has been noted as generating effective barriers to job search as much as the actual quality of the service (Grieco, 1989). Moreover, inner-city residents have been found to be almost totally dependent on buses to search in less familiar areas of the city and to be hampered by their knowledge of 'known' bus routes. This is in contrast to suburban residents who generally have more choice of travel modes, including car use, and have a greater spatial awareness of the city (Quinn, 1986). There is also evidence of higher emergency admissions relating to distance from hospital in areas where deprivation levels are high (Chishty and Packer, 1995).

Poor land-use planning has contributed to transport inequalities. Relocation of hospital and other healthcare facilities to edge-of-town sites, poorly served by public transport, favours car users as opposed to those without access to a car. It also shifts costs on to users who are disproportionately represented by the disadvantaged (Mohan, 1992). A prime example of this is reflected in changing patterns of food shopping. Total distance travelled for food shopping increased by 60% between 1975/76 and 1989/91, and miles travelled by car drivers during the same period more than doubled. This increased use of car trips for food shopping has been a response to the growth of out-of- and edge-of-town food and retail stores. These stores offer a wide range of cheap foods, attractive to households with a car, adequate cash-flow and storage facilities, who can drive to the stores and bulk buy. High-income households and those with access to a car spend 79% and 73% respectively of their expenditure on food in supermarkets compared to 62% among pensioners

and 60% among households with no car (CSO, 1996). Indeed, Sainsbury's, for example, claims that "new sites are located where safe and convenient access is obtainable by car", and that "today we would not open a store which did not have a large surface level car park" (Raven et al, 1995, p 10).

While some local shops have been forced to close due to the competition from superstores, others have been forced to increase prices and reduce the range of stock in order to compete. The cost of shopping at local corner stores has been found to be up to 60% higher than shopping at major stores, equivalent to £10-£20 a week for an average pensioner couple (Piachaud and Webb, 1996).

Rural

There has been a marked increase in the rural population in the last two decades – mostly consisting of car owners; indeed present circumstances in rural areas almost preclude living there if you cannot afford to run a car. In part, this is reflected by the fact that motor traffic levels are rising fastest in the countryside (Countryside Commission, 1992). Table 5 shows that fewer households in rural than urban areas have no car (and this holds true among the lower-income groups). Facilities are further away, bus services are likely to be inadequate and distances too great for cycling or walking. For example, 20% of rural households with the lowest incomes have to travel about 25 miles a week to shop, compared to 12 miles a week for similar households in urban areas.

Table 5: Car ownership in rural and urban areas (1992/94)

	No car	I car	2+ cars
London	39	43	18
Urban	34	44	21
Rural	22	44	34

Source: DoT (1995a); Crown Copyright

Access to healthcare in remote areas may be poorer, making car ownership especially important (Watt et al, 1994). Few rural parishes have medical facilities and the total number of facilities continues to decline (Rural Development Commission, 1998). When local buses provide the only means of transport, shopping is likely to be infrequent and in bulk, which may create load-carrying problems (for older people or mothers with small children) or cash-flow difficulties (for those on low incomes). There is a polarisation of opportunity between those with and without access to a car (Bannister, 1989). Non-car-owning households have been found to visit only 31% of the destinations of members of households with two or three cars, indicating less access to facilities than car-owning households (Root et al, 1996), essentially a form of 'social exclusion'.

Two key issues that can disadvantage rural residents are the high cost of car dependence, and the low and declining levels of public transport (Rural Development Commission, 1998). High levels of car ownership in rural areas, taken by some to reflect wealth, may instead indicate an extra burden on those on low incomes and any attempt to increase fuel taxes will have little or no effect on traffic volumes. For example, the perceived need for private motor transport may have a negative impact on household expenditure to the extent that savings may be sought in food expenditure (Bannister, 1980). For economically inactive households journeys to shops by car may account for about 20% of the weekly budget for running a car (Root et al, 1996).

Significant sections of the rural population are recognised as being particularly dependent on public transport provision, including many women, older people and young people (Rural Development Commission, 1997). Declining levels of public transport services in rural areas also exacerbate a decline in walking and cycling as most people will turn to the motor car as the main alternative and so increase the danger to the remaining pedestrians and cyclists. The higher average speeds on uncongested country roads is directly associated with higher severity rates of casualties for all types of road users on such roads.

Ethnic groups

Transport has a 'race' dimension though there is very little research into minority ethnic use of transport services, not least because of a lack of relevant data (Gardiner and Hill, 1996; Jones, 1997). Many of the highest rates of unemployment in UK cities are experienced by ethnic minority groups in inner-urban areas, where the ethnic minority populations

are relatively high (Owen, 1994). These are often areas marked by multiple disadvantages. For example, the increased risk of traffic accidents among child pedestrians of Asian origin living in inner-city areas has been associated with high levels of 'on-street' parking, higher traffic volumes including 'rat-running', narrow streets and absence of play areas (Lawson and Edwards, 1991).

Car ownership among ethnic groups is illustrated in Table 6. In some ethnic minority groups car ownership may be attained through car sharing within households with costs being shared despite low incomes (J, Nazroo, personal communication, March 1998). Licence holding among women from some ethnic minority groups is minimal and access to cars likewise limited.

Table 6: Percentage of households in Great Britain with no car by ethnic group of household head

White	33.0
Black Caribbean	54.8
Black African	61.9
Indian	23.2
Pakistani	36.2
Bangladeshi	60.9
Chinese	29.4
Asian	32.4

Source: Derived from 1991 Census Report for Great Britain

Gender

Women and men often have quite different travel needs, the former typically involving more complex scheduling but with less adequate facilities to meet them. Needs change through the life-cycle, but at all stages women are more reliant on buses. Yet the cost of public transport, and the problems it presents for travellers with children, lead many women to prefer to walk. As a result, women with children, as with pensioners, become heavily reliant on local facilities (Graham, 1984, p 145). Women as carers have greater difficulties in accessing health services, particularly those reliant on public transport (Hamilton et al, 1991). Overall average distance walked is now greater for women than men (DETR, 1997e). However, they are less likely to cycle, feeling more vulnerable to traffic danger, personal attack, sexual harassment and embarrassment than men (Transport Research Laboratory, 1997).

In 1994/96 81% of males over the age of 16 were full car-driving licence holders compared with 56% for women. The lowest level for men was 50% for those aged 17-20. The lowest level for women was 19% for those aged 70+. At all ages more men hold full licences than women but the difference is more marked as age rises, so that, for example, twice as many men aged 60-69 hold full licences as do women within the same age group, 82% compared with 41% respectively (ONS, 1997a). More men than women own cars, at 64% and 35% respectively, but ownership among women has risen far more sharply in recent years than for men. Men are also more likely to use company cars than women (on the basis of licence holders and workforce profile). Company cars form a significant amount of the UK vehicle fleet with 52% of vehicles registered in recent years being company-owned cars (DoT, 1995b).

Fear for personal safety, especially at night, has become an important deterrent to the use of public transport among women (and older people). Surveys in a number of UK cities have established that around two thirds of women are afraid to go out at night alone and significant numbers will not use public transport (Atkins, 1989). Perceived fear imposes a significant psychological cost and seriously inhibits the behaviour of a large number of women (Trench et al, 1992), effectively excluding them from involvement in some evening activities. Any health benefits that might otherwise have been gained through this travel will have been lost.

Children

Children's needs in terms of transport policy are an area of neglect and their independent mobility and access are severely restricted by contemporary urban environments (Davis and Jones, 1996a, 1996b).

Accidents

An accident is the most common cause of hospital admission for children between ages 5 and 16 in the UK. Of these admissions traffic injuries feature most prominently. Indeed, in the UK, death rates for child pedestrians are the second highest in Europe (Jarvis et al, 1995). Social deprivation is a key determinant of child road accidents (Sharples et al, 1990). Children living in deprived areas have a high road

accident rate and there is a dose response (ie, the greater the degree of deprivation the higher the accident rate) between degree of deprivation and accident rates (Kendrick, 1993): this area association has been reported widely (Dougherty et al, 1990; Joly et al, 1991; Durkin et al, 1994). Socio-economic inequalities in child injury rates have increased between 1981-91 (Roberts and Power, 1996). The child pedestrian death rates for social class V is over four times that of children in social class I and is a contemporary disease of childhood poverty (Roberts et al, 1996). This has been associated with levels of car ownership. Children from families without a car have been noted to cross a greater numbers of roads than those from car-owning households. Children from households with two or more cars cross least roads as pedestrians (Roberts et al, 1996).

The proportion of vehicles exceeding speed limits in low socio-economic areas is also higher than in more affluent areas (Stevenson et al, 1995), with higher traffic volumes (Mueller et al, 1990), despite lower car ownership. Children living in an environment marked by multiple social disadvantage are likely to acquire vulnerable characteristics, such as inpulsivity and poor cognitive skills in relation to their environment (Bagley, 1992). The risk of pedestrian injury is over 50% higher for children of single mothers compared with children with two parents in the household (Roberts and Power, 1995). Yet it appears likely that the willingness or ability to advocate for child safety varies inversely with the need for it, mirroring Tudor Hart's inverse care law for medical care (Roberts, 1995).

Independent mobility

Mirroring adult reductions in physical activity (Health Education Authority and Sports Council, 1992), levels of physical activity among children are declining (Cale and Almond, 1992; Armstrong and McManus, 1994). Conditions of modern society appear to inhibit children from physically active life-styles (Sleap and Warburton, 1996). This can encourage sedentary life-styles with their attendant increases in risk factors for illnesses such as coronary heart disease. For example, year on year more children are travelling to school by car. Nationally, 65% of 5- to 10-year-olds in the years 1989 to 1994 travelled less than one mile to school. Even for this distance car travel has doubled since 1975/76 (DoT, 1995a).

Older people

The current transport system is largely hostile to older people. Of all UK pedestrian deaths, 46% involve people aged 60 years and over, largely in urban areas (DETR, 1997a). Older people are also over-represented in serious pedestrian injuries and older females are 2.5 times more at risk of injury as pedestrians than are males of the same age for the same distance walked or number of roads crossed (Ward et al, 1994). This indicates a high level of risk per unit of exposure compared with other age groups. One calculation estimates that the fatality rate for young pensioners per kilometre walked is approximately twice that among children and the rate for old pensioners about 10 times as high (Hillman, 1991).

Roads are often perceived as barriers to the day-to-day movements of older people, and studies of pedestrian crossing behaviour indicate that children and older people are particularly delayed as traffic volumes rise (Hine and Russell, 1996; Langlois et al, 1997). Road traffic can lead to a perceived danger of travel which causes feelings of insecurity, anxiety and stress. This could in turn lead to restricted travel with a consequent loss of any health benefit that might otherwise have been gained, such as contact with neighbours. A low-quality environment such as one with high volumes of motor traffic undermines social support and can leave older people feeling isolated (Appleyard, 1981). Deteriorating neighbourhoods tend to promote distrust of others among older adults (Krause, 1993).

The decline in public transport has had a detrimental effect on the independent mobility of older people but where inexpensive and regular services exist older people appear to 'enjoy a high level of mobility' (Goodwin et al, 1983). Bus deregulation has had particularly negative effects on older women's ability to reach basic services, making journeys 'traumatic'. Some women have found themselves isolated because levels of public transport provision do not enable them to visit their friends and relatives, reducing feelings of freedom, self-sufficiency and independence (Hamilton et al, 1991). A survey in the Cotswolds found significant proportions of both independent and dependent older people to be unable to travel far from their parish, and a sizeable minority to be truly housebound (Grant and Smith, 1988).

While car ownership is a function of age, access to a car among older people is allied with other indicators of advantage in material circumstances which are associated with better health (Arber and Ginn, 1993). However, the gender gap between car ownership among those over 65 has not narrowed in recent years unlike among younger adults (DoT, 1993). Those over 65 are also less likely to have access if they live alone. For 65- to 74-year-olds living alone, 29% have access to a car. This drops to 15% for those aged 75 years and upwards (General Household Survey, 1996).

Recommendations

The key aim of any recommendation must be to improve access for all in order to reduce inequalities. The most equitable mode of road transport is walking and the least is the car. Most measures targeted to reduce car use will improve access for those without access or with only limited access to cars. This can only be achieved, however, if walking, cycling and public transport are seen as more attractive to car users than use of the car for most journeys. This will require an unprecedented level of support for alternative modes of transport, backed up by vigorous traffic restraint measures and removal of fiscal incentives which engender habitual car use.

An overriding goal will be, therefore, for the Department of the Environment, Transport and the Regions (DETR) to establish motor traffic reduction targets (as proposed in the Road Traffic Reduction [UK Targets] Bill) and to develop complementary targets for increases in walking and public transport. The DETR should establish a Traffic Reduction Unit, headed by a senior civil servant, reporting directly to the Secretary of State, to coordinate action to achieve the traffic reduction targets.

Policy   **Decentralise funding and responsibility for local transport from central government while providing an overall policy framework and monitoring of local authority policies. At present over 80% of local transport funding is controlled by central government.**

Benefits   • Greater autonomy for local authorities to develop integrated transport strategies which meet local access needs within a national policy framework.

Evidence   European countries with the best records regarding provision for and use of alternative modes to the car have the most decentralised systems of government in the world. Denmark and the Netherlands are examples, having had major decentralisation programmes beginning in the 1970s.

Policy   **Accelerate the implementation of 20 mph schemes through doubling the Local Safety Scheme annual funding from central government by 2002, and again by 2006, and give local authorities greater discretion is the application of 20 mph zones. Also, introduce trials of low-speed areas (under 30 mph).**

Benefit   • Increased independent mobility for pedestrians and cyclists, but particularly children and the elderly, and a decrease in road accident casualties.

Evidence   Transport Research Laboratory research shows that in 20 mph zones there is, on average, a 61% drop in pedestrian casualties and a 67% drop in child pedestrian and cyclist casualties. Significantly there was a 6.2% reduction in accidents for each mile per hour reduction in vehicle speed (DETR, 1997b). In Denmark, in 1978, 'living areas' (or Section 40 areas) were introduced with 15 kmph limits. These have pedestrian priority and speed reducing measures. Studies revealed a 78% drop in KSI casualties (Engel and Thomsen, 1992).

Policy   **Target traffic calming schemes in housing estates with high levels of child pedestrian and cycle accidents. Create informal play space alongside traffic calming measures.**

Benefits   • Reduced road accidents among children, but especially those in poorer neighbourhoods. More informal play space near homes. Noise levels can also be reduced by traffic calming.

Evidence   Research has found that estates with traffic calming and good space at the front of the houses provide the best environment for children. Where streets had these features, nearly one child in four engaged in active play, such as running, walking, ball games, and use of bicycles and play equipment (Wheway and Millward, 1997). Research into the noise impact of traffic calming measures shows that the lower speeds obtained result in reductions in noise where traffic flows largely exclude heavy goods vehicles (DoT, 1996).

Policy   **Allow local police forces to make an administrative charge for speeding offences by which speed cameras can be financed.**

Benefit   • This has the potential to offer a very effective, low-cost way of enforcing speed limits. It could also lead to reductions in accidents.

Evidence   Speed cameras bring a typical casualty reduction of 28%, and it has been calculated that they bring an annual economic return of five times the fixed cost (currently £12,000) and running costs (currently £8,500 per year) (DETR, 1997b).

Policy   **Enforce current speed limits and review all speed limits.**

Benefit   • For most pollutants, emissions increase as speed rises but reduce with slower and smoother driving. Likewise, accident risk and severity of injures rise with higher speeds. Enforcing speed limits would be beneficial to pedestrians and cyclists who are disproportionately at risk per mile travelled.

Evidence The Transport Research Laboratory has found that for every mile per hour decrease in average speed there is a corresponding 5% decrease in accidents and a 7% decrease in deaths. Air and noise pollution increase as speed rises.

Policy **Provide suitable powers for statutory partnerships between transport operators, local authorities and traffic commissioners to set and monitor standards for all modes of public transport, focusing, in particular, on fares, ticketing systems for through travel, comprehensive and easily accessible information, and total quality in service provision.**

Benefit • Increased access and mobility for children, women, the unemployed, those on low incomes and older people.

Evidence South Yorkshire cheap fares policy 1975-86.

Policy **In urban areas, reallocate road space to provide more infrastructure for pedestrian and cycle route networks. Between 1999 and 2005 year-on-year funding for such measures should be increased by 20%.**

Benefit • Increased access and mobility at the least financial cost to individuals. Reduction in casualties while also promoting public health.

Evidence In cities such as York (Table 1) and continental cities, use of these modes has increased while accidents have decreased (House of Commons, 1996). Some continental cities invest more funds in cycling each year than has been spent in the UK as a whole: Groningen in the Netherlands is one example. Also, where cycle use becomes popular and safer, evidence shows that increases in use are proportionately greater among women (Cyclists' Touring Club, 1995).

Policy **Encourage large employers to restrict workplace parking for employees living less than 1.5 miles from driving to work and promote alternatives through Green Commuter Plans.**

Benefits • Increased viability of public transport from those switching and increased site facilities for cyclists.

Evidence Southampton University Hospital which developed a Green Commuter Plan, achieved a reduction of 700 cars per day and a 60% increase in cycle use with more people cycling and walking than prior to the introduction of the Green Commuter Plan (Cyclists' Touring Club, 1997). Thames Water in Swindon negotiated a 50% discount on rail travel with Great Western Trains in a special arrangement designed to switch business travel from car to rail on specific routes. The discount makes rail travel cheaper than paying the car mileage allowance (Transport 2000/ London First, 1997).

Policy **Recommend that transport operators provide bicycle parks at all public transport interchanges. Consider legislating for this if 80% of such interchanges not achieved by 2002.**

Benefit • Increase modal share for bicycles and public transport use.

Evidence Forty per cent of all rail trips in the Netherlands, where secure bicycle parking facilities are provided at railway sations, start or finish as a bicycle trip.

Policy **Establish a Children's Unit within the DETR to promote safe routes to schools, and targeted funding and guidance to local authorities.**

Benefits • Promotes independent mobility for children, regular physical activity and habitual pattern which can, if encouraged, be carried on into adult life-style.

Evidence   Development of safe routes to schools programmes in Denmark during the 1980s and some schemes in the UK in the past few years which have achieved increases in walking and cycling and declines in car use (Davis and Osborne, 1996).

Policy   **End company car subsidies.**

Benefit   • An increase in the use of alternative modes of transport to the car and, therefore, a reduction in road accidents and pollution.

Evidence   It is calculated that from stopping use of company cars for private mileage alone a reduction of 175 deaths and 10,585 injuries could be obtained (IEEP, 1995). Some of these deaths would be among pedestrians and cyclists.

Policy   **Introduce road pricing in urban areas if the government agrees to hypothecation of funds to help pay for substantive improvements in public transport, and for walking and cycling.**

Benefit   • Those without cars or direct access to cars would gain considerably if funding for alternatives to cars were improved.

Evidence   An area road pricing scheme was introduced in Singapore in 1975. In 1974 the public transport share in the city was 46%, by 1988 it had risen to 63% and car use decline from 43% to 22%. This modal share has remained stable since (Royal Commission on Environmental Pollution, 1994).

Notes

[1] I am indebted to Dr Barbara MacGibbon for the draft of her paper on the subject.

[2] This figure is now likely to be higher as it was based on transport statistics for 1976.

References

Abdalla, I., Barker, D. and Raeside, R. (1997) 'Road accident characteristics and socio-economic deprivation', *Traffic Engineering and Control*, December, pp 672-6.

Appleyard, D. (1981) *Livable streets*, Berkeley, CA: University of California Press.

Arber, S. and Ginn, J. (1993) 'Gender and inequalities in health in later life', *Social Science and Medicine*, vol 36, no 1, pp 33-46.

Armstrong, N. and McManus, N. (1994) 'Children's fitness and physical activity – a challenge for physical education', *British Journal of Physical Education*, Spring, pp 20-6.

Atkins, S. (1989) *Critical paths – Designing for secure travel*, London: Design Council.

Automobile Association (1993) *Cycling motorists: How to encourage them*, Basingstoke: Automobile Association.

Bagley, C. (1992) 'The urban environment and child pedestrian and bicycle injuries: interaction of ecological and personality characteristics', *Journal of Community and Applied Social Psychology*, vol 2, no 4, pp 281-9.

Banister, D. (1980) *Transport mobility and deprivation in intra-urban areas*, Farnborough: Gower.

Banister, D. (1989) *The reality of the rural transport problem*, Rees Jeffreys Road Fund 'Transport and Society' Papers, Discussion Paper 1, Oxford: Transport Studies Unit, University of Oxford.

Benzeval, M., Judge, K. and Whitehead, M. (eds) (1995) *Tackling inequalities in health: An agenda for action*, London: King's Fund.

Bicycle Association (1997) *Britain by cycle*, Coventry: Bicycle Association.

Bradshaw, W. (1996) 'Ten turbulent years – the effects on the bus industry of deregulation and privatisation', *Policy Studies*, vol 17, no 2, pp 125-36.

British Lung Foundation (1998) *Transport and pollution – The health costs*, London: British Lung Foundation.

BMA (British Medical Association) (1995) *Inequalities in health*, London: BMA.

Cale, L. and Almond, L. (1992) 'Physical activity levels of secondary-aged children: a review', *Health Education Journal*, vol 51, no 4, pp 192-7.

Chishty, V. and Packer, C. (1995) 'Age, distribution from hospital, and level of deprivation are influential factors', Letter to *British Medical Journal*, vol 310, no 1, April, p 867.

Countryside Commission (1992) *Trends in transport and the countryside*, Cheltenham: Countryside Commission.

CSO (Central Statistical Office) (1996) *Social trends*, London: HMSO.

Cyclists' Touring Club (1995) *More bikes – Policy into best practice*, Godalming: Cyclists' Touring Club.

Cyclists' Touring Club (1997) *Reaping the benefits*, Godalming: Cyclists' Touring Club.

Davis, A. and Jones, L. (1996a) 'Children and the urban environment: an issue for the new public health agenda', *Health and Place*, vol 2, no 2, pp 107-13.

Davis, A. and Jones, L. (1996b) 'Environmental constraints on health: listening to children's views', *Health Education Journal*, vol 55, no 4, pp 363-74.

Davis, A. and Osborne, P. (1996) 'Safe routes to schools demonstration project', Planning and Transport Research and Computation of Hammersmith.

DETR (Department of the Environment, Transport and the Regions) (1997a) *Road accidents Great Britain 1996 – The casualty report*, London: HMSO.

DETR (1997b) *Road safety strategy: Current problems and future solutions*, London: DETR.

DETR (1997c) *Vehicle speeds in Great Britain 1996*, Statistical Bulletin (97)11, London: DETR.

DETR (1997d) *Digest of environmental statistics No 19*, London: HMSO.

DETR (1997e) *National travel survey 1994/96*, London: The Stationery Office.

DoH (Department of Health) (1998) *Quantification of the effects of air pollution on health in the United Kingdom*, London: HMSO.

DoT (Department of Transport) (1993) *National travel survey 1989/1991*, London: HMSO.

DoT (1994) *Bus and coach statistics 1993-1994*, London: HMSO.

DoT (1995a) *National travel survey 1992/94*, London: HMSO.

DoT (1995b) *Transport statistics Great Britain, 1994*, London: HMSO.

DoT (1996) *Traffic calming: Traffic and vehicle noise*, Traffic Advisory Leaflet 6/96, London: DoT.

Dougherty, G., Pless, B. and Wilkins, R. (1990) 'Social class and the occurrence of traffic injuries and deaths in urban children', *Canadian Journal of Public Health*, vol 81, May/June, pp 204-9.

Duhme, H., Weiland, S., Keil, U., Kraemer, B., Schmid, M., Stender, M. and Chambless, L. (1996) 'The association between self-reported symptoms of asthma and allergic rhinitis and self-reported traffic density on street of residence in adolescents', *Epidemiology*, vol 7, no 6, pp 578-82.

Durkin, M., Davidson, L., Kuhn, L., O'Connor, P. and Barlow, B. (1994) 'Low-income neighbourhoods and the risk of severe pediatric injury: a small-area analysis in Northern Manhattan', *American Journal of Public Health*, vol 84, no 4, pp 587-92.

Eberhardt, J. (1988) 'The influence of road traffic noise on sleep', *Journal of Sound and Vibration*, vol 127, no 3, pp 449-55.

Edwards, J., Walters, S. and Griffiths, R. (1994) 'Hospital admissions for asthma in preschool children: relationship to major roads in Birmingham, United Kingdom', *Archives of Environmental Health*, vol 49, no 4, pp 223-7.

Engel, U. and Thomsen, L. (1992) 'Safety effects of speed reducing measures in Danish residential areas', *Accident Analysis and Prevention*, vol 24, no 1, pp 17-28.

Engwicht, D. (1992) *Towards an eco-city: Calming the traffic*, Sydney: Envirobook.

Fox, J. (1988) 'Social network interaction: new jargon in health inequalities', *British Medical Journal*, no 297, pp 373-4.

Gant, R. and Smith, J. (1988) 'Journey patterns of the elderly and disabled in the Cotswolds: a spatial analysis', *Social Science and Medicine*, vol 27, no 2, pp 173-80.

Gardiner, C. and Hill, R. (1996) 'Analysis of access to cars from the 1991 UK Census samples of anonymised records: a case study of the elderly population of Sheffield', *Urban Studies*, vol 33, no 2, pp 269-81.

Gaster, S. (1991) 'Urban children's access to their neighbourhood: changes over three generations', *Environment and Behaviour*, vol 23, no 1, pp 70-85.

Gillies, P. (1997) 'Social capital: recognising the value of society', *Healthlines*, September, pp 15-17.

Goodwin, P. (1990) 'Demographic impacts, social consequences, and the transport policy debate', *Oxford Review of Economic Policy*, vol 6, no 2, pp 76-90.

Goodwin, P. , Bailey, J., Brisbourne, R. Clarke, M., Donnison, J., Render, T. and Whiteley, G. (1983) *Subsidised public transport and the demand for travel: The South Yorkshire example*, Oxford Studies in Transport Series, Aldershot: Gower.

Graham, H. (1984) *Women, health and the family*, Brighton: Harvester.

Grant, R. and Smith, J. (1988) 'Journey patterns of the elderly and disabled in the Cotswolds: a spatial analysis', *Social Science and Medicine*, vol 27, no 2, pp 175-80.

Greenwood, D., Muir, K., Packham, C. and Madeley, R. (1996) 'Coronary heart disease: a review of the role of psychosocial stress and social support', *Journal of Public Health Medicine*, vol 18, pp 221-31.

Grieco, M. (1989) 'Low income families and inter-household interdependency: the implications for transport policy and planning', Paper to 'Transport and urban deprivation' workshop, Liverpool, University of Liverpool.

Hamilton, K., Jenkins, L. and Gregory, A. (1991) *Women and transport: Bus deregulation in West Yorkshire*, Bradford: University of Bradford.

Health Education Authority and Sports Council (1992) *Allied Dunbar National Fitness Survey*, London: Health Education Authority/Sports Council.

Hillman, M. (1991) *Uses and abuses of transport and road safety statistics in policy formulation*, Manchester: Statistical Society.

Hillman, M., Adams, J. and Whitelegg, J. (1990) *One false move: A study of children's independent mobility*, London: Policy Studies Institute.

Hine, J. and Russell, J. (1996) 'The impact of traffic on pedestrian behaviour: assessing the traffic barrier on radial routes', *Traffic Engineering and Control*, February, pp 81-5.

House of Commons (1996) *Risk reduction for vulnerable road users*, Transport Committee Third Report, London: HMSO.

IEEP (Institute for European Environmental Policy) (1995) *Company car taxation*, London: IEEP.

Jarvis, S., Towner, E. and Walsh, S. (1995) 'Accidents', in B. Botting (ed) *The health of our children*, OPCS, London: HMSO.

Joly, M., Foggin, P. and Pless, B. (1991) 'Geographical and socio-ecological variations of traffic accidents among children', *Social Science and Medicine*, vol 33, no 7, pp 765-9.

Jones, L. (1997) 'Putting transport on the social policy agenda', in M. May, E. Brunsdon and G. Craig (eds) *Social Policy Review 8*, London: Social Policy Association.

Kendrick, D. (1993) 'Prevention of pedestrian accidents', *Archives of Disease in Childhood*, vol 68, no 5, pp 669-72.

Klæboe, R. (1992) 'Measuring the environmental impact of road traffic in town areas', Paper to PTRC Summer Annual Meeting, Seminar B, London: Planning and Transport Research Computation.

Krause, N. (1993) 'Neighbourhood deterioration and social isolation in later life', *International Journal of Aging and Human Development*, vol 36, no 1, pp 9-38.

Langlois, J., Keyl, P., Guralnik, J., Foley, D., Marottoli, R. and wallace, R. (1997) 'Characteristics of older pedestrians who have difficulty crossing the street', *American Journal of Public Health*, vol 87, no 3, pp 393-7.

Lawson, S. and Edwards, P. (1991) 'The involvement of ethnic minorities in road accidents: data from three studies of young pedestrian casualties', *Traffic Engineering and Control*, January, pp 12-19.

Lercher, P. and Kofler, W. (1996) 'Behavioural and health responses associated with road traffic noise exposure along Alpine through-traffic routes', *Science of the Total Environment*, no 189/190, pp 85-9.

Mohan, J. (1992) 'Who foots the bill?', *Health Service Journal*, vol 27, August, pp 22-3.

Mueller, B., Rivara, F., Lii, S. and Weiss, N. (1990) 'Environmental factors and the risk for childhood pedestrian–motor vehicle collision occurrence', *American Journal of Epidemiology*, vol 132, no 3, pp 550-60.

Nicholl, J., Freeman, M. and Williams, B. (1987) 'Effects of subsidising bus travel on the occurrence of road traffic casualties', *Journal of Epidemiology and Community Health*, vol 41, pp 50-4.

Nottinghamshire County Council (1995) *School travel: Health and the environment*, Nottingham: Cleary Hughes Associates for NCC.

Ohrstrom, E. (1991) 'Psycho-social effects of traffic noise exposure', *Journal of Sound and Vibration*, vol 151, no 3, pp 513-17.

Oldfield, R. (1979) *Effects of car ownership on bus patronage*, LR 872 Crowthorne: Transport Road Research Laboratory.

Ong, P. and Blumenberg, E. (1998) 'Job access, commute and travel burden among welfare recipients', *Urban Studies*, vol 35, no 1, pp 77-93.

ONS (Office of National Statistics) (1997a) *Social trends 28*, London: Stationery Office.

ONS (1997b) *Health inequalities*, Decennial Supplement No 15, London: The Stationery Office.

OPCS (1996) *Living in Britain: Results from the General Household Survey 1994*, OPCS, London: HMSO.

Oosterlee, A., Drijver, M., Lebret, E. and Brunekreef, B. (1996) 'Chronic respiratory symptoms in children and adults living along streets with high traffic density', *Occupational and Environmental Medicine*, vol 53, pp 241-7.

Owen, D. (1994) 'Spatial variations in ethnic minority group populations in Great Britain', *Population Trends*, vol 78, pp 23-33.

Piachaud, D. and Webb, J. (1996) *The price of food*, London: London School of Economics.

Poloniecki, J., Atkinson, R., Ponce de Leon, A. and Anderson, H. (1997) 'Daily time series for cardiovascular hospital admissions and previous day's air pollution in London, UK', *Occupational and Environmental Medicine*, vol 54, pp 535-40.

Power, A. (1996) 'Area-based poverty and resident empowerment', *Urban Studies*, vol 33, no 9, pp 1535-64.

Quinn, D. (1986) 'Accessibility and job search', *Regional Studies*, vol 20, no 2, pp 163-73.

Raven, H., Lang, T. and Dumonteil, C. (1995) *Off our trolleys: Food retailing and the hypermarket economy*, London: Institute for Public Policy Research.

Roberts, I. (1995) 'Who's prepared for advocacy? Another inverse law', *Injury Prevention*, vol 1, no 1, pp 152-4.

Roberts, I. and Power, C. (1995) 'Social policy as a cause of childhood accidents: the children of lone mothers', *British Medical Journal*, no 311, pp 925-8.

Roberts, I. and Power, C. (1996) 'Does the decline in child injury mortality vary by social class?', *British Medical Journal*, no 313, pp 784-6.

Roberts, I., Norton, R. and Taua, B. (1996) 'Child pedestrian injury rates: the importance of "exposure to risk" relating to socio-economic and ethnic differences, in Auckland, New Zealand', *Journal of Epidemiology and Community Health*, vol 50, no 1, pp 162-5.

Root, A., Boardman, B. and Fielding, W. (1996) *The cost of rural travel*, Oxford: Environmental Change Unit.

Royal Commission on Environmental Pollution (1994) *18th report: Transport and the environment*, London: HMSO.

Rural Development Commission (1997) *Disadvantages in rural areas*, Salisbury: Rural Development Commission.

Rural Development Commission (1998) *1997 survey of rural services*, Salisbury: Rural Development Commission.

Scottish Office (1996) *Linking road traffic accidents statistics to census data in Lothian*, Edinburgh: Central Research Unit.

Sergent, J. and Fothergill, L. (1993) *The noise climate around our homes*, Information Paper IP21/93, Watford: Building Research Establishment.

Sharples, P., Storey, A., Aynsley-Green, A. and Eyre, J. (1990) 'Causes of fatal accidents involving head injury in the Northern region, 1979-86', *British Medical Journal*, no 301, 24 November, pp 1193-7.

Sheffield City Council (1986) *The bus booklet*, Sheffield: Sheffield City Council.

Sleap, M. and Warburton, P. (1996) 'Physical activity levels of 5-11-year-old children in England: cumulative evidence from three direct observation studies', *International Journal of Sports Medicine*, vol 17, pp 248-53.

Stevenson, M., Jamrozik, K. and Spittle, J. (1995) 'A case-control study of traffic risk factors and child pedestrian injury', *International Journal of Epidemiology*, vol 24, no 5, pp 957-64.

Townsend, P. and Davidson, N. (eds) (1982) *Inequalities in health: The Black Report*, London: Penguin.

Townsend, P., Phillimore, P. and Beattie, A. (1988) *Health and deprivation: Inequality in the North*, London: Croom Helm.

Transport 2000/London First (1997) *Changing journeys to work: An employers guide to Green Commuter Plans*, London: Transport 2000.

Transport Research Laboratory (1997) *Attitudes to cycling: A qualitative study and conceptual framework*, Report 266, Crowthorne: Transport Research Laboratory.

Trench, S., Oc, T. and Tiesdell, S. (1992) 'Safer cities for women', *Town Planning Review*, vol 63, no 3, pp 279-96.

Ward, H., Cave, J., Morrison, A., Allsop, R., Evans, A., Kuiper, C. and Willumsen, L. (1994) *Pedestrian activity and accident risk*, Farnborough: AA Foundation for Road Safety Research.

Watt, I., Franks, A. and Sheldon, T. (1994) 'Health and health care of rural populations in the UK: is it better or worse?', *Journal of Epidemiology and Community Health*, vol 48, pp 16-21.

Weiland, S., Mundt, K., Ruckmann, S. and Keil, U. (1994) 'Self-reported wheezing and allergic rhinitis in children and traffic density on street of residence', *Annals of Epidemiology*, vol 4, pp 243-7.

Wheway, R. and Millward, A. (1997) *Child's play: Facilitating play on housing estates*, Coventry/York: Chartered Institute of Housing/Joseph Rowntree Foundation.

Wjst, M., Reitmeir, P., Dold, S., Wulff, A., Nicolai, T., von Loeffelholz-Colberg, E. and von Matius, E. (1993) 'Road traffic and adverse effects on respiratory health in children', *British Medical Journal*, vol 307, no 4, September, pp 596-600.

World Health Organisation (1995) *Concern for Europe's tomorrow: Health and the environment in the WHO European region*, Stuttgart: European Centre for Environment and Health.

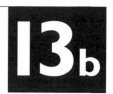

Inequalities in health[1] related to transport[2]

Barbara MacGibbon

Introduction

The need for transport includes travel for school, work, health services, shopping, leisure and green space. The increased use of private cars, for all these purposes, has been accompanied by a decline in the use, and therefore in the provision of, public transport. Furthermore, the cost of using public transport has increased at a greater rate than that of running a car. Thus the less well off, who do not have access to a car but are dependent on public transport, are doubly disadvantaged. Privatisation and deregulation have aggravated the situation in some areas.

In addition to availability and cost of public transport there is the question of accessibility. Elderly people, disabled people and mothers with small children may be unable to make use of public transport without assistance.

The volume and speed of traffic has led to a decrease in the number of cyclists on the roads, and restricted the independent mobility of young children and elderly or disabled pedestrians.

Although mortality from road traffic accidents is declining, premature deaths from this cause show a marked (and increased) social class gradient.

There are two important areas where research is still needed to establish whether transport-related inequalities in health exist. The first concerns transport associated air pollutants and whether there is evidence of a socio-economic gradient in their adverse effects on health. The second is why house tenure and car access are so strongly linked to good health and longevity.

Transport-related inequalities

Availability of public transport

In the decade since deregulation was introduced in 1986 the number of passenger journeys by local bus, outside London, has decreased by 29%. The price index for bus travel increased by 89% – nearly three times faster than petrol prices (DoT, 1996a). In London (where there is no deregulation and additional reasons for using public transport) passenger journeys have increased by 5% and fares by 38% over this period.

Table 1 illustrates changing patterns in bus use between 1985/86 and 1992/94. As local bus use has declined, so has the service provided. The position in 1996 is summarised in Table 2. Privatisation and (outside of London) deregulation of bus services has resulted in loss of control over routes, timetables and fares, unless a local authority subsidises a particular route. Such subsidies have decreased by more than 50% in real terms since deregulation. But reimbursement of concessionary fares for children, elderly people and disabled people has increased, from 2% to 5% in different parts of England (DETR, 1997a).

Table 1: Bus use in England and Wales

	1985/86	1989/91	1992/94	% change 1985/86-1992/94
Other English metropolitan	164	127	119	-27
South East, excluding London	43	37	34	-21
Rest of England and Wales	59	58	48	-19
London	127	114	113	-1

Source: DoT (1995); Crown Copyright

Table 2: Frequency of bus service by population density in Great Britain (% of households)

Frequency of service	Built-up areas	Towns over 25k	Towns 3-25k	Rural
15 mins or less	53	38	12	7
About every 30 mins	31	35	32	18
About every 60 mins	5	10	25	21
Less frequent daily service	–	2	10	29
No daily service	–	–	2	8

Note: "Don't knows" account for the remaining households.

Source: DoT (1996b); Crown Copyright

An important cause of the decline in public transport use and services is the increase in the use of private cars (see Table 3). For journeys of over one mile, cars are by far the most frequently used means of travelling for leisure and other personal purposes: to and from work, business, shopping and education (school journeys comprise 20% of peak-hour travel). In its *20th Report* (RCEP, 1997), the Royal Commission on Environmental Pollution (RCEP) quote a report commissioned by the RAC (ESRC Transport Studies Unit et al, 1995) which concluded that up to 80% of car trips are unnecessary and need not be made by car, but also drew attention to the unattractiveness of alternative modes of transport. While rail and local bus fares have increased by nearly one third in real terms since 1980, motoring costs have decreased by 5% (Stokes, 1995). As is to be expected, there is a clear socio-economic gradient in relation to car ownership (see Table 4). It is the less well off who are dependent on local bus use in rural and urban areas (see Table 5).

Table 3: How people get about (1993/95)

	Proportion of journeys	Proportion of distance travelled
On foot	29	3
By cycle	2	1
By car	59	81
By local bus	6	4
By rail	1	5
In other ways	3	7
All modes	100	100

Source: RCEP (1997, p 55, Table 4.1); DoT (1996b, Tables 2aii and 2bii); Crown Copyright

Table 4: Percentage ownership of cars, by household income, Great Britain 1993/95 (1993/95)

	No car	1 car	2+ cars
Lowest quintile	69	28	4
Second quintile	52	42	7
Third quintile	24	53	23
Fourth quintile	13	55	31
Highest quintile	6	46	49
Total	**33**	**45**	**22**

Source: DoT (1996a, p 61); Crown Copyright

Table 5: Use of public transport in relation to income (1994-96 survey)

Mode of transport	Lowest	Second	Third	Fourth	Highest	All
Local bus	100	92	72	60	36	70
Non-local bus	1	3	1	2	3	2
London Transport Underground	10	3	7	8	24	9
National rail	12	4	9	10	26	11

Source: DETR (1997a, p 38); Crown Copyright

Rural areas

There has been a marked increase in the rural population in the last two decades – mostly consisting of car owners. Indeed, present circumstances in rural areas almost preclude living there if you cannot afford to run a car. Table 6 shows that fewer households in rural areas than urban areas have no car (and this holds true among the lower income groups). Table 7 explains the need: facilities are further away, bus services are likely to be inadequate and distances too great for cycling or walking. For example, 20% of rural households with the lowest incomes have to travel about 25 miles a week to shop, compared to 12 miles a week for similar households in urban areas (Bentham and

Haynes, 1985). When local buses provide the only means of transport, shopping is likely to be infrequent and in bulk – which may create load-carrying problems (for elderly people or mothers with small children) or cash-flow difficulties (for those on low incomes).

Table 6: Car ownership in rural and urban areas, Great Britain (1992-94)

	% no car	% I car	% 2+ cars
London	39	43	18
Urban	34	44	21
Rural	22	44	34

Source: DoT (1995); Crown Copyright

Table 7: Parishes without services

	1991 (%)	1994 (%)
Permanent shop of any kind	41	42
General store	71	70
Post Office	42	43
Village hall	30	28
School (for 6-year-olds)	53	50
School (for any age)	50	49
Pub	–	29
Daily bus service	72	75
GP (based in parish)	84	83
Dentist	91	91
Pharmacy of any kind	81	79
Jobcentre	–	99
Library (permanent or mobile)	12	12
Public nursery	96	93
Private nursery	93	86
Police station	89	92

Source: Rural Development Commission (1995)

Provision of medical facilities in rural areas may also depend on transport (see Table 8); use of services often declines in proportion to distance. A study in Norfolk (Macintyre et al, 1993) found that:

- more remote rural households without access to a car were three times less likely to visit their GP, given similar levels of need, than urban households with cars;
- rural households were generally less inclined to visit their GP than urban dwellers;
- there was an association between low use of hospital services and households in villages without a GP's surgery, suggesting that access to a GP is crucial to hospital use.

Table 8: Provision of medical facilities in rural parishes (1994)

	Parishes containing service (%)
Hospitals with Accident & Emergency and outpatient facilities	1
Hospitals with Accident & Emergency but with no outpatient facilities	–
Hospitals with no Accident & Emergency but with outpatient facilities	1
Hospitals with no Accident & Emergency or outpatient facilities	–
GP practices based in the parish	17
GP practices based elsewhere	15
Post-natal clinics based in the parish	8
Visiting clinics	13
Dental surgeries	9
Opticians	5
Other specialist practitioners	10
Pharmacies at a doctor's surgery	12
Pharmacies not at a doctor's surgery	10
Prescription delivery services run by a pharmacy	7
Prescription delivery services run by volunteers	8
Homes for the mentally handicapped or physically disabled	8
Residential and nursing homes for the elderly	24

Source: Rural Development Commission (1995)

In addition to the obvious implications for health, if transport for healthcare or food shopping is inadequate, well-being and mental health may be adversely affected by enforced loneliness or isolation due to lack of transport for social purposes. The Environmental Change Unit at Oxford University found that households in rural areas without cars visited only half the places visited by households with cars. Lifts with a friend, and public transport accounted for 21% of trips, the remainder were by foot, bike, taxi, and so on.

Also, the general health and well-being of lower income groups of rural residents who feel obliged to run a car to survive, may be reduced because of the need to cut back on other expenditures.

Urban areas

Similar problems may exist in urban areas, particularly in deprived inner-city areas and outlying housing estates. A study in the west of Scotland found that an area where 75% of households had no car had less public transport provision than an area where 53% of households had no car (Piachaud and Webb, 1996). Considerable variations exist in the extent to which local authorities subsidise bus routes between less affluent residential areas and, for example, shopping centres and hospitals. In a few areas Tesco and Asda have provided free buses to their supermarkets. However, for many women without cars the choice is between complicated journeys by bus, or walking long distances, often through run-down areas and with young children.

The problem for those living on low incomes – who include many elderly and disabled people as well as mothers (particularly lone parents) with young children, dependent on state benefits – is as likely to be related to cost and accessibility, as availability of public transport. For all these groups, the presence of steps create difficulties in getting onto a bus when handicapped by chronic illness, a walking stick or frame, or a pushchair and small children. Public transport may only be a realistic option if assistance can be provided. Low income may preclude travelling by bus for those not entitled to subsidised travel. Whatever the reasons for restricted bus travel, the resulting need to shop locally is likely to mean spending more for less varied and less wholesome food than would be available more cheaply in the town centre or supermarket (Roberts and Power, 1996).

It also results in isolation, particularly for those living on a housing estate, with small children. Bus concessions for long-term income support and family credit recipients would be very costly, and would not cover people not on benefit but with a low income.

Considerations of safety may also limit the use of public transport, especially in the case of elderly women. Although buses themselves are a very safe mode of travel, there may be problems getting to and from the bus, particularly at night.

Road traffic accidents

The Black Report (Townsend and Davidson, 1982) showed steep social class gradients for accident mortality in children. Although the death rates in 1981 and 1991 showed a fall in each social class the decline in rates for children in social classes IV and V (21% and 2% respectively) was smaller than for children in social classes I and II (32% and 37%). Road traffic accidents are the cause of approximately half the accidental deaths in children, and show an

approximately fivefold social class gradient (Di Giuseppe and Roberts, 1997).

In 1992 over 44,000 children were reported injured in road accidents. Nearly two thirds of the deaths and serious injuries involve child pedestrians. For both boys and girls, casualty rates increase from birth to peak at 12 years, but, particularly between ages 6-10 years, boys (who tend to play more in the street) are at greater risk than girls. About 200 child and teenage pedestrians are killed by motor vehicles each year in England and Wales (Di Giuseppe and Roberts, 1997). In 1994 the average death rate per 100,000 population, for child pedestrians in European countries was 0.9; the rate in Great Britain was 1.4. Among seven northern European countries, Great Britain had the second highest rate for 0- to 4-year-olds, the third highest for 5- to 9-year-olds and the highest for 10-14 and 15-17 age groups. Part of the explanation may be the greater degree of urbanisation and of old residential road layouts in this country (Harland et al, 1996).

Research in Scotland suggests that pedestrian casualties are largely due to increased exposure (Scottish Office Central Research Unit, 1996). Rates are higher in areas of high population density with a high proportion of rented dwellings, residents from social class V and with low levels of car-ownership, particularly in relation to young children, and to male pedestrians injured at night. Attention has been drawn to the role of inadequate parental supervision (Christie, 1995a) often associated with atypical marital status (eg single parenthood) (Sharples et al, 1990), lack of safe play areas, and lack of understanding of road safety in social classes IV and V compared with I and II, particularly with ethnic minorities where language difficulties may exist (Lawson, 1990; Christie, 1995a).

Most child pedestrian deaths or serious injuries occur on minor roads in built-up areas (Christie, 1995b). Measures such as road humps and narrowing have been introduced to lower car speeds, but insufficient attention has been paid to the responsibilities of car drivers in residential areas. Despite the existence of the Department of Transport's campaign 'Kill your speed, not a child', a survey in 1996 showed that 72% of cars exceeded the 30 mph speed limit (DETR, 1997b). Speeding is also more common in low socio-economic than affluent areas (Stevenson et al, 1995). Many drivers do not alter their mode of driving if children are around (Christie, 1995a).

While educational and traffic calming measures have contributed to the fall in the number of child pedestrian deaths despite large increases in traffic volume, a major component has been a substantial reduction in children's traffic exposure, particularly among higher social classes. Here there has been a marked increase in the number of children taken to school by car, or accompanied by their parents. There was an almost fourfold increase in the proportion of junior-school children driven to school between 1971 and 1990. However, children in low-income families are not only without access to a car but are also more likely to walk to school unaccompanied (Roberts et al, 1996) and so be exposed to the risk associated with the increased number of cars on the roads.

The social class gradient for deaths from road traffic accidents persists into adult life, though the gradient is less marked than in children (see Figure 1). Table 10 shows the number of lives and working-man years of life which could be saved if death rates were equalised. The explanation of the social class gradient is not clear. A total of 42% of the 1,700 deaths in 20 -to 64-year-olds were among drivers of vehicles other than motorcycles; motor cyclists and pedestrians each ran at about half this rate, while cyclists constituted a small percentage of deaths (and a small proportion of road users in general). However, no analysis by social class was available for individual categories of accident, to indicate whether there is a preponderance of deaths among social class V adult male pedestrians.

Figure 1: Differential in mortality from motor vehicle traffic accidents (1991-93) (European age-standardised mortality rates)

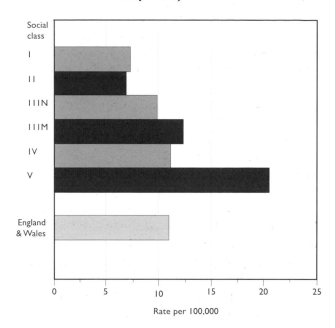

Notes: Mortality from motor vehicle traffic accidents is nearly three times higher in men in class V compared to men in class 1. (In the early 1970s, class V had just over twice the mortality of class 1.) The mortality rate from accidents in class 1 is eight per 100,000 men; in England and Wales, 11 per 100,000 and in class V, 21 per 100,000.

Source. ONS (1998), Crown Copyright

Table 9: Mortality from motor vehicle accidents, England and Wales (1991-93)

- There are about 1,700 deaths each year to men aged 20-64 from motor vehicle traffic accidents.
- This could be reduced by 600 if all men had the same death rates as those in classes I/II (370 would be at ages under 35).
- This becomes 18,000 working man-years of life saved.

Source: ONS (1998)

Another type of health inequality is related to road traffic – the volume of motor vehicles on the roads has limited the healthy activities of non-car owners/ users such as cyclists and pedestrians. Even in country lanes it may no longer be considered safe to walk, cycle, ride a horse or push a pram.

Although ownership of bicycles is higher than ever before (ONS, 1997) they are used for less than 2% of journeys (DoT, 1996b) (although in some British cities bicycles are more commonly used for getting to work) compared with 18% in Denmark and 27% in the Netherlands (DoT, 1996c), where cycling is safer than in Britain. The high risk of injury or death in this country is a deterrent. Even with the small number of cyclists, there were about 200 deaths and 3,500 serious injuries in 1996 (DETR, 1997c).

Pedestrian deaths are falling, but this is as much due to a decline in walking as improved safety. Between 1989-91 and 1993-95 the average annual distance walked fell by 16% (DoT, 1996b). Nevertheless, there were approximately 1,000 deaths and 10,000 serious injuries in 1996 (DETR, 1997c).

Given the social class distribution of car ownership (see Table 4) the impact of these car-related restrictions/risks of alternative (and healthier) modes of transport, falls unequally on lower income groups.

Traffic-related air pollution

Road traffic emissions are now the major source of ambient air pollutants. Studies using proximity to busy roads as a surrogate for exposure to pollutants have produced inconclusive results about effects on respiratory health. Better measures of exposure are available, for example, from the London Research Centre (based on modelling) and from the South East Institute of Public Health (based on monitoring). But these data have not been examined in relation to the socio-economic characteristics and health status of areas with different patterns of exposure. Such research would provide stronger evidence for, or against, a socio-economic gradient in exposure to traffic-associated air pollution and effects on health. (Proposals for such research have been/are being developed by the Small Area Health Statistics Unit (SAHSU)/ Department of Epidemiology, Imperial College, at St Mary's Hospital Medical School.)

No information was available on whether a socio-economic gradient exists among emergency hospital admissions after air pollution episodes. Even if the greater prevalence of smoking in social classes IV and V, and the associated predisposition to cardio-respiratory disease were the underlying cause of vulnerability to air pollution episodes, the existence of a socio-economic gradient in associated hospital admissions would still constitute evidence of inequalities in health outcome related to pollutants from road traffic.

Housing tenure and car access

People living in rented houses and in households with no car are at greater risk of ill-health and premature death (Fletcher et al, 1997). It has generally been assumed that the relationship is indirect reflecting income and psychological characteristics. However, should there be a *direct* link between, for example, car access (to services) and health, then there would be important implications for public health, including the reduction of transport-related inequalities. An ESRC Research Programme at the MRC Medical Sociology Unit ('Housing tenure and car ownership: why do they predict health and longevity?') will be completed at the beginning of 2000.

Possible interventions

The two components in reducing transport-related inequalities in health and well-being – improving public transport services and decreasing car dependency – are inextricably linked. Unless public transport can be seen as an attractive alternative to the car, significant changes in the patterns of car use are unlikely. However, some of the requirements for improving public transport (particularly buses) – greater punctuality and speed of travel – are dependent on reducing the number of cars (parked as well as moving) on the roads. Furthermore, without such a reduction, cycling is likely to remain a minor mode of transport. It is therefore essential that measures to improve public transport and to decrease car dependency proceed in parallel.

Policy   **Development of an integrated public transport system in urban and rural areas which will include reliable connections between bus and rail services, and provision for cycle, as well as car, parking at transport intersections and work places. (In its *20th report*, the RCEP discusses in detail the requirements of an integrated public transport system [RCEP, 1997].) This will encourage a decrease in car dependency and so reduce accident risks to pedestrians and cyclists.**

Possible interventions for policy implementation

Measures to improve local bus services:

- legislation to allow local authorities greater control over the routes and frequency of privatised bus services;
- central government support for less profitable bus routes (fuel duty rebate to operators and grants to local authorities to subsidise such routes or to provide community buses);
- local authorities to be allowed to keep revenue from, for example, motoring fines, to use for promotion of alternative modes of transport, including by means of subsidies;

- encouragement of supermarket free-bus schemes or subsidies;
- wider adoption of low-threshold buses to improve accessibility and extension of transport helper, dial-a-ride and taxi-voucher schemes for disabled people.

Measures to decrease car dependency: once a substantial increase in the use of (improved) public transport has been established, greater stability of fares may provide an economic incentive for switching from private cars to public bus/train services. Initially, however, disincentives will be necessary:

- regular increases in fuel tax (with protection of those on low incomes in rural areas where car use is essential);
- abolition of tax benefits for company cars; abolition of free car parking at work;
- increase in rush-hour parking charges in urban centres;
- restrictions on single-occupant car access to major city centres during rush hours;
- stricter enforcement of parking laws;
- provision of adequate car-parking facilities at bus/ train intersections and adoption of public transport routes and schedules to meet passenger needs;
- improved provision of jobs and services in villages and small towns.

Measures to decrease road traffic accidents involving pedestrians and cyclists and to promote cycling and walking as modes of travelling. In addition to reducing the number of cars on the road:

- wider use of video cameras for enforcing speed limits;
- greater use of traffic-calming measures in residential areas;
- wider adoption and enforcement of 20 mph speed limits in high-density residential areas and pedestrian routes to schools;
- introduction of 'safe zones', with a speed limit of 10 mph, in deprived housing areas with no access to play areas;

- make drivers more aware of their responsibility to drive with greater care when children are around;
- continue road-safety awareness campaigns for parents and children, particularly targeting areas with a high proportion of social class IV and V residents and ethnic minorities;
- greater provision of monitored and traffic-calmed 'safe routes' to encourage children's unaccompanied walking to school;
- encourage parents who accompany their children to school to adopt alternative means of travel to their own car (eg car sharing, public transport, walking);
- greater priority for needs of pedestrians: clean, safe pavements; adequate pedestrian-operated traffic lights for road crossing; traffic-calmed safe routes linking residential areas with local shops and buses, and so on;
- provision of networks of designated cycle tracks, with priority for cyclists at traffic lights and roundabouts.

Evidence for benefits from proposed interventions to reduce transport-related inequalities

Benefits to health

Fewer cars: When traffic severance measures were introduced in urban redevelopment in Coventry, 'rat-run' traffic was reduced by 68% and this was accompanied by a 50% reduction in accidents, particularly to children (King et al, 1987). When the New Zealand government introduced restrictions on car use (because of the energy crisis) there was a 46.4% reduction in child pedestrian mortality (Roberts et al, 1987).

Slower cars: Introduction of (200) 20 mph zones resulted in a 70% reduction in child pedestrian accidents and a 48% reduction for child cyclists. For each one mile per hour reduction there was a 6.2% decrease in accidents (MacKie et al, 1993; Transport Research Laboratory, 1996). A study in Birmingham (Lawson, 1990) showed that in almost half of the fatal accidents involving young pedestrians, drivers were exceeding the speed limit.

Targeting traffic management to deprived areas would reduce the socio-economic inequalities in child pedestrian deaths.

Road safety education: Children's behaviour on the road can be altered by training – particularly in small groups in real situations (O'Reilly, 1993) – but there is evidence that children and parents in social classes IV and V may have less understanding of the risks. This is especially the case for ethnic minorities where language difficulties may exist (RoSPA, 1993). In Birmingham Asian pedestrians under nine years of age were more than twice as likely to be killed on the road as their white counterparts (Lawson, 1990). The need to involve disadvantaged communities in setting the agenda for local action has been stressed in other contexts, but is also true for road safety measures.

Road safety should be a compulsory component in the school curriculum, as it is in other European countries, where child pedestrian death rates are lower (Harland et al, 1996).

There is little evidence of benefit from campaigns to make speeding as socially unacceptable as drinking and driving (see earlier).

Decrease in car dependency: Apart from the benefits associated with a reduction in the number of cars on the road, a switch to public transport would result in fewer accidents since buses are much safer. They are involved in far fewer (about 15-fold) fatal accidents or serious injuries to pedestrians and cyclists than cars (DETR, 1997c, Table 23) (see Tables 10(a) and 10(b). However, motorists are unlikely to switch from use of their own cars and strong disincentives will be needed. In the past, a 10% increase in the price of petrol has only produced a 3% decrease in consumption (DoT, 1994). Hence the tougher measures suggested here.

Cycling and walking: People are put off cycling and walking because of the risk of accidents. Fewer/slower cars, together with the provision of segregated cycle tracks and pedestrian-friendly traffic management schemes, would encourage the adoption of these healthier modes of travelling (Cyclists' Touring Club/Pedestrians' Association, 1995) which would be of particular benefit to lower income groups. These measures would also facilitate increased mobility of elderly and disabled people, and

Table 10(a): Pedestrians killed, seriously injured (1995)

Colliding vehicle	Single-vehicle accident (SVA)	Multiple-vehicle accident	Total	%	Vehicle casualties in SVA	Pedestrian casualties over vehicle casualties
Pedal cycle	93	11	104	0.8	20	5.2
Motorcycle	381	36	417	3.4	65	6.4
Car	9,627	683	10,310	83.9	88	117.2
Bus or coach	405	619	424	3.4	10	42.4
Light goods	544	69	613	5.0	6	102.2
Heavy goods	248	43	219	2.4	5	58.2
Other	112	6	118	1.0	2	59.0
Total	**11,424**	**869**	**12,293**	**100.0**	**196**	**62.7**

Table 10(b): Cyclists killed, seriously injured (1995)

Colliding vehicle	Single-vehicle accident (SVA)	Multiple-vehicle accident	Total	%	Vehicle casualties in SVA	Pedestrian casualties over vehicle casualties
Pedal cycle	43	12	55	1.5	–	–
Motorcycle	63	11	74	2.1	34	2.2
Car	2,681	131	2,992	83.1	50	59.8
Bus or coach	49	3	52	1.4	3	17.3
Light goods	192	6	198	5.5	3	66.0
Heavy goods	162	11	173	4.8	5	34.6
Other	34	5	39	1.1	3	13.0
Total	**3,406**	**194**	**3,600**	**100.0**	**98**	**36.7**

Source: BMA (1997, Tables 5 and 6); DoT (1996d); Crown Copyright

young children – who have particular difficulty in crossing roads under heavy traffic conditions (Hine and Russell, 1996).

Improved local bus services: The problems and needs of rural and urban lower income groups, dependent on public transport (especially local buses) are described earlier. Many of the suggested interventions are concerned with mitigating the adverse impacts of deregulation.

Necessary improvements include changes in affordability and accessibility as well as in routes and frequency. The British Medical Association's report (1997), *Road transport and health*, quotes evidence from Yorkshire, that an increase in distance travelled by bus occurred when fares were frozen (Nicholl et al, 1987) and, after deregulation, when bus fares rose by 250%, there was a reduction in bus journeys, particularly among unemployed and elderly people (Hamilton et al, 1991). Similar evidence exists for the effect of fares on passenger journeys in London

and other English metropolitan areas (DETR, 1997a). The British Medical Association report stresses the importance of mobility for social contact, as well as access to basic services, for health and well-being, particularly of vulnerable groups such as elderly people (Fox, 1988; Hamilton et al, 1991). The inadequacy/inaccessibility of public transport for disabled people is well documented (GL ADP, 1996).

Cost benefits

Improving public transport to reduce inequalities in health can be cost-effective. The decline in social networking caused by inadequate local bus services results in an increase in requests for statutory domiciliary services (Sheffield City Council, 1986). The potential cross-sector benefits of improving accessibility for disabled people have been estimated to be between £256m and £1,161m (1990-91) – as a result of decreasing costs of domiciliary care and of state benefits by enabling travel for training and possible employment (Fowkes et al, 1994). A

Transport Research Laboratory report (Fowkes et al, 1994) states that, given the reasonably low cost of providing accessible transport, there could be cross-sector benefits of between £30,000 and £40,000 per annum (1991) for 1,000 people.

In one study, difficulties in travelling was the reason given for not applying for jobs by one third of the unemployed people in two Oxfordshire villages (Root et al, 1996).

Road traffic accidents: The annual cost of child pedestrian accidents is over half a billion pounds (Harland et al, 1996), so there is considerable potential for cost benefits from interventions to reduce the number of speeding cars. In its *20th Report* (RCEP, 1997) the RCEP quotes two estimates for the annual cost of road accidents (at 1994 prices): £4.5-7.5bn (Newbery, 1995) and £2.9-9.4bn (Maddison et al, 1996). These estimates are for all road traffic accidents, not just fatal accidents involving children and male adults, for which socio-economic gradients are documented. The measures suggested for decreasing inequalities in premature deaths from road accidents would result in an overall decrease.

A correlation has been demonstrated between low bus fares and a decrease in road traffic accidents, and vice versa. An increase in fares in London in 1982 was associated with an increase in accidents, at a cost of £20m (Controller of Transport and Development, 1983). Subsidising fares may therefore be a cost-effective measure.

Other cost benefits: Revenue would accrue from, for example, proposed changes in taxation of petrol and company cars; also from motoring fines and municipal parking charges. These revenues could offset the costs of improving alternative modes of transport to the car, including subsidies.

Conclusion

Government departments tend not to see the problem of transport-related inequalities as a whole, but to separate costs (for the DETR, of interventions) from cost-savings (for the Department of Health, from benefits to health and well-being). An integrated approach would make clearer the

likely overall budgetary benefits from tackling these inequalities.

Acknowledgements

Thank you to Dr Brenda Boardman of the Enviromnental Change Unit, University of Oxford, for information about transport in rural areas. Also to Lisa Bostock (forthcoming PhD: 'It's catch-22 all the time' for information on mothers' experiences of caring for pre-school children on low incomes in the 1990's and Chapter 5: 'Caring routines in disadvantaged circumstances').

Notes

[1] Using the World Health Organisation definition of health: not merely the absence of disease or disability but complete physical, psychological and social well-being.

[2] Unless otherwise states, transport refers to road transport.

References

Bentham, G. and Haynes, R. (1985) 'Health, personal mobility and the use of health services in rural Norfolk', *Journal of Rural Studies*, vol 1, no 3, pp 231-9.

BMA (British Medical Association) (1997) 'Health impacts of road transport', Chapter 4 in *Road transport and health*, London: BMA.

Christie, N. (1995a) *The high risk child pedestrian: Socio-economic and environmental factors in their accidents*, Project report 117, Crowthorne: Transport Research Laboratory.

Christie, N. (1995b) *Social, economic and environmental factors in child pedestrian accidents: A research review*, Project Report 116, Crowthorne: TRL.

Confederation of Passenger Transport (1997) *Facts '97*, London: Confederation of Passenger Transport.

Controller of Transport and Development (1983) *Report to the Transport Commission of the GLC*, Item T937, London, October.

Cyclists' Touring Club/Pedestrians' Association (1995) *Joint statement on providing for walking and cycling as transport and travel*, Godalming: Cyclist's Touring Club.

DETR (Department of the Environment, Transport and the Regions) (1997a) *Bus and coach statistics, Great Britain 1996/97*, London: HMSO.

DETR (1997b) *Vehicle speeds in Great Britain 1996*, London: HMSO.

DETR (1997c) *Road accidents Great Britain 1996 – The casualty report*, London: HMSO.

Di Giuseppi, C. and Roberts, I. (1997) 'Child and adolescent injury mortality', *Injury Prevention*, vol 3, pp 47-9.

DoT (Department of Transport) (1994) *18th Report: Transport and the environment*, Evidence to RCEP, London: HMSO.

DoT (1995) *National travel survey, 1992/94*, London: HMSO.

DoT (1996a) *Transport statistics Great Britain, 1995*, London: HMSO.

DoT (1996b) *National Travel Survey 1993/95: Transport statistics report*, London: HMSO.

DoT (1996c) *National Cycling Strategy*, London: DoT.

DoT (1996d) *Road safety casualty reduction: Targeting the future*, London: DoT.

ESRC Transport Studies Unit, Oxford University and RDC Inc (1995) *Car dependence*, A report for the RAC Foundation for Motoring and the Environment, RAC.

Fletcher, A. et al (1997) *Socio-economic and demographic circumstances in middle aged and older people and subsequent health outcomes*, Office for National Statistics Longitudinal Study, Update 17, London.

Fowkes, A., Oxley, P. and Helsen, B. (1994) *Cross-sector benefits of accessible public transport*, Cranfield: University School of Management.

Fox, J. (1988) 'Social network interaction: new jargon in health inequalities', *British Medical Journal*, no 297, pp 373-4.

GLADP (Greater London Association of Disabled People) (1996) *All change 2000*, London: GLADP.

Hamilton, K., Jenkins, L. and Gregory, A. (1991) *Women and transport: Bus deregulation in West Yorkshire*, Bradford: University of Bradford.

Harland, G. (1996) 'Research into vulnerable road users: planning for safer child pedestrians', Paper presented to Federation of Road Safety Research Institutions conference, Crowthorne: TRL.

Hine, J. and Russell, J. (1996) 'The impact of traffic on pedestrian behaviour: assessing the traffic barrier on radial routes', *Traffic Engineering and Control*, vol 32, no 2, pp 81-5.

King, D.M. et al (1987) 'Child pedestrian accidents in inner areas: patterns and treatment', PTRC Summer Annual Meeting, Seminar D, University of Bath.

Lawson, S. (1990) 'Accidents to young pedestrians: distribution, circumstances, consequences and scope for counter measures', Foundation for Road Safety Research.

Macintyre, S., Maciver, S. and Soomans, A. (1993) 'Area, class and health: should we be focusing on places or people?', *Journal of Social Policy*, vol 22, no 2, pp 213-34.

MacKie, A.M. et al (1993) 'Traffic calming: the design and effectiveness of 20 mph zones', London: Public Transport Research and Computation.

Maddison, D. et al (1996) *Blueprint 5: The true costs of road transport*, London: Earthscan Publications Limited.

Newbery, D.M. (1995) 'Royal Commission Report on Transport and the Environment: economic effects of recommendations', *Economic Travel*, 105, September.

Nicholl, J., Freeman, M. and Williams, B. (1987) 'Effects of subsidising bus travel on the occurence of road traffic casualties', *Journal of Epidemiology and Community Health*, vol 41, pp 50-4.

ONS (Office for National Statistics) (1997) *Social Trends 27*, London: HMSO.

O'Reilly, D. (1993) 'Child pedestrian safety in Great Britain', in DoT, *Road accidents Great Britain 1993*, London: HMSO.

Piachaud, D. and Webb, J. (1996) *The price of food: Missing out on mass consumption*, London: Suntory and Toyota International Centre for Economics and Related Disciplines/London School of Economics.

RCEP (Royal Commission on Envrionmental Pollution) (1997) *20th Report: Transport and the environment – Developments since 1994*, London: The Stationery Office.

Roberts, I. and Power, C. (1996) 'Does the decline in child injury mortality vary by social class?', *British Medical Journal*, no 313, pp 784-6.

Roberts, I. et al (1987) 'Child pedestrian mortality and traffic volume in New Zealand', *British Medical Journal*, no 305, p 283.

Roberts, I., Norton, R. and Taua, B. (1996) 'Child pedestrian injury rates: the importance of "exposure to risk" relating to socio-economic and ethnic differences, in Auckland, New Zealand', *Journal of Epidemiology and Community Health*, vol 50, pp 162-5.

Root, A., Broadman, B. and Fielding, W.J. (1996) *Rural travel and transport corridors (interim report). Sustainable mobility and access in rural transport*, Energy and Environment Programme, Oxford: Environmental Change Unit, University of Oxford.

RoSPA (Royal Society for the Prevention of Accidents) (1993) *Safety and minority ethnic communities*, RoSPA.

Rural Development Commission (1995) *1994 Survey of rural services*, Salisbury: RDC.

Scottish Office Central Research Unit (1996) Development Department Research Programme, Research Findings No 19 and No 27.

Sharples, P.M., Stoey, A., Aynsley-Green, A. and Eyre, J. (1990) 'Causes of fatal childhood accidents involving head injury in the Northern Region 1976-86', *British Medical Journal*, no 301, pp 1193-7.

Sheffield City Council (1986) *The bus booklet*, Sheffield: Sheffield City Council.

Stevenson, M., Jamrozik, K. and Spittle, J. (1995) 'A case-control study of traffic risk factors and child pedestrian injury', *International Journal of Epidemiology*, vol 24, pp 959-64.

Stokes, G. (1995) Papers on rural transport for the Transport Studies Unit, University of Oxford.

Townsend, P. and Davidson, N. (eds) (1982) *Inequalities in health: The Black Report*, London: Penguin Books.

Transport Research Laboratory (1996) *Review of traffic calming schemes in 20 mph zones*, Report No 215, Crowthorne: TRL.

14

Gender

Sara Arber

Executive summary

The health experiences of women are different from those of men. Women and men have differing patterns of mortality and morbidity, and differing roles in the provision of health and social care. These differences primarily reflect gender roles relating to the social, cultural and economic circumstances of women's and men's lives. It is essential that the health service is sensitive to how gender roles affect health and the ways in which changes in gender roles over time relate to health needs.

Policy recommendations

1 **There is a greater need for gender sensitivity and awareness in all aspects of healthcare provision.** This would be assisted by policies which:
   - increased the proportion of women in positions of influence within trusts and commissioning bodies;
   - made health services staff at all levels more aware of gender issues and how these relate to health needs through training programmes and publicity material.

2 **There is a need to monitor healthcare provision to ensure equality for men and women with equivalent conditions, for example, in treatment for heart disease. This policy would be assisted by:**
   - the routine collection and reporting of statistics separately for men and women.
   - all clinical trials and epidemiological investigations including women as well as men

(except for those relating to reproductive medicine).

3 **Policies should be designed to reduce the high mortality of men in youth and young adulthood, especially in areas of economic deprivation:**
   - policies which reduce unemployment, poverty and urban deprivation are of particular relevance.

4 **Older women suffer considerably more functional impairment because of chronic ill-health than older men. Policies should be adopted which minimise the adverse effects of such impairments, so reducing the likelihood that older women will become dependent and socially isolated.**
   Policies need to:
   - provide an adequate income for older women, preferably through increasing the basic state pension to above the Income Support level. Only a quarter of older women have any form of non-state pension, and this situation is unlikely to improve for the next generation of older women;
   - increase public expenditure on transportation, health and social care. Cuts in these areas of service provision hit older women harder than older men, both because of older women's lower income and because older women are more likely to live alone and therefore have to rely on more distant relatives or the state to provide care to enable them to continue to live in the community.

5 **There is a need for more research on inequalities in women's health and inequalities in the health of older people.** Evidence presented suggests that socio-economic inequalities are almost as great among men and women in their seventies and eighties as among those in mid-life:

- data should routinely be collected on the individual's last main occupation for men and women of *all* ages in surveys and the Census;
- other measures of socio-economic status should be routinely collected and analysed, such as highest educational qualifications and employment status.

6 **There has been a lack of concern about health promotion issues relating to older women and men:**

- policies are needed which emphasise the promotion of healthy life-styles among older people. These should be targeted at all levels of health practitioners, as well as through media campaigns.

Evidence for each of the above policies is provided in this chapter, using section numbers which correspond to the policy recommendations identified above.

Introduction

The topic of *gender* in relation to inequalities in health is exceptionally large and potentially overlaps with aspects included in all the input papers. This report identifies six issues relating to gender which are of particular importance for addressing inequalities in health.

1 Gender sensitivity in health service provision

The health experiences of women are different from those of men. Women and men have differing patterns of mortality and morbidity, and have different roles in the provision of health and social care. These differences primarily reflect gender roles relating to the social, cultural and economic circumstances of women's and men's lives. It is essential that health service practitioners are sensitive to how gender roles affect health and the ways in which changes in gender roles over time impact on changing health needs. A prerequisite is gender-sensitive planning which is informed by the needs of all users.

Biological (or sex) differences and healthcare provision

The provision of health services should build on a clear understanding of both the biological and social differences between women and men and the impact these differences have on their health needs. Hitherto, the health service has primarily paid attention to biological differences. Attention to women's distinctive reproductive system has resulted in extensive specialised services focusing on women's reproductive needs, including childbirth, contraceptive services, abortion and infertility services. The welcome establishment of 'well woman' clinics has largely developed around women's distinctive biology, including screening programmes associated with women's reproductive organs (such as breast and cervical screening). There has been much less specialist health attention focused on men's distinctive reproductive biology, and little parallel development of 'well men' clinics or screening for prostate or testicular cancer.

Gender and healthcare needs

There has been little awareness among healthcare providers of the ways in which social, cultural and economic differences between women and men affect needs for healthcare and the ways in which health services are used (Doyal, 1998). It is important to understand how women's and men's health experiences are intricately intertwined. Gender roles and relationships affect both women's and men's health outcomes. Examples include violence against women, the unpaid family caring undertaken by women (which may be absent for men without a partner), the lack of economic resources of lone mothers and the effect this has on the health of their children, the ways in which unemployment of young men affects their self-identity and adverse psychological effects when it is not possible to take on a 'breadwinning role'.

To take just one example, women provide major caring roles for their children and partners, both in health and in sickness. Caring for frail or disabled relatives has been shown to place a major burden on carers, which may have both physical and mental health consequences (Braithwaite, 1990; Taylor et al, 1995). The contribution of unpaid carers at home is becoming increasingly significant within healthcare provision, as length of stay in hospital has shortened, shifting the costs of care to the private domain of the family. Parallel to the adverse health and financial costs of caring are the difficulties faced by men and women who live alone, and therefore do not have a potential carer living in the same household. Men living alone face added problems because they are less likely to maintain good contact with family members than women (Arber and Ginn, 1991). On average men have different sorts of friendships compared to women, and these may be less easy to rely on in times of ill-health.

A gendered approach is needed which sees both women's and men's health within the wider context of relations between women and men. The failure to think of men's bodies and illnesses as sexed has been bad for men's health as well as for women's. Thus, the health system has failed to take gender seriously (Doyal, 1998). Rather than focusing on women's health issues, such as breast cancer, and men's health issues, such as prostate cancer, there is a need to be sensitive to the health impacts of gender and the gender impacts of ill-health. Thus, planning and provision of healthcare with greater gender sensitivity and awareness will benefit both men and women in better meeting their health needs.

2 Lack of attention to women in mainstream healthcare and clinical research

Women's health issues have been dominated by a concern with reproductive healthcare. There has been a relative lack of attention devoted to women in mainstream areas of health, for example, in clinical research and the failure to audit gender differences in treatment procedures and outcomes.

In epidemiological research and clinical trials in many mainstream areas of healthcare, there has been a failure to include women in sufficient numbers. In some studies, women have been excluded altogether (Sharp, 1994; Rosser, 1994), for example, in research on coronary heart disease and on AIDs.

Older people have also been excluded from epidemiological studies and trials of clinical interventions. The MRC (1994) found a lack of medical knowledge about to what extent older people benefit from various procedures, because they have largely been excluded from clinical trials. This has an adverse effect on the healthcare of older people because clinicians are more likely to make inappropriate decisions due to lack of available research evidence. The MRC recommended that research studies in the future should have no upper age limit and that chronological age should not be used as a proxy for biological fitness.

With the move to greater 'evidence-based medicine', it is essential that research evidence is based on trials which include both women and men, and trials which involve all age groups. For example, there may be gender and age differences in appropriate diagnostic procedures and therapeutic outcomes in relation to coronary heart disease (Sharp, 1994).

An important issue is the extent to which men and women with the *same* medical conditions are treated differently; for example, there is evidence that women with coronary artery disease are less likely to be offered coronary artery bypass operations or angioplasty (Petticrew et al, 1993; Sharp, 1994), and women in the US with kidney failure are less likely to receive a kidney transplant than men. Researchers need to assess whether there is sex discrimination in the provision of medical procedures and treatments. Thus clinical audit should pay attention to differences in treatment between men and women, and routinely collect and present data separately for men and women.

3 Gender inequalities in mortality

There is a vast literature on gender inequalities in mortality and morbidity, how these trends have changed over time and to what extent they vary across the life-course. In this brief review it is impossible to do justice to this extensive literature, so I will simply highlight some key issues.

It is well known that women outlive men, and that the gender difference in expectation of life this century had increased to over six years by 1971. Since then it has fallen somewhat to 5.2 years in 1992 (ONS, 1996). Men's higher mortality rate occurs at all ages across the life-course, and is particularly pronounced in youth and early adulthood, for example, the death rate is 2.8 times higher for men than women aged 20-24 (see Table 1).

Table 1: Death rates per 1,000 for men and women by age group, England and Wales (1995)

Age group	Men	Women	Sex ratio* men/women
Under 1 year	6.9	5.3	1.30
1-4	0.3	0.2	1.12
5-9	0.2	0.1	1.33
10-14	0.2	0.1	1.43
15-19	0.6	0.3	2.11
20-24	0.9	0.3	2.81
25-34	1.0	0.4	2.13
35-44	1.7	1.0	1.58
45-54	4.0	2.7	1.49
55-64	12.2	7.3	1.67
65-74	35.9	21.3	1.69
75-84	88.8	56.6	1.57
85+	194.3	151.8	1.28

Note: * calculated from exact death rates.

Source: Derived from ONS (1996, Tables 6 and 7)

Gender differences in mortality in youth and early adulthood largely reflect social and cultural differences between men and women. This can be seen from the cause-specific mortality rates of men and women (see Table 2). Men from age 15 to 44 have a three to four times higher mortality rate from accidents and from suicide/violence than women. Thus policies to reduce gender differences in mortality in youth and early adulthood must address the social and cultural roles, and risk-taking behaviour of men. Men have a much higher mortality rate from AIDS than women, but in 1992 AIDS accounted for under 5% of male deaths at age 30-34 and a smaller proportion among other age groups.

A key concern of the Independent Inquiry should be that over the past 20 years, when mortality rates have fallen for women across the age range, there has been an increase in the mortality rate of men aged 25-39 (see Table 2 and Figure 1). This increase for young adult men was previously reported by Dunnell (1991).

Table 2: Standardised mortality rates per 100,000 for five-year age groups from 15-44 in 1992, and change between 1982 and 1992, men and women in the UK

	15-19	20-24	25-29	30-34	35-39	40-44
All causes						
Men 1992	63	86	88	102	142	206
Change 1982-92	–18	–3	+2	+1	+6	–32
Women 1992	28	33	37	52	83	133
Change 1982-92	–2	–2	–6	–10	–11	–24
Accidents						
Men 1992	29	33	25	23	20	22
Change 1982-92	–19	–12	–5	–3	–4	–4
Women 1992	9	8	5	6	6	7
Change 1982-92	–3	–2	–2	–1	–1	0
Suicides/violence						
Men 1992	11	27	27	26	27	28
Change 1982-92	+3	+10	+6	+5	+6	+5
Women 1992	4	7	8	7	8	9
Change 1982-92	+1	+1	0	–1	–2	-2

Source: Derived from Tickle (1996, Tables 10 and 11)

Figure 1: Improvement in mortality rate 1982 to 1992 (% of 1982 rate) by age in five-year bands for UK males and females

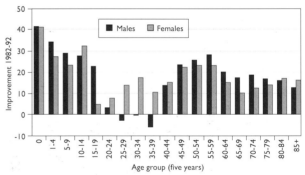

Source: Tickle (1996, Figure 3); Crown Copyright

There has been less improvement in men's mortality rate in areas of economic deprivation, such as Manchester, Liverpool and inner London, than in more affluent areas, such as Surrey. In addition, the gender difference in mortality is smaller in areas of relative affluence and greater in the most economically deprived areas. Raleigh and Kiri (1997), based on a comparison of life expectancy in district health authority (DHA) areas in 1984-86 and 1992-94, report a gender differential in life expectancy of 4.8 years in Cambridge (81.4 for women and 76.6 for men) compared with 6.8 years for Manchester (76.7 for women and 69.9 for men). They show that the average gender differential in life expectancy for the five DHAs with the highest male expectation of life was 4.7 years compared with 6.8

years for the five DHAs with the lowest male expectation of life. The latter DHAs comprised Manchester, Liverpool and three inner London DHAs. Thus, gender differences in mortality are greatest in areas of economic deprivation, with high levels of unemployment and urban degeneration. Living in such areas is likely to affect the economic and cultural roles of men with resulting adverse health consequences.

Gender differences in morbidity

In the past it was assumed that women reported higher levels of morbidity than men, and research addressed the apparent paradox of men's higher mortality rate but women's higher rate of morbidity (eg Nathanson, 1977). However, more recent survey data suggest that gender differences in global measures of health and well-being are relatively modest, and of much less importance than hitherto thought (Macintyre et al, 1996, 1999). Even among the oldest age groups, there is little difference in the proportion of older men and women who rate their health as 'good' (see Figure 2).

Figure 2: Percentage of men and women reporting good health by age

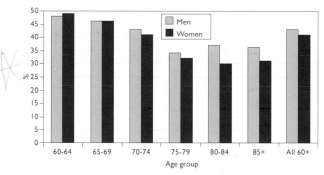

Source: General Household Survey, 1992/93, 1993/94, 1994/95 (authors' analysis)

However, despite the lack of gender difference in global measures of ill-health, there are major differences in certain areas, particularly in mental health and well-being (Macintyre et al, 1996). Women are more likely to report a range of conditions reflecting poor mental health, for example, anxiety and depressive disorders, but men report much higher rates of alcohol and drug dependence (Miles, 1991). These gender differences relate to the social and cultural roles of men and women. Recent increases in alcohol and cigarette consumption by women reflect changes in gender role expectations.

4 Gender differences in functional disability and need for care

Despite the lack of gender difference on global measures of ill-health, women are severely disadvantaged in terms of their greater level of functional disability, especially at older ages (Martin et al, 1988).

Good health is essential to independence, especially the individual's capacity to carry out personal self-care, such as bathing, eating, negotiating stairs and walking outside the home. Chronic illness and disability tend to restrict the individual's independence, as well as generating extra costs for a special diet, additional heating, laundry, or nursing care. People with higher levels of functional disability or cognitive impairment will require more practical support and personal care from either informal carers or the state.

Older women are more likely than older men to suffer from conditions which are non-fatal but result in chronic and disabling illnesses hindering their activities of daily living. The 1994 General Household Survey showed that older women were more likely to experience restrictions of mobility, self-care and ability to perform household tasks than older men (Bennett et al, 1996; see Table 3). Under a fifth of men over 85 were unable to go out and walk down the road, compared with nearly half of the women. Under 10% of men over 85 were unable to go up and downstairs, compared with 29% of women. By combining together six measures of functional impairment (ability to get up and down stairs, walking outside, getting around the house, ability to bath or wash oneself, to cut toenails and to get in and out of bed), we show that in 1994, nearly twice as many women as men over 65 suffered from functional impairments sufficient to require help on a daily basis to remain living in the community – 15% of women and 8.5% of men (Arber and Cooper, 1999). Figure 3 shows that this gender difference in 'severe disability' occurs for each age group of older people, but is particularly stark at ages above 85, among whom nearly 40% of women and 21% of men suffer from severe impairment.

Table 3: Gender differences in % unable to perform various activities of daily living by age group, 65+

	65-69	70-74	75-79	80-84	85+	65+
a) *Going out and walking down the road*						
Men	4	6	8	18	18	8
Women	9	10	16	23	44	16
b) *Going up and down stairs*						
Men	6	4	5	8	9	5
Women	5	9	11	16	29	11
c) *Bathing, washing all over*						
Men	3	5	6	12	17	6
Women	5	7	9	15	23	10
d) *Household shopping*						
Men	7	7	9	21	26	10
Women	7	14	23	29	55	21

Source: Derived from Bennett et al (1996, Tables 6.23, 6.28 and 6.30)

Figure 3: Percentage reporting severe disability by age and sex

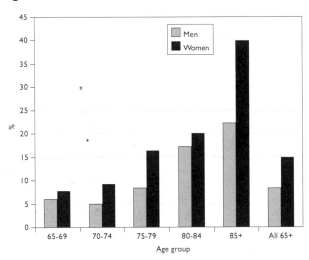

Source: General Household Survey, 1994/95 (authors' analysis)

A key concern of the health service should be to minimise the adverse effects of functional impairment, and maximise the ability of older women and men to live independently. Thus, older women have a far greater threat to their quality of life because of their higher level of functional impairment. This threat can be reduced if financial resources are sufficient to provide aids and adaptations, run a car or take taxis rather than rely on public transport, and so on. However, older women are more likely to live in poverty than older men (Arber and Ginn, 1991; Ginn and Arber, 1991).

Income is vital to the health of older people. Not only is it necessary to provide the basic health needs of heating, an adequate diet and decent housing, but it is also increasingly important because of the need to pay for social and healthcare. An adequate income maximises the likelihood of an older person remaining autonomous and independent within a given level of functional impairment, by allowing the purchase of home aids and adaptations, moving to more suitable accommodation, or paying for private transportation when required. Cutbacks in public transportation have had particularly adverse effects on older women, because they are less likely to drive. Even if they can drive, most older women have insufficient financial resources to run a car.

Government policies since 1979 have had negative consequences for the income of older people, especially women. The state National Insurance pension since 1980 has been uprated in line with prices instead of earnings. This has led to a decline in the real value of the state pension, which is worth only 16% of average male earnings, and is projected to fall to only 10% by 2021 (Evandrou and Falkingham, 1993). In 1997, the state pension was £5,187pa for a married couple and £3,247pa for a single older person. This was below the means-tested Income Support level, so older people who only have a state pension are by definition in poverty. Older women are more adversely affected than men, because most are solely reliant on the state pension. Two thirds of older men also have an occupational or personal pension, but this is the case for only a quarter of older women (Arber and Ginn, 1994).

The greater the movement towards individual provision for retirement through occupational and personal pensions, the greater will be the income inequality between older women and men and between those with an intermittent, or low paid employment history and those with an advantaged position in the labour market. Current government policies relating to pensions are leading to growing inequality among older people, linked to their previous occupation and the continuity of their employment career. Thus the opportunities to enjoy a Third Age of health and autonomous action are likely to become increasingly gendered, as well as class-divided, with financial dependency acting as an obstacle to citizenship rights (Arber and Ginn, 1995).

Gender differences in access to social care

Changes in community care policies in the early 1990s made it more difficult for older people to obtain local authority-funded residential care and home care (Walker, 1993). Although, such policies are put forward as gender-neutral, they have greater adverse effects on older women. Older men not only have more financial resources to pay for care, but are more likely to be married and have a wife who can provide care should they need it, whereas older women tend to live alone (Arber and Ginn, 1991, 1995).

Older people with severe functional disability need help with activities of daily living or personal self-care on a daily basis. Older disabled women are twice as likely as men with a comparable level of disability to live alone (see Table 4), and therefore are more reliant on family members living elsewhere, other informal carers in the community, and state-provided domiciliary services. Nearly two thirds of severely disabled older men can rely on support/care provided by their wife (Table 4).

Table 4: Household structure by disability level of men and women, aged 65+

	Not disabled (0-5)		Severe disability (6-8)		Very severe disability (9-12)	
	Men	**Women**	**Men**	**Women**	**Men**	**Women**
Lives alone	24	48	27	60	22	40
Lives with spouse	61	37	63	20	62	33
Lives with others	15	15	10	20	16	27
	100%	100%	100%	100%	100%	100%
N =	1,312	1,725	91	196	32	106

Source: General Household Survey, 1994/95 (authors' analysis)

The greatest threat to an older person's autonomy and independence is generally considered to be entry into a nursing or residential home. The 1991 Census found that twice as many women as men over 65 lived in communal establishments, 3% of men and 6.4% of women (OPCS, 1993). This gender differential in communal residence is particularly pronounced over the age of 85, when 26% of women and 15% of men are residents (see Figure 4). Figure 5 shows that the greater proportion of older women than men living in residential settings

primarily reflects that more women are widowed, and so do not have a partner to provide care should they become disabled (Arber and Cooper, 1999).

Figure 4: Percentage of older men and women in communal establishments by age group (1991)

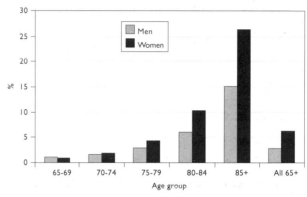

Source: Derived from OPCS (1993, Table 2)

Figure 5: Percentage of older men and women resident in communal establishments in 1991 by marital status and age group

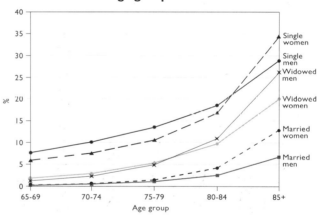

Source: OPCS (1993, derived from Table 2)

Although older women have a longer expectation of life than men, they also have more years in which they can expect to be disabled or live in a residential setting. The gender differential in disability means that older women are more likely to require both informal care and support from state health and welfare services (Arber and Ginn, 1991, 1992). Nearly half of disabled older women live alone, which, while promoting independence, means they are reliant on state domiciliary services, mainly home care services and community nurses. They are also heavily dependent on the unpaid work of relatives and other informal carers, and are more likely to enter residential care. Older women's disadvantage is compounded by their lower average income than that of older men; a poor deal for the majority of women who have spent a lifetime of unpaid work looking after children, husband and others, often in addition to waged work.

5 Gender differences in the nature of inequalities in health

Much research on inequalities in health focuses on men, with less attention devoted to inequalities in the health of women. Research on occupational and class differences in mortality, has been dominated by analyses of inequalities in mortality of men aged 20-64. Little attention has been paid to inequalities in the health of older people, which is particularly ironic given the greater health needs and ill-health of the older population. One reason for this relative neglect is that the conventional measures of class are often considered inapplicable for sections of the population that are not currently in paid employment (Rose and O'Reilly, 1997). However, our research (Arber and Ginn, 1993; Arber and Cooper, 1999) shows stark inequalities in health based on the last main occupation of women and men for each age group, including age 85 and over (see Figure 6).

Arber (1997a, 1997b) provides extensive evidence of the nature of health inequalities between men and women of working age and among older men and women. These papers argue for the importance of using a clear conceptual model of the relationship between socio-economic measures such as educational qualifications, occupational class, employment status and material resources (housing, car ownership and income) in order to fully understand inequalities in health. It is necessary to simultaneously analyse all these factors using multi-variate models, and when analysing women with partners to take into account both their own characteristics and the socio-economic characteristics of their partner.

It is essential to analyse inequalities in health for women as well as men, and for older people as well as people of working age. In this way it will be possible to understand whether different or similar factors influence inequalities in women's and men's health, and to what extent the socio-economic inequalities of working life are mirrored by parallel

Figure 6: Percentage reporting good health by social class and age

Men

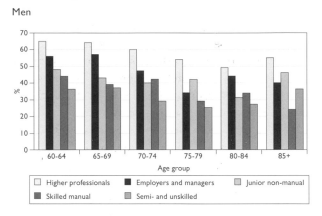

Women

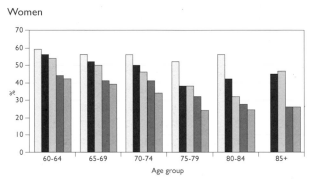

Source: General Household Survey, 1992/93, 1993/94, 1994/95 (authors' analysis)

inequalities in later life. The recommendation from Arber (1997a, 1997b) is that data on the individual's last main occupation should be collected for all people not currently in paid employment, and this should be used in analyses of inequalities in health among the non-employed.

6 Health promotion needs of older women and men

When considering the health of older people it is important to make explicit the nature and extent of gender differences in later life. The higher level of mortality of men than women at each age (Table 1) means that women became numerically dominant to a greater extent with advancing age. There are nearly 50% more women than men aged 65 and over, and by the age of 85, women outnumber men by nearly three to one. The stark gender differences in marital status also need to be continually borne in mind: half of older women are widowed, but this is the case for under a fifth of older men (Arber and Ginn, 1991, 1994).

Ageism within society has led to a tendency to consider older people as an homogenous group, emphasising their ill-health, disability and poverty. As well as the ageism inherent within contemporary society, it is important to consider whether health providers are explicitly or implicitly ageist in their priorities and policies, and if so, how this might have a differential effect on older women and men (Arber and Ginn, 1998). Henwood states "not only is there widespread discrimination against older people in the provision of healthcare, but they are also the victims of restricted assumptions about the quality of health care which can be expected in old age" (Henwood, 1990, p 43).

The provision of healthcare in the 1990s has been dominated by a concern to achieve the objectives specified in the *Health of the nation* document (DoH, 1992). However, this provides little comfort for older people, because the emphasis is on reducing 'premature death'. The main targets specify upper age limits, for example, to reduce rates of coronary heart disease (CHD) and stroke among those under 65 and 65-74, and to reduce lung cancer under the age of 75. Since CHD and stroke are the major causes of death among women and men over 75, it is anomalous and discriminatory that they are excluded from such targets. Only one target specifically mentions older people, and this is to reduce the death rate from accidents among people over 65. This target may be considered of particular benefit to the NHS, since setting broken bones and the rehabilitation costs following falls and accidents represents a significant part of NHS expenditure.

These restrictive assumptions about older people have also been prevalent in the Health Education Authority, for example, a recent survey of the health attitudes and life-styles of the general population (HEA, 1992) was restricted to the age range 16 to 74 years. Similarly, the HEA Health Education and Monitoring Survey (HEMS) has excluded people aged 75 and over (Bridgwood et al, 1996). The maximum age criterion used in these surveys is based on the implicit assumption that health promotion among people aged 75 and over is less relevant or not needed. Ginn et al (1997) challenge these restricted assumptions about the possibilities of

improving the health of all older people, which, given the numerical gender distribution in later life, affects women to a much greater extent than men.

References

Arber, S. (1997a) 'Comparing inequalities in women's and men's health: Britain in the 1990s', *Social Science and Medicine*, vol 44, no 6, pp 773-87.

Arber, S. (1997b) 'Insights about the non-employed, class and health: evidence from the General Household Survey', in D. Rose and K. O'Reilly (eds) *Constructing classes. Towards a new social classification for the UK*, Swindon: ESRC/ONS, pp 78-92.

Arber, S. and Cooper, H. (1999) 'Gender differences in health in later life: a new paradox?', *Social Science and Medicine*, vol 48, no 1, pp 63-78.

Arber, S. and Ginn, J. (1991) *Gender and later life: A sociological analysis of resources and constraints*, London: Sage Publications.

Arber, S. and Ginn, J. (1992) 'In sickness and in health: care-giving, gender and independence of elderly people', in C. Marsh and S. Arber (eds) *Families and households: Divisions and change*, London: Macmillan, pp 86-105.

Arber, S. and Ginn, J. (1993) 'Gender and inequalities in health in later life', *Social Science and Medicine*, vol 36, no 1, pp 33-46.

Arber, S. and Ginn, J. (1994) 'Women and ageing', *Reviews in Clinical Gerontology*, vol 4, pp 93-102.

Arber, S. and Ginn, J. (1995) *Connecting gender and ageing: A sociological approach*, Buckingham: Open University Press.

Arber, S. and Ginn, J. (1998) 'Health and illness in later life', in D. Field and S. Taylor (eds) *Sociological perspectives on health, illness and health care*, Oxford: Blackwell Scientific, pp 134-52.

Bennett, N., Jarvis, L., Rowlands, O., Singleton, N. and Haselden, L. (1996) *Living in Britain: Results from the 1994 General Household Survey*, OPCS, London: HMSO.

Braithwaite, V. (1990) *Bound to care*, Sydney: Allen and Unwin.

Bridgwood, A., Malbon, G., Lader, D. and Matheson, J. (1996) *Health in England 1995: What people know, what people think and what people do*, London: HEA.

DoH (Department of Health) (1992) *The health of the nation*, Cmd 1986, London: HMSO.

Doyal, L. (1998) *Women and health services: An agenda for change*, Buckingham: Open University Press.

Dunnell, K. (1991) 'Deaths among 15-44 year olds', *Population Trends, 64*, London: HMSO, pp 38-43.

Evandrou, M. and Falkingham, J. (1993) 'Social security and the life course: developing sensitive policy alternatives', in S. Arber and M. Evandrou (eds) *Ageing, independence and the life course*, London: Jessica Kingsley, pp 201-33.

Ginn, J. and Arber, S. (1991) 'Gender, class and income inequalities in later life', *British Journal of Sociology*, vol 42, no 3, pp 369-96.

Ginn, J., Arber, S., and Cooper, H. (1997) *Researching older people's health needs and health promotion issues*, London: HEA.

HEA (Health Education Authority) (1992) *Health and lifestyles survey*, London: HEA.

Henwood, M. (1990) 'No sense of urgency: age discrimination in health care', in E. McEwen (ed) *Age: The unrecognised discrimination*, London: Age Concern, pp 43-57.

Macintyre, S., Hunt, K. and Sweeting, H. (1996) 'Gender differences in health: are things really as simple as they seem?', *Social Science and Medicine*, vol 42, pp 617-24.

Macintyre, S., Ford, G. and Hunt, K. (1999) 'Do women "over-report" morbidity? Men's and women's responses to structured prompting on a standard question on long standing illness', *Social Science and Medicine*, vol 48, no 1, pp 89-98.

Martin, J., Meltzer, H. and Elliot, D. (1988) *The prevalence of disability among adults: Report 1*, London: HMSO.

Miles, A. (1991) *Women, health and medicine*, Buckingham: Open University Press.

MRC (Medical Research Council) (1994) *The health of the UK's elderly people*, London: MRC.

Nathanson, C. (1977) 'Sex, illness and medical care. A review of data, theory and method', *Social Science and Medicine*, vol 11, pp 13-25.

OPCS (Office of Population Censuses and Surveys) (1993) *Communal establishments, 1991 Population Census*, London: HMSO.

ONS (Office for National Statistics) (1996) *Population Trends, 86*, London: The Stationery Office.

Petticrew, M., McKee, M. and Jones, J. (1993) 'Coronary artery surgery: are women discriminated against?', *British Medical Journal*, vol 306, pp 1164-6.

Raleigh, V.S. and Kiri, V. (1997) 'Life expectancy in England: variations and trends by gender, health authority and level of deprivation', *Journal of Epidemiology and Community Health*, vol 51, no 6, pp 649-58.

Rose, D. and O'Reilly, K. (eds) (1997) *Constructing classes. Towards a new social classification for the UK*, Swindon: ESRC/ONS.

Rosser, S. (1994) 'Gender bias in clinical research: the difference it makes', in A. Dan (ed) *Reframing women's health: Multidisciplinary research and practice*, London: Sage Publications, pp 253-65.

Sharp, I. (1994) *Coronary heart disease: Are women special?*, London: National Heart Forum.

Taylor, R., Ford, G. and Dunbar, M. (1995) 'The effects of caring on health: a community-based longitudinal study', *Social Science and Medicine*, vol 40, no 10, pp 1407-15.

Tickle, L. (1996) 'Mortality trends in the United Kingdom, 1982 to 1992', *Population Trends, 86*, London: The Stationery Office.

Walker, A. (1993) 'Community care policy: from consensus to conflict', in J. Bornat, C. Pereira, D. Pilgrim and F. Williams (eds) *Community care: A reader*, London: Macmillan, pp 204-26.

15

Mental health

David Goldberg

The new government's 'Welfare to Work' programme, and the commitment to reducing extremes of poverty, will both – if effective – go a long way towards remedying the social class inequalities referred to in this document. The following five policy changes are now recommended.

Executive summary

Policy 1

Resource allocation formula to be adjusted to take account of much greater mental health needs of deprived inner-city areas. (At present, resource is imperfectly distributed according to mental health need – see Johnson et al, 1998). **Resource for mentally disordered offenders** to be removed from regional allocations and provided from top-sliced monies, otherwise inequities of provision in deprived inner-city areas are accentuated. It would also be helpful if the Department of Health now implemented their February 1996 directive in full: "24 hour nursed care for people with Severe and Enduring Mental Illness" (NHS Executive HSG (96)6/LASSL (96)16), since we know that about 30% of our present acute beds are used by long-term patients.

Inequality: poor services in socially deprived inner-city areas across country; unequal access to specialist mental healthcare across country: social class V, with highest rates, unlikely to be admitted unless suicidal or homicidal. Those with dementia, and those with neuroses and miscellaneous psychiatric disorders are less likely to be admitted in London. Conditions especially bad in socially deprived areas (Johnson et al, 1998; see Table 1).

Table 1: The diagnoses of hospitalised patients in inner London compared to other parts of the UK (%)

Diagnosis	Inner London	Other cities	Rest of country
Males			
Dementia	7.0	11.0	16.0
Schizophrenia and other psychosis	**50.0**	35.0	**29.0**
Neurosis and other psychiatric	18.0	29.0	**32.0**
Females			
Dementia	12.0	18.0	21.0
Schizophrenia and other psychosis	**41.0**	29.0	**30.0**
Neurosis and other psychiatric	**23.0**	32.0	**34.0**

Note: diagnoses without marked differences *not* shown; outer London nearly identical with 'Other cities' and therefore *not* shown.

Source: Derived from DoH data showing Finished Care Episodes by diagnosis for three parts of the country (Sylvia Kingaby, Mental Health Statistics, Dept 2C)

Likely benefits: overcrowding of wards, and long waits for basic items of service for those in deprived inner cities would be lessened; premature discharge of dangerous patients into the community would be reduced; higher quality community care might be made available; low morale and high staff burnout would be addressed so that problems of staffing the mental health services (all professions) would be addressed.

Evidence favouring effectiveness: waiting times, and overcrowding, is less evident in those services with a less striking mismatch between available resources and demand (Johnson et al, 1998).

Policy 2

Improve facilities for working women: greater use of flexible hours, more crèche facilities, equitable promotion for women. Greater flexibility for working fathers would also take some of the strain of childcare from overstretched mothers. The 'after-school clubs' announced in the Green Budget are a step in the right direction.

Inequality: gender differences in rates for neurotic illness: female rates are higher than male rates; the female preponderance mainly due to excess rates in lower social classes (ONS – data provided by Frances Drever; OPCS – notably Meltzer et al, 1995a, 1995b).

Likely benefits: these social changes would remedy the large discrepancies, since gender differences are less evident when social factors are controlled out (Jenkins, 1985; Wilhelm and Parker, 1989).

Evidence favouring effectiveness: this evidence is indirect: the female preponderance found by OPCS in 1993 was 1.58 to 1.0; while that found by Rawnsley and colleagues in industrial Wales in 1972 was 1.92 to 1.00; or by Wing et al in Camberwell (1980) in 1979 was 2.1 to 1.0. It is argued that modest progress has been made between the 1970s and the 1990s in respect of ameliorating working conditions for women, and this may account for the differences in ratios. Studies of students at the beginning of their studies often fail to show any sex difference (Hammen and Padesky, 1977; Parker, 1979; Lloyd and Gartrell, 1981).

Policy 3

Provide preschool teaching to disadvantaged children from ethnic minorities: for example, African Caribbean children.

Inequality: high rates of disorder in ethnic minorities; partly related to unemployment, lower scholastic achievement and high drug use.

Likely benefits: improved scholastic performance during school years; a decrease in delinquency and crime and use of welfare assistance; a lower incidence of teenage pregnancy; more frequent success in open employment.

Evidence favouring effectiveness: the Perry School Project involved 123 black youths from low socio-economic families who were randomly assigned to a high quality preschool programme of early childhood education at the ages of three and four, with no treatment controls who received usual education. Information on these youths was collected annually to age 11, then at ages 14, 15 and 19. This preschool programme altered outcome variables at aged 19 by a factor of 2, including all those mentioned above (Berrueta-Clement et al, 1984; Schweinhart and Weikart, 1988). The cost per child of this education was US$1,589; the economic benefits exceeded costs by a factor of 7 to 1!

Policy 4

Increasing taxes on tobacco and alcohol; introducing 'parent monitoring' of drug use in primary school children; introducing 'drug abuse prevention programmes' in secondary schools. Smoking banned in public places; severe restrictions to be put on tobacco advertising.

Inequality: social class difference in alcohol and drug problems among males: increased rates in lower social classes.

Likely benefits: increased taxation will decrease alcohol and tobacco use in the population as a whole; prevention in primary schools leads to decreased rates of drug dependency by school children. (Drug interventions need to be introduced very early to be effective – by the time an adolescent is using a drug regularly it is too late for prevention. Interventions must aim either to prevent first use, or to intervene between first use and regular use. Drugs are spread to other users in second and subsequent years after regular use.)

Evidence favouring effectiveness: several studies by economists document the relationship between alcohol consumption and taxation (Richardson and

Crowley, 1994; Edwards et al, 1994; Ponicki et al, 1997). 'Parent monitoring' has been shown to reduce drug use by primary schoolchildren (Chilcoat et al, 1995; Chilcoat and Anthony, 1996) and effective drug and tobacco programmes have been shown to reduce use of these agents by schoolchildren (Pentz et al, 1989a, 1989b; Ellickson and Bell, 1990). The recent Home Office paper suggests that this policy would also be effective in the United Kingdom (Hurry and Lloyd, 1997).

Policy 5

Mental health public information campaign targeted at various subsets of the population. (1) Ethnic minority populations stressing (i) importance of consulting GPs when symptoms of depression, psychosis or drug dependence appear; (ii) symptoms of depression (especially Asians); (iii) hazards of drug dependence (especially African-Caribbeans). **(2) Low social class elderly population** in cardiovascular risk factors (dementia prevention – Prince et al, 1994; Hofman et al, 1997) and handicaps associated with depression.

Inequality: high rates of psychosis and drug problems among second generation immigrants; high suicide and attempted suicide rates among Asians; low detection rates for depression in ethnic minorities. High rates for dementia in low social classes; unequal distribution of elderly depression by region, probably due to differing levels of social support.

Likely benefits: reduction in illness rates.

Evidence favouring effectiveness: **there appears to be very little**. One study showed that giving Asian patients information about depression resulted in higher detection rates by GPs (Jacob, 1997). However, the inequality is an important one, and an experimental intervention is justified.

Part I: The inequalities

Socio-economic

For **neurotic illness** (with a female excess), there is a pronounced social class gradient for females, but not for males. For **alcohol and drug dependence** (with a male excess), there is a clear social class

gradient for men, but not for women (ONS, Annex SG).

There is a social class gradient for **suicide**: the rate in class V is four times higher than that in class I in 1993 (ONS); this differential is increasing – the rate in class V was double that of class I in 1970 (ONS).

There is a large excess of deaths due to **cerebrovascular disease** in social class V, rising from 14 (class I) to 45/100K (class V) (ONS). Cardiovascular risk factors are risk factors for *all* dementias (including Alzheimer's Disease), not merely for multi-infarct dementia.

Overcrowding of wards ('high bed occupancy' – rates well in excess of 140%) and **severe delays** in obtaining basic elements of mental healthcare are found mainly in deprived inner cities, where too many inpatient beds have been closed to pay for community care, so that patients have to be cared for (expensively and often far from their homes) in the private sector (Johnson et al, 1998).

Unemployed people have double the rates for neurotic illness than employed people (OPCS).

Poverty is strongly related both to psychiatric morbidity and to suicide. The mean weekly gross income of all adults in the General Household Survey for 1993 was £150; this may be compared with £90 for those with neurotic or psychotic illnesses, and only £70 for those with suicidal thoughts. (A total of 71% of those without psychiatric disorder were working, to be compared with 56% of those with psychiatric disorders and 27% of those with suicidal thoughts.) The association between suicide and economic deprivation is also demonstrated by other surveys (Gunnell et al, 1995; McLoone, 1996).

The inequality in the provision of **primary care services** documented in the Black Report still continues despite major investment in primary care in London (Johnson et al, 1998).

Gender

Female rates for neurotic disorders greatly exceed male rates, and are especially marked for anxiety/depression, obsessive compulsive disorder (OECD) and phobias; by contrast, male rates exceed female rates for alcohol and drug dependence (OPCS, 1995). Female rates for mental disorders treated by doctors exceed male rates by 2,260 to 1,241/10,000 at risk. The female excess for neurotic illness disappears if social factors are controlled (Jenkins, 1985; Wilhelm and Parker, 1989).

Suicide is becoming more common among young males, not females.

The proportion of boys drinking at least once a week is rising, and the number of units of alcohol taken is increasing (HEA and ONS surveys, 1988-94). Over all ages, government policies have not reduced the proportions of males or females drinking heavily or very heavily (ONS, 1986-94).

Regular smoking is becoming more common among girls, but remaining constant among boys (HEA and ONS surveys 1982-96).

Exposure of children to drugs, especially lysergic acid, ecstasy, cannabis and amphetamines, are rising sharply with time for both sexes. The female rate for amphetamines is rising faster than the male rate (HEA and ONS surveys).

Ethnicity

The rates for **neurotic** illness are higher among Asian women than among either white or black women; the rates for black men are higher than either white or Asian men (OPCS).

The rates for **psychotic illnesses** are much higher for African Caribbeans than for whites, and this effect is most marked in the second generation (OPCS; and Carpenter and Brockington, 1980; Harrison et al, 1988; King et al, 1994; Huchinson et al, 1996; Bhugra et al, 1997; Johnson et al, 1998).

Africans and West Indians have nine times higher rates of **drug dependence**, Asians four times whites (OPCS).

Pathways into care: black men and women are less likely to bring psychotic symptoms to the attention of their GPs (Bhughra, 1997, personal communication; Thomas et al, 1993; Commander et al, 1997); having consulted, their GP is less likely to

detect disorder among both black men and women and Asians (Thomas et al, 1993); although having detected disorder, black men and women were more likely to be referred to mental health services rather than being cared for by the GP (Thomas et al, 1993).

Region

There do not appear to be major remediable differences between regions: however, deprived urban areas have higher rates for mentally disordered offenders (Johnson et al, 1998), for common mental disorders are for psychotic illnesses requiring hospital treatment (OPCS).

There are marked differences between the diagnoses of hospitalised patients in inner London compared to other parts of the country, summarised in Table 1.

There are interesting regional differences of depression among elderly people, even when social class is controlled, and these are probably due to differences in social networks and social support available for elderly people in different parts of the country.

Part II: Likely beneficial interventions based upon evidence

In general, it is better to intervene for whole populations than it is to identify high risk groups. Such measures as increasing the mean income of the population and thus indirectly improving the housing stock and the nutrition of the population, as well as general public health measures such as cleaner air and better public transport, may be expected to have beneficial effects. However, in the case of health promotion the middle class tends to listen to and to act upon the message, and focused interventions are therefore justified. The two examples recommended here (ethnic minorities and low social class elderly) are both cases where an urgent public health message needs to be focused on particular groups within the population. In the case of drug dependence, much of the efforts are misdirected because they are applied to adolescents who are already using drugs regularly: the interventions needs to go in, much earlier, to primary schools (Berrueta-Clement et al, 1984). The 'Welfare to Work' programme of the present government may be expected to have major effects upon inequalities if it is successful. Any measures which make single parents poorer can be confidently expected to exacerbate the inequalities with which we have been concerned. Evidence for the efficacy of the individual policy recommendations are to be found in the Executive summary. There are many inequalities that can only be partly ameliorated.

References

Berrueta-Clement, J.R., Schweinhart, L.J., Barnett, W.S., Epstein, A.S. and Weikart, D.P. (1984) *Changed lives: The effects of the Perry pre-school program on youths aged 19*, Ypsilanti, MI: High Scope Press.

Bhugra, D., Leff, J., Mallet, R., Der, G., Corridon, B. and Rudge, S. (1997) 'Incidence and outcome of schizophrenia in whites, African-Caribbeans and Asians in London', *Psychological Medicine*, vol 27, pp 791-8.

Carpenter, L. and Brockington, I. (1980) 'A study of mental illness in Asians, West Indians and Africans living in Manchester', *British Journal of Psychiatry*, vol 137, pp 201-5.

Chilcoat, H.D. and Anthony, J.C. (1996) 'Impact of parent monitoring on initiation of drug use through late childhood', *Journal of American Academy Child Adolescent Psychiatry*, vol 35, no 1, pp 91-100, January.

Chilcoat, H.D., Dishion, T.J. and Anthony, J.C. (1995) 'Parent monitoring and the incidence of drug sampling in urban elementary school children', *American Journal of Epidemiology*, vol 141, no 1, pp 25-31, 1 January 1.

Commander, M., Sashi Dharan, S.P. et al (1997) 'Access to mental health care in an inner city mental health district, II Association with demographic factors', *British Journal of Psychiatry*, vol 170, pp 317-20.

Edwards, G., Anderson, P., Babor, T. et al (1994) *Alcohol policy and the public good*, Oxford: Oxford Medical Publications.

Ellickson, P.L. and Bell, R.M. (1990) 'Drug prevention in junior high: a multi-site longitudinal test', *Science*, vol 247, no 4948, pp 1299-305, 16 March.

Gunnell, D., Peters, T., Kammerling, R. and Brooks, J. (1995) 'Relation between parasuicide, suicide, psychiatric admission and socio-economic deprivation', *British Medical Journal*, vol 311, pp 226-30.

Hammen, C. and Padesky, C. (1977) 'Differences in the expression of depressive responses on the Black Depression Inventory', *Journal of Abnormal Psychology*, vol 86, pp 609-14.

Harrison, G., Owens, D., Holton, A., Neilson, D. and Boot, D. (1988) 'A prospective study of severe mental disorder in Afro-Caribbean patients', *Psychological Medicine*, vol 18, pp 643-57.

Hofman, A., Ott, A. and Bots, M. et al (1997) 'Atherosclerosis, apolipoprotein A, and prevalence of dementia in the Rotterdam study', *Lancet*, vol 349, pp 151-4.

Hurry, J. and Lloyd, C. (1997) 'A follow up evaluation of Project Charlie: a life skills drug education programme for primary schools', Paper 16, London: Home Office Drug Prevention Unit.

Hutchinson, G., Takei, N., Fahy, T., Bhugra, D. et al (1996) 'Morbid rates of schizophrenia in first degree relatives of white and African-Caribbean patients with psychosis', *British Journal of Psychiatry*, vol 169, pp 776-80.

Ingham, J., Rawnsley, K. and Hughes, D. (1972) 'Psychiatric disorder and its declaration in contrasting areas of South Wales', *Psychological Medicine*, vol 2, pp 281-92.

Jacob, K.S. (1997) 'A RCT of the effect of patient education on explanatory models and common mental disorders in primary care', PhD thesis, University of London.

Jenkins, R. (1985) 'Sex differences in minor psychiatric morbidity', *Psychological Medicine*, Monograph supplement no 7.

Johnson, S., Ramsay, R., Thornicroft, G. et al (1998) *London's mental health*, London: The King's Fund.

King, M., Coker, E., Leavy, G. et al (1994) 'Incidence of psychotic illness in London – comparison of ethnic groups', *British Medical Journal*, vol 309, pp 1115-19.

Lloyd, C. and Gartrell, N. (1981) 'Sex differences in medical student health', *American Journal of Psychiatry*, vol 138, pp 1346-51.

McLoone, P. (1996) 'Suicide and deprivation in Scotland', *British Medical Journal*, vol 312, pp 543-4.

Meltzer, H., Gill, B., Petticrew, M. and Hinds, K. (1995a) *The prevalence of psychiatric morbidity among adults living in private households*, Report 1, London: HMSO.

Meltzer, H. Gill, B., Petticrew, M. and Hinds, K. (1995b) *Economic activity and social functioning of adults with psychiatric disorders*, Report 3, London: HMSO.

Parker, G. (1979) 'Sex differences in non clinical depression in Dip Ed students in Sydney Teachers College', *Australian and New Zealand Journal of Psychiatry*, vol 13, pp 127-32.

Pentz, M.A., MacKinnon, D.P., Flay, B.R., Hansen, W.B., Johnson, C.A. and Dwyer, J.H. (1989a) 'Primary prevention of chronic diseases in adolescence: effects of the Midwestern Prevention Project on tobacco use', *American Journal of Epidemiology*, vol 130, no 4, pp 713-24, October.

Pentz, M.A., Dwyer, J.H., MacKinnon, D.P., Flay, B.R., Hansen, W.B., Wang, E.Y. and Johnson, C.A. (1989b) 'A multicommunity trial for primary prevention of adolescent drug abuse. Effects on drug use prevalence', *Journal of the American Medical Association*, vol 261, no 22, pp 3259-66.

Ponicki, W., Holder, H.D., Gruenewald, P.J. and Romelsjo, A. (1997) 'Altering alcohol price by ethanol content: results from a Swedish tax policy in 1992', *Addiction*, vol 92, no 7, pp 859-70, July.

Prince, M., Cullen, M. and Mann, A. (1994) 'Risk factors for Alzheimer's Disease', *Neurology*, vol 44, pp 97-104.

Richardson, J. and Crowley, S. (1994) 'Optimum alcohol taxation: balancing consumption and external costs', *Health Economics*, vol 3, no 2, pp 73-87, March-April.

Schweinhart, L.J. and Weikart, D.P. (1988) 'The High Scope Perry Preschool programme', in R.H. Price, E.L. Cowen, R.P. Lorion and J. Ramos-McKay (eds) *14 ounces of prevention*, Washington, DC: American Psychological Association.

Thomas, C., Stone, K., Osborn, M. et al (1993) 'Psychiatric morbidity and compulsory admission among UK-born Europeans, Afro-Caribbeans and Asians in central Manchester', *British Journal of Psychiatry*, vol 163, pp 91-3.

Wilhelm, K. and Parker, G. (1989) 'Is sex necessarily a risk factor for depression?', *Psychological Medicine*, vol 19, pp 401-13.

Wilhelm, K. and Parker, G. (1994) 'Sex differnces in life time depression rates: fact or artefact?', *Psychological Medicine*, vol 24, pp 97-111.

Wing, J.K. Nixon, J., Mann, S. and Leff, J. (1980) 'Reliability of the PSE used in a general population study', *Psychological Medicine*, vol 7, pp 505-12.

16

Smoking, drinking, physical activity and screening uptake and health inequalities

Jane Wardle, Michael Farrell, Melvyn Hillsdon, Martin Jarvis, Stephen Sutton and Margaret Thorogood

Inequalities in health behaviours

Behaviours such as smoking, exercise, diet and alcohol consumption make a major contribution to levels of disability and death in the UK today. Insofar as these behaviours also vary by socio-economic status, they contribute to health variations, and therefore have implications for government policy to reduce health inequalities. This paper summarises the evidence related to socio-economic, and to a lesser extent gender, differences in smoking, exercise, alcohol consumption, and participation in cancer screening, and considers the policy implications of the findings.

Socio-economic variations in health-related behaviours have not attracted the rigorous analysis that might be expected in the epidemiological literature. Unfounded assumptions about the patterning of socio-economic distributions, or the implications for health, are commonplace. Political and ethical issues may have played a part in this, since in the debate on the contribution of health behaviours to health inequalities, there appears to be a view that documenting socio-economic differences in life-style is synonymous with 'victim blaming'. This is not the perspective taken in this paper. To the extent that there are associations between deprivation and patterns of health-related behaviours, these may provide proximal explanations of health inequalities, but also raise deeper questions about the mechanisms through which health-compromising life-styles are perpetuated and changed in contemporary Britain.

Summary of the evidence relating health behaviours to socio-economic status

Good data are available on smoking, which provide a clear picture of a graded association with socio-economic position. Deprivation is linked to a higher prevalence of smoking, higher smoke intake, and lower cessation, with the most deprived groups in the population having been almost entirely excluded from what is otherwise a strong trend towards reducing smoking. As smoking is the principal cause of lung cancer and makes a significant contribution to heart disease, it clearly contributes substantially to inequalities in chronic disease and death. Furthermore, smoking may exacerbate economic hardship among poorer groups through the substantial costs associated with sustaining nicotine addiction. There has been a vigorous debate on gender differences in smoking uptake and cessation. The evidence is examined in Appendix A of this chapter, which indicates that while smoking levels were higher in men than women for many years, in the younger cohorts smoking parity appears to have become established over the past decade, with no real evidence for gender differences in trends in uptake or cessation.

Alcohol consumption is more complex to evaluate since its adverse effects may be related to the dose, its patterning, and the context of consumption, yet many existing sources of data are not informative at this level of detail. At all ages, women are less likely than men to be drinkers and much less likely to be heavy drinkers. Socio-economic deprivation is associated both with higher levels of abstinence (or very infrequent drinking) and with higher levels of excessive drinking and problems with drunkenness.

It is this latter pattern which may have most adverse effects on health, which fits with data showing that alcohol-related diseases and deaths are higher in men, and higher in the more economically deprived groups.

Physical activity poses even more problems of data collection, and any conclusions can only be tentative in view of the problems of measurement. There appear to be consistent gender differences, with women reporting lower levels of general activity and less participation in active leisure pursuits. Socio-economic differentials vary in a complex fashion for different activity indicators. When the activity indicators cover all aspects of moderate to vigorous activity, including occupational, there is a general trend towards higher levels of activity at intermediate levels of deprivation, with lower activity levels among the most and least deprived groups. An alternative strategy is to examine differences in inactivity, which is accepted to be a risk factor for overweight. The lower socio-economic groups are more likely to report being sedentary, and it is likely that this contributes to the matching social gradient in obesity.

Health screening participation is a very different kind of behaviour, being related to disease detection rather than health promotion. It is also more likely to be motivated entirely by health-related considerations, whereas drinking, sports and smoking are woven into patterns of everyday living, being subject to a range of different motivations. Data on screening participation by socio-economic status have not been explored much in relation to the UK national screening programmes, but the analyses presented in Part 1 suggest that there is lower participation, particularly for cervical screening, among more deprived women or women living in more deprived areas.

Synergies and interactions between health behaviours

The interrelationship between health behaviours, both in terms of life-style patterns (ie clustering of risk behaviours) and in terms of magnification of adverse effects (eg smokers with poor nutritional status have a greater risk of lung cancer) is another important issue. The data presented here suggest that the most disadvantaged sectors of the community are more likely to smoke, have problems with drink and be inactive. It is likely that these risks are additive or even interactive. The effects of clustering and amplification of risk need to be explored critically in analyses of the contribution of health behaviours to health inequalities.

Policy implications

This review suggests that the association between smoking and socio-economic disadvantage makes a major contribution to health inequalities. Policy initiatives to promote smoking cessation among the more deprived sectors of the community should be a priority. Several suggestions, including making nicotine replacement therapy reimbursable under the NHS, would appear to be viable and cost-effective strategies to combat inequalities.

The contribution of alcohol consumption to health inequalities is less easy to establish. The evidence points to a link between socio-economic status, binge drinking (or drunkenness) and costs to health and society, but not one which is likely to be as significant for health inequalities as smoking. A focus on alcohol is therefore a lower priority in terms of policy initiatives to reduce health inequalities. One implication of the findings is that patterns of drinking rather than overall intake might be the target of intervention, which implicates strategies to promote safer ways to handle alcohol. Health education initiatives may be able to make a contribution in terms of 'safer drinking' advice, although this is unlikely to be a simple message to put across. Control of availability of alcohol in some settings, or even of some varieties of alcoholic drinks, may also play a part.

The situation is similar for physical activity. Overall levels of physical activity are not strikingly lower among the lower socio-economic status groups, probably because of the higher rate of manual occupational activity. But the most disadvantaged are the most likely to be entirely inactive. There is an emerging consensus that encouraging walking is likely to be a significant part of promoting a more active nation, and this may have different implications for different sectors of the community. In the more deprived areas, promoting walking for pleasure is likely to require improving the safety and appearance of the physical environment.

Health screening is a specifically health-related behaviour and one which is nationally organised to reduce cancer deaths. The striking social class differences in cervical cancer death rates implicate socio-economic differentials in screening participation as one factor, and this is confirmed in data from surveys. As more new screening methods are introduced, it is essential that the problems of ensuring equitable access for all sectors of the community should be a priority, and should be built into the organisation of screening programmes.

PART 1: CIGARETTE SMOKING AND HEALTH INEQUALITIES

The extent of the association

Smoking-related disease and health inequalities

As illustrated in Table 1(a) and (b), there is wide variation in death rates from the main smoking-related diseases, with Standardised Mortality Ratios in unskilled male workers three times higher than in professionals for heart disease, five times higher for lung cancer, six times higher for emphysema, and 14 times higher for chronic airways obstruction. Similar but somewhat smaller variations are seen in women. Alternative indicators of socio-economic status such as housing tenure or access to a car are additionally predictive of death rates (Goldblatt, 1990; Carroll et al, 1993; Smith and Harding, 1997). Quantitative estimates of the proportion of this variation caused by smoking are not currently available, although there is general acceptance that at least 90% of lung cancer deaths are attributable to smoking, and that overall risk of death in continuing smokers is 1 in 2 (Doll et al, 1994). In view of factors such as earlier age of starting to smoke in deprived smokers, higher average smoking dose and poorer diet, it would be anticipated that risk per smoker would be higher in poor than in affluent smokers. The methodology of Peto and Lopez (Peto et al, 1992, 1994) for

estimating smoking-attributable deaths in different countries could in principle be applied to different socio-economic groups within countries. The application of such a methodology would seem to be a priority for the UK.

Table 1

a) Standardised Mortality Ratios by social class for some major smoking-related diseases, men aged 20-64, England and Wales (1991-93)

	Lung cancer	Ischaemic heart disease	Chronic airways obstruction	Bronchitis and emphysema
I Professional	45	63	21	44
II Managerial	61	73	42	43
IIINM Skilled	87	107	78	81
IIIM Skilled	138	125	131	125
IV Semi-skilled	132	121	146	137
V Unskilled	206	182	298	268

Source: Drever et al (1997); Crown Copyright

b) Mortality Rate Ratios by social class from longitudinal study cohort: women aged 35-64, England and Wales (1986-92)

	Lung cancer	Ischaemic heart disease	Respiratory diseases
I /II	0.47	0.50	0.47
IIINM	0.50	0.66	0.50
IIIM	1.00	1.00	1.00
IV/V	1.35	1.33	1.23

Note: Reference class is III Manual.

Source: Harding et al (1997); Crown Copyright

Cigarette smoking prevalence and socio-economic disadvantage

Cigarette smoking prevalence is closely associated with socio-economic status, with a gulf between rich and poor that has widened substantially over the past 20 years. The question of gender differences in smoking, which has attracted much attention recently, is addressed in Appendix A of this chapter. Occupational class has been the main indicator of socio-economic status used in publications of national smoking statistics. Table 2, which is drawn from the General Household Survey, shows cigarette smoking for men and women by social class over the period 1974 to 1994. Among both men and women prevalence in professional groups declined by a half, while among unskilled manual workers there was a smaller decline of about one third, with the result

Table 2: Prevalence of cigarette smoking by sex and socio-economic group (1974-79)

Persons aged 16 or over   Great Britain

Socio-economic group*	Percentage smoking cigarettes											Base 1994 =100%
	1974	1976	1978	1980	1982	1984	1986	1988	1990	1992	1994	
Men												
Professional	29	25	25	21	20	17	18	16	16	14	16	538
Employers and managers	46	38	37	35	29	29	28	26	24	24	20	1566
Intermediate and junior non-manual	45	40	38	35	30	30	28	25	25	25	24	1372
Skilled manual and own account non-professional	56	51	49	48	42	40	40	39	36	34	33	2541
Semi-skilled manual and personal service	56	53	53	49	47	45	43	40	39	39	38	1040
Unskilled manual	61	58	60	57	49	49	43	43	48	42	40	387
Total non-manual	45	37	36	33	28	28	26	24	23	22	21	3476
Total manual	56	52	51	49	44	43	40	40	38	36	35	3968
All aged 16 and over	51	46	45	42	38	36	35	33	31	29	28	7642
Women												
Professional	25	28	23	21	21	15	19	17	16	13	12	475
Employers and managers	38	35	33	33	29	29	27	26	23	21	20	1722
Intermediate and junior non-manual	38	35	33	34	30	28	27	27	27	27	23	2349
Skilled manual and own account non-professional	46	42	42	42	39	37	36	35	32	31	29	2204
Semi-skilled manual and personal service	43	41	41	41	41	36	33	39	36	35	34	1533
Unskilled manual	43	38	41	41	41	36	33	39	36	35	34	525
Total non-manual	38	35	32	32	29	27	26	25	25	23	21	4565
Total manual	45	41	41	41	38	37	36	36	34	33	31	4262
All aged 16 and over	41	38	37	37	33	32	31	30	29	28	26	9108

Source: Bennett et al (1996)

that by 1994 unskilled groups were two to three times more likely to smoke than professionals. Nevertheless, by 1994 smokers were comfortably in the minority in all social class groups, with the highest rates being observed in unskilled men and women, at 40% and 34% respectively.

Social class is only one measure of socio-economic status, and numerous commentators have pointed out that indicators such as unemployment, housing tenure and access to a car independently predict both smoking prevalence and health inequalities (Moser et al, 1988; Pugh et al, 1991). Table 3, which uses data from the 1996 General Household Survey, explores a range of measures of disadvantage additional to class as predictors of cigarette smoking. Among both men and women, current smoking is predicted by rented housing tenure, lack of access to a car, unemployment, and crowded living conditions, as well as by lone parenthood and divorced or

separated marital status. This illustrates what might be proposed as a general law of British society, namely that any marker of disadvantage that can be envisaged and measured, whether personal or material, is likely to have an independent association with cigarette smoking.

To obtain an indication of how overall smoking prevalence relates to disadvantage, an index of deprivation has been created incorporating information on occupational class, housing tenure, car access, employment status, and the extent of crowding in the home. Respondents score 1 for each of the following: manual occupation; rented housing; no car; unemployed; crowded living conditions (one or more persons per room). The resulting index, with scores ranging from 0 among the affluent to 5 among the most deprived, is similar to the indices employed by Townsend and by

Table 3: Socio-economic predictors of current cigarette smoking

	Men		Women		All	
	OR	95%CI	OR	95%CI	OR	95%CI
Social class						
I	1.00		1.00		1.00	
II	2.29	1.68-3.12	2.13	1.54-2.95	2.19	1.75-2.74
IIINM	1.89	1.35-2.65	2.39	1.70-3.34	2.18	1.72-2.76
IIIM	2.99	2.19-4.07	3.12	2.25-4.32	3.04	2.43-3.80
IV	3.53	2.56-4.86	3.44	2.46-4.80	3.45	2.74-4.35
V	3.24	2.23-4.69	3.05	2.10-4.42	3.12	2.40-4.05
Rented tenure	2.20	1.93-2.50	1.95	1.74-2.20	2.07	1.89-2.25
No car	1.37	1.18-1.60	1.39	1.21-1.60	1.38	1.24-1.52
Unemployed	1.55	1.26-1.90	1.64	1.28-2.08	1.61	1.38-1.88
Crowding	1.25	1.03-1.51	1.01	.84-1.21	1.12	.98-1.28
Lone parent	1.21	.93-1.58	1.62	1.35-1.96	1.44	1.24-1.67
Divorced or separated	1.64	1.31-2.05	1.37	1.11-1.69	1.53	1.32-1.78

Note: Odds for each variable control for all the other variables in the model.
   OR: odds ratio; CI: confidence interval.

Source: General Household Survey (1996); Thomas et al (1998); Crown Copyright

Carstairs (Townsend et al, 1988; Carstairs and Morris, 1989; Morris and Carstairs, 1991), but is applied to individuals rather than areas.

Table 4 gives cigarette smoking prevalence by deprivation score for the years since 1973 using data from the General Household Survey. In each year, for both men and women, there is an approximately linear increase in cigarette smoking with increasing deprivation. What is particularly striking is that, while smoking rates have more than halved among the affluent, there has been increasingly less decline over time with increasing levels of deprivation. Among the most deprived, 70% or more were smokers in 1973, and that still remains the case some 23 years later. The widening gulf in cigarette smoking by deprivation closely parallels the widening in health inequalities over the same period. The extraordinarily high rates of smoking shown by this index for the most deprived sectors of the community are confirmed by surveys of particular groups: 84% cigarette smoking among prisoners (Bridgwood and Malbon, 1995); and 90% among homeless people sleeping rough (Gill et al, 1996).

Smoking cessation and socio-economic disadvantage

Table 5 gives rates of smoking cessation by deprivation over the years since 1973 (M.J. Jarvis, 1997a). Mirroring the observations in Table 4, it

shows that while rates of cessation have more than doubled among affluent people, from 25 to 55%, among the poorest groups there has been little or no change, with 10% or less of ever-regular smokers giving up.

Nicotine dependence and socio-economic disadvantage

There is strong emerging evidence that the level of nicotine dependence among smokers increases systematically with deprivation. This is evident both from questionnaire indicators of dependence in the General Household Studies (eg time to first cigarette of the day), and from studies with quantitative measures of smoke intake. Figure 1 shows plasma and saliva cotinine concentrations among smokers from the *Health Survey for England* (Colhoun and Prescott Clarke, 1996) and the Health and Lifestyle Survey (Cox et al, 1993) respectively. Both surveys show increasingly high levels of nicotine intake with increasing deprivation, with average intake being close to 50% higher in the most deprived than in the most affluent smokers. These observations carry the implication that the risk of smoking-related disease per smoker should also be higher in deprived than affluent smokers; and that interventions to increase rates of smoking cessation among poor people will need to take appropriate account of the dependence issue.

Table 4: Percentage cigarette smoking prevalence by deprivation

Men

	Deprivation score						
	0	1	2	3	4	5	All
1973	38.7	47.2	55.4	63.4	72.3	74.2	52.6
1974	38.8	45.2	55.2	61.1	70.4	89.2	51.2
1976	31.8	40.4	49.6	59.0	65.6	81.2	46.1
1978	31.2	40.2	48.5	56.6	66.9	82.7	44.5
1980	28.5	37.4	48.3	54.4	65.0	72.1	42.4
1982	25.2	31.3	41.9	52.2	61.9	74.2	37.9
1984	23.4	31.8	41.1	50.0	65.0	80.6	36.3
1986	22.6	32.7	40.3	47.6	65.4	56.9	34.6
1988	20.3	31.6	39.4	50.7	65.7	63.6	32.9
1990	19.9	29.9	39.0	46.6	64.7	60.7	31.0
1992	18.4	27.3	37.2	48.0	60.1	77.8	29.4
1994	17.2	25.4	36.7	46.4	61.8	73.2	28.2
1996	17.6	26.6	39.4	45.5	64.0	90.9	28.6

Bases	0	1	2	3	4	5	All
1973	2,069	2,770	2,958	2,163	538	49	10,546
1974	2,115	2,599	2,543	2,079	476	37	9,849
1976	2,358	2,925	2,843	2,127	517	85	10,855
1978	2,537	2,902	2,521	1,995	472	52	10,479
1980	2,504	2,964	2,600	1,876	448	61	10,453
1982	2,317	2,518	2,204	1,644	423	93	9,199
1984	2,278	2,547	1,799	1,347	383	72	8,426
1986	2,671	2,826	1,777	1,190	350	58	8,872
1988	2,829	2,834	1,604	1,100	268	22	8,657
1990	2,763	2,738	1,474	902	201	28	8,106
1992	2,843	2,931	1,472	912	223	36	8,417
1994	2,605	2,602	1,356	821	217	41	7,642
1996	2,549	2,452	1,258	719	172	22	7,172

Women	0	1	2	3	4	5	All
1973	35.4	37.7	42.8	46.8	66.8	66.7	41.5
1974	33.2	38.5	40.7	46.8	66.9	58.3	40.5
1976	31.7	36.1	38.8	42.4	61.6	63.2	37.9
1978	28.9	32.0	38.7	45.5	65.7	85.7	36.6
1980	27.5	35.2	39.7	44.6	61.1	40.0	36.8
1982	26.3	29.6	35.7	41.1	60.1	61.5	33.2
1984	23.7	29.8	35.7	43.4	55.8	70.0	32.1
1986	24.2	28.2	34.8	41.7	56.6	64.3	31.0
1988	21.9	29.0	37.0	42.8	53.4	100.0	30.4
1990	20.2	28.4	37.0	41.4	59.5	75.0	29.1
1992	20.4	26.7	33.9	40.0	57.0	33.3	27.6
1994	17.1	23.8	32.0	37.6	55.2	50.0	25.6
1996	17.4	26.2	35.8	42.2	61.2	100.0	27.5

Bases	0	1	2	3	4	5	All
1973	2,758	3,158	3,213	2,561	419	8	12,115
1974	2,672	3,052	2,967	2,367	396	12	11,466
1976	3,025	3,374	3,162	2,505	414	19	12,499
1978	3,182	3,220	3,002	2,341	394	14	12,153
1980	3,300	3,170	2,939	2,323	352	15	12,099
1982	3,012	2,852	2,456	1,987	308	26	10,641
1984	3,054	2,721	2,181	1,608	226	10	9,800
1986	3,432	2,877	2,188	1,572	221	14	10,304
1988	3,646	2,872	2,007	1,419	161	6	10,111
1990	3,551	2,736	1,757	1,249	148	4	9,445
1992	3,832	2,765	1,833	1,186	142	6	9,764
1994	3,004	2,959	1,785	1,160	192	8	9,108
1996	2,959	2,712	1,657	1,047	121	5	8,501

Source: General Household Survey (1973-96)

Table 5: Percentage smoking cessation by deprivation

Men

	Deprivation score						
	0	1	2	3	4	5	All
1973	25.1	22.2	19.4	16.3	8.8	11.8	19.8
1974	26.1	24.6	18.7	17.5	9.7	2.9	20.8
1976	30.3	28.0	24.4	19.0	14.5	1.4	24.5
1978	34.6	30.1	26.4	22.4	10.0	6.4	27.3
1980	41.0	35.6	30.4	25.9	11.7	11.8	32.1
1982	44.6	42.1	35.4	29.6	15.7	9.0	36.6
1984	48.1	41.6	37.0	31.7	16.1	9.2	38.5
1986	45.1	39.9	35.7	30.6	13.0	10.3	37.5
1988	52.3	41.5	37.3	29.2	11.1	11.1	40.7
1990	53.5	43.7	36.9	33.1	15.2	10.5	42.8
1992	54.1	46.3	41.3	32.5	19.4	3.4	44.6
1994	58.4	50.4	40.6	34.1	18.7	14.3	47.1
1996	58.7	48.7	38.3	34.8	15.3	0.0	46.7

Bases	0	1	2	3	4	5	All
1973	1,390	1,970	2,287	1,767	443	43	7,899
1974	1,418	1,851	1,964	1,687	392	34	7,346
1976	1,519	2,028	2,175	1,733	428	71	7,954
1978	1,583	2,011	1,885	1,574	371	47	7,471
1980	1,521	1,987	1,937	1,471	343	51	7,310
1982	1,369	1,624	1,563	1,292	324	78	6,250
1984	1,311	1,600	1,260	1,024	305	65	5,565
1986	1,536	1,863	1,265	914	276	39	5,893
1988	1,614	1,787	1,134	849	207	18	5,609
1990	1,517	1,680	1,019	680	158	19	5,073
1992	1,513	1,737	1,040	698	170	29	5,187
1994	1,307	1,527	907	607	166	35	4,549
1996	1,299	1,471	864	529	131	20	4,314

Women	0	1	2	3	4	5	All
1973	25.1	22.6	17.1	13.8	8.3	16.7	19.0
1974	28.5	20.8	20.3	15.0	6.3	0	20.3
1976	29.4	26.2	23.8	19.6	10.2	14.3	24.1
1978	37.3	31.0	23.7	19.6	6.8	7.7	27.1
1980	37.6	29.3	25.2	21.6	13.0	14.3	27.9
1982	39.3	35.5	29.6	26.7	11.9	15.8	32.1
1984	44.9	35.2	29.3	27.9	16.0	12.5	34.4
1986	44.8	38.7	33.0	27.1	15.5	0	36.4
1988	48.2	38.6	32.0	27.0	18.9	0	37.7
1990	50.7	39.6	31.6	29.9	11.1	0	39.3
1992	50.7	44.2	36.1	32.1	17.3	0	42.4
1994	55.9	47.4	38.4	32.8	11.7	20.0	44.5
1996	53.8	43.2	35.2	29.7	10.8	0	41.5

Bases	0	1	2	3	4	5	All
1973	1,325	1,550	1,662	1,399	306	6	6,247
1974	1,265	1,492	1,526	1,309	285	7	5,884
1976	1,390	1,658	1,615	1,324	284	14	6,285
1978	1,494	1,502	1,526	1,325	279	13	6,139
1980	1,466	1,582	1,565	1,321	247	7	6,188
1982	1,316	1,310	1,248	1,116	210	19	5,219
1984	1,327	1,256	1,111	968	150	8	4,820
1986	1,524	1,330	1,143	900	148	9	5,054
1988	1,556	1,362	1,093	836	106	6	4,959
1990	1,468	1,284	950	739	99	3	4,543
1992	1,607	1,329	973	698	98	2	4,707
1994	1,170	1,342	930	649	120	5	4,216
1996	1,122	1,256	920	629	83	5	4,015

Source: General Household Survey (1973-96)

218

Emergence of the association between smoking and disadvantage among young people

There is rather little information available on the relationship between deprivation and smoking in teenagers, as the regular ONS surveys of schoolchildren's smoking do not incorporate measures of socio–economic status. Nevertheless, there is evidence that smoking is a measure of social trajectory, with prevalence being more closely related to people's destination than to their circumstances of origin (Glendinning et al, 1994). In the 1958 birth cohort, cigarette smoking at age 16 increased from 24% among those from the most affluent households to 48% among the most deprived. But the gradient at age 16 was much sharper (80% among the most deprived) when

cohort members were categorised by deprivation measured seven years later at age 23 by their own achieved position, rather than by characteristics of the parental household (Figure 2). This implies that factors conferring an increased risk of smoking at age 16 also have a bearing on subsequent downward social mobility.

Why do poor people smoke more?

Consideration of policy initiatives to lower rates of smoking among disadvantaged groups in society requires us to have some understanding of why poor people are more likely to smoke. If smoking serves some useful function in people's lives, our approach to the issue must be different than if it is seen as a purely destructive force. It could be seen as socially counterproductive to knock away a valued prop, even if its effects on health are serious.

The most common functional explanation of smoking is that it is self–medication. Cigarette smoking is seen as a means of regulating mood, of managing stress, and of coping with all the hassles and strain resulting from material deprivation

Figure 1: Quantitative measures of smoke intake in smokers by deprivation

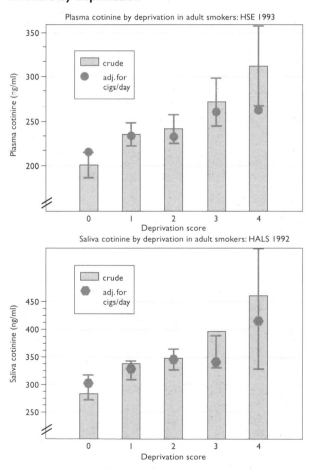

Figure 2: Smoking at 16 by deprivation measured at 16 and 23

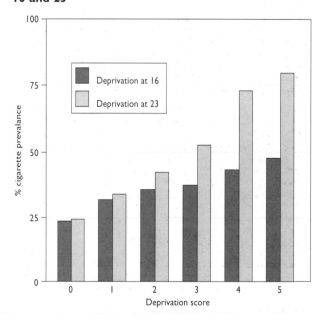

Source: Data from Health Survey for England (HSE) (top) Colhoun and Prescott-Clarke (1996); and the Health and Life-style Survey (HALS) (bottom) Cox et al (1993)

Source: Data from the National Child Development Study, Ferri (1993)

(Graham, 1987; Davey Smith and Morris, 1994). This account chimes with smokers' self-reports of calming effects from cigarettes and with poor women's observation that smoking is the one thing they do for themselves, that gives them some space from the difficult task of caring for young children in poverty (Graham, 1994). This view has achieved wide currency in recent years, but it is open to several major objections. The most serious of these is the nature of nicotine as a drug. Nicotine is a stimulant, similar to drugs such as amphetamine. Sedative or anxiolytic effects, if they exist at all, are very hard to find either in animals or humans. Smoking is closely associated with adverse mood states, but there is no evidence that it ameliorates them other than through withdrawal relief (Schoenborn and Horm, 1993). Stress modulation over the course of the day suggests that mood-elevating effects of cigarettes are attributable to relief of adverse mood from incipient withdrawal rather than any absolute benefits (Parrott, 1995). Smoking cessation is associated with lowered, rather than higher, levels of perceived stress, consistent with the idea that smoking may provoke stress rather than relieve it (Cohen and Lichtenstein, 1990).

An alternative view is that poor people smoke because they are on an addictive treadmill. They start smoking because they grow up in a culture in which most adult role models smoke and smoking is the norm. They quickly become nicotine dependent, and smoking is then maintained by negative reinforcement: continued smoking averts the unpleasentness of not smoking. On this view, what needs explaining is why poor people are less able to achieve cessation than more priviledged groups. Possible explanations are either that poor people are less motivated to give up, because they are less well informed and concerned about smoking's effects; or that the stresses arising from material deprivation make it harder for them to cope with the additional difficulty of going without cigarettes, which is acknowledged to be very hard for most people to achieve. The evidence that poor people's motivation to stop smoking is low is not strong. Self-report items from the General Household Survey show that the proportion of smokers who express a desire to give up smoking altogether is rather constant, at about two thirds across the whole range of socio-economic deprivation.

Policy initiatives to reduce smoking in disadvantaged groups

There can be little doubt that policies to reduce cigarette smoking must be at the heart of any initiatives to address health inequalities. Equally, if they are to be effective, new policies should amount to more than just an intensification of current approaches, which, while helpful in achieving an overall reduction in smoking prevalence, have not been successful in reducing smoking in disadvantaged groups.

The main planks of current policy are interventions designed to increase people's motivation to quit: price; restrictions on smoking in public places; and health education campaigns. Addressing dependence/addiction has received less attention. Year-on-year increases in the real cost of cigarettes are easily implemented, command widespread support, and should be continued, although there is some uncertainty about the impact on poor people, for whom tobacco expenditure amounts to a high proportion of disposable income (Marsh and McKay, 1994). Some economists have argued that poor smokers respond equally as much or more to price than do affluent smokers (Townsend et al, 1994), while others are less certain. The very low rates of smoking cessation seen in disadvantaged groups are inconsistent with the idea that for them price is an effective means of promoting cessation. Price increases may influence poor people to switch to cheaper and higher yielding brands (M.J. Jarvis, 1998), to roll their own cigarettes, and to cut down on the number of cigarettes they smoke, rather than to quit altogether. Because of the phenomenon of nicotine compensation, lowering cigarette consumption is unlikely to confer any benefit in lowering risk of smoking-related disease.

Make nicotine replacement therapy reimbursable under the NHS

Many influences conspire to make smoking cessation hard to achieve for poor people. Living in a culture where smoking continues to be the norm and where your partner is likely to be a smoker powerfully militates against cessation (M.J. Jarvis, 1997), as do the stresses from living in impoverished material circumstances. However, these factors are not easily open to change. The key factor amenable to intervention would appear to be nicotine dependence, and poor people are likely to be more strongly dependent than are affluent smokers. Nicotine replacement therapy (NRT) has been shown to be an effective treatment aid, approximately doubling success rates from both brief and intensive treatments (Fiore et al, 1994, 1996; Silagy et al, 1994; Tang et al, 1994), and with evidence that its efficacy is maintained in real world settings (Pierce et al, 1995; Sonderskov et al, 1997). NRT specifically targets the dependence problem. Making NRT prescribable under the NHS would have the effect of making it available free to the groups most needing help (Fowler, 1997). It would also have the desirable effect of increasing doctors' involvement in smoking treatment after years in which the move to over-the-counter status has greatly reduced their perception that they have something effective to offer. Since smokers contribute about £2.40 to the exchequer with each pack of 20 cigarettes they buy, there is a strong argument from equity that they have earned some help when they wish to stop. Since the likelihood of success in a quit attempt is largely determined in the first one or two days (Westman et al, 1997), the cost to the NHS could be limited by issuing a prescription for only one week in the first instance, with continued supplies for up to six weeks being contingent on abstinence at a one week follow-up. No full-scale trial of free versus commercially priced NRT has yet been conducted, but preliminary evidence points to better compliance and outcome when the smoker does not have to pay (Hughes et al, 1991).

Harm reduction as a policy to reduce smoking-related disease

The advent of novel forms of nicotine delivery, as in NRT and some innovative products from tobacco companies (Sutherland et al, 1993), has focused attention on harm reduction as a potentially important new arm of policy (Warner et al, 1997). There is compelling evidence that people smoke for nicotine, but much of the burden of smoking-related disease is attributable to other smoke components, particularly the tar fraction. Smoking cigarettes has been likened to injecting drugs through a dirty syringe. The potential benefit of shifting the market toward safer forms of nicotine delivery than the cigarette is illustrated by the case of Sweden, where

20% of adult males use oral moist snuff, a non-combustible form of nicotine delivery which carries considerably less risk than cigarettes (Bolinder, 1997). Linked to this, Sweden has the lowest rates of male lung cancer in Europe and also the lowest cigarette smoking prevalence.

The Food and Drug Administration (FDA) in the US has recently asserted its jurisdiction over tobacco as both a drug and a drug delivery device. This opens up the possibility of regulations which will strictly limit permissible emissions from cigarettes, and perhaps force their eventual replacement by non-combustible forms of nicotine delivery. In the UK, product modification policy has so far focused on a series of voluntary agreements with tobacco companies on reducing tar deliveries of cigarettes. These have now been overtaken by action at a European level restricting maximum tar yields to no more than 12 mg. The weakness of this approach is that nominal tar yields have little bearing on smokers' actual exposure: lower tar yield is associated with lower nicotine yield, and smokers simply compensate by larger and more frequent puffs and deeper inhalation.

A new regulatory body

An idea that needs serious consideration in the UK is the establishment of a nicotine regulatory authority or some such body (perhaps under the aegis of the Medicines Control Agency or perhaps freestanding), with regulatory powers similar to those of the FDA. Strict controls on specified carcinogens in cigarette smoke could force the tobacco industry toward less toxic forms of nicotine delivery which would still be acceptable to users. The advantage of this kind of approach in the context of health inequalities is that it would side-step the intractable problem of achieving higher cessation in disadvantaged groups, but if vigorously implemented could have great potential for reducing smoking-related disease. This idea, like making NRT prescribable on the NHS, was put forward for government consideration from the July 1997 Tobacco Summit.

PART 2: ALCOHOL AND HEALTH INEQUALITIES

The association of alcohol with health inequalities

Deaths from diseases caused by alcohol show a clear gradient with socio-economic position. Among men, standardised mortality ratios for cirrhosis and other chronic liver disease in England and Wales in 1991–93 ranged from 67 in professional groups to 242 in unskilled workers (Table 6). There was a similar gradient in deaths associated with the much rarer diagnosis of Alcohol Dependence Syndrome. Corresponding figures for women are not available. In addition to these direct effects, drinking makes a substantial contribution to deaths from accidents, which varied fourfold from professional to unskilled groups in the same period (Table 6). UK data are limited, but a study from Finland showed a clear class gradient in alcohol-related mortality. Almost half of the excess mortality from accidents and violence in manual compared with non-manual workers was accounted for by alcohol-related deaths (Makela et al, 1997).

Table 6: Standardised Mortality Ratios by social class for alcohol-related diseases, men aged 20-64, England and Wales (1991-93)

	I	II	IIINM	IIIM	IV	V	No deaths
Alcohol dependence syndrome	73	58	89	95	110	253	227
Chronic liver disease and cirrhosis	67	75	115	97	119	242	3,270
Accidents	54	57	74	107	106	226	10,275

Source: Drever and Whitehead (1997); Crown Copyright

As well as the overall quantity consumed, the impact of alcohol on health may be determined by the drinking patterns. In a prospective study of Finnish men, those who had a pattern of binge drinking had a relative risk of 3.01 for all deaths, 7.10 for deaths from injury, poisoning, violence and suicide, and 6.50 for fatal myocardial infarction (Kauhanen et al, 1997). This was after adjustment for total alcohol consumption.

Consideration of the health consequences of alcohol consumption should take into account the putative protective effect of moderate drinking on cardiovascular disease. However, there is no existing evidence to show that this modifies alcohol's association with health inequalities.

Patterns of alcohol consumption and problems by deprivation

Numerous factors have to be considered if patterns of alcohol consumption are to be adequately characterised. Overall levels of drinking are important, but so is the patterning over time, the quantity of alcohol consumed on a single drinking occasion, and the social context of consumption. The proportion of complete abstainers may vary substantially by age, gender and socio-economic position, so average consumption figures must be interpreted cautiously. In view of the peaking of alcohol consumption in the young, with the associated risks of accidents and violence, drinking habits in young adults need to be considered separately from those in older people.

Higher levels of consumption of alcohol have been consistently observed in certain deprived groups including the unemployed (Forcier, 1988; Catalano, 1991; Hammarstroem, 1994) and the homeless living in hostels (Gill et al, 1996; Hall and Farrell, 1997).

Data on the association between various indicators of socio-economic status and alcohol consumption are available from a number of sources. The 1994 *Health Survey for England* (Colhoun and Prescott-Clarke, 1996) has the same drinking questions as the General Household Survey, but also includes the CAGE screening items on alcohol problems, and questions on the frequency of being drunk (which may give an indication of binge drinking occasions). Table 7 shows associations between deprivation (indexed by a summary score with a score of one for each of the following: manual occupation; rented housing; no access to a car; and current unemployment) and various indices of alcohol consumption.

Among men aged less than 30 there was little variation by deprivation in the proportion who abstained completely or drank very rarely, but a modest gradient in women, such that the poorest women were about 50% more likely not to drink than the most affluent (21.9% versus 14.0%). Among drinkers there was little overall variation in the average number of units consumed per week or in the proportion drinking above recommended limits. But despite this, there was a gradient in alcohol problems, with twice as many problem drinkers in the poorest as in the most affluent among both men and women (16.9% versus 8.5%; and 6.1% versus 3.3% respectively). In line with this, the incidence of regular drunkenness increased substantially with level of deprivation.

In older adults there was a sharper gradient in never/ rarely drinking, which was much commoner in deprived than in more affluent people. About a quarter of the most deprived men and a half of the most deprived women were abstainers or drank only

rarely. There was again no marked variation by deprivation in average weekly units among drinkers or in the proportion drinking above recommended limits in men. However, problem drinking was twice as common among the most deprived than the most affluent men (11.2% versus 6.2%), and there was three times the incidence of regular drunkenness (12.9% versus 4.0%). Affluent women consumed more alcohol on average than deprived women, and were nearly twice as likely to drink above recommended limits, but had no higher incidence of problem drinking and were much less likely to report being drunk (1.5% versus 5.2%).

These observations suggest that alcohol is likely to contribute to health inequalities in the UK more through the patterning of drinking than through total consumption. Poor drinkers seem to be more likely to get drunk and to encounter drinking problems. This could be because they are more likely to drink a large quantity on a single occasion, to drink on an empty stomach, or to drink in social settings (eg outside) which lead to difficulties.

Table 7: Alcohol consumption and problems

| | Deprivation score | | | |
	0	1	2	3 +
Age <30				
Men				
% never/rarely drink	10.2	8.2	10.3	11.5
mean weekly units*	18.4	25.1	24.8	24.8
% above 21 units*	32.5	41.5	41.4	37.9
% drunk at least once/week*	20.5	31.6	34.9	25.2
% problem drinkers	8.5	12.6	11.9	16.9
Women				
% never/rarely drink	14.0	18.5	22.7	21.9
mean weekly units*	8.5	9.3	10.5	8.2
% above 14 units*	19.3	20.4	20.7	17.2
% drunk at least once/week*	8.8	15.2	18.0	16.8
% problem drinkers	3.3	4.6	6.2	6.1
Age 30+				
Men				
% never/rarely drink	7.5	11.2	24.3	26.5
mean weekly units*	18.2	17.3	18.2	19.2
% above 21 units*	32.1	27.7	29.6	28.1
% drunk at least once/week*	4.0	7.0	9.0	12.9
% problem drinkers	6.2	5.9	5.9	11.2
Women				
% never/rarely drink	15.9	28.0	42.0	48.0
mean weekly units*	7.5	6.4	4.7	5.3
% above 14 units*	17.2	13.9	9.5	11.7
% drunk at least once/week*	1.5	3.0	4.1	5.2
% problem drinkers	3.5	3.0	2.7	3.4
Bases	0	1	2	3 +
Men: <30	460	679	316	187
30+	2,086	2,030	844	569
Women: <30	738	603	366	228
30+	2,973	1,922	1,076	683

Note * base=drinkers only.
Source: HSE (1994)

Drinking problems and alcohol dependence: the OPCS Psychiatric Morbidity Survey

The 1995 OPCS Psychiatric Morbidity Survey (Meltzer et al, 1995), which examined neurotic and psychotic illness in the general population, included extensive assessment of both alcohol-related problems and alcohol dependence. A range of problems including belligerence, problems with a spouse, relatives or friends, job problems, problems with the police, accidents, financial problems and health problems were explored using standardised survey instruments (Hilton, 1991). A total of 19% of men and 5% of women reported encountering at least one alcohol problem in the previous 12 months. There was a graded increase in the incidence of alcohol problems from affluent to poor, with 15.1% and 3.5% of affluent men and women reporting at least one alcohol problem in the past 12 months, rising to 36.7% and 9.9% among the most deprived men and women.

Alcohol dependence was assessed through 12 questionnaire items which followed earlier work in the US (Clark and Hilton, 1991) and were designed to measure three components of dependence: symptomatic behaviour; loss of control of drinking; and binge drinking. Overall 8% of men and 2% of women reported dependence (Meltzer et al, 1996), with predictors being similar to those for problem drinking. Farrell et al (in preparation) have analysed the psychiatric morbidity dataset, looking at the association of dependence on alcohol, nicotine and drugs with scores on a deprivation index similar to that employed in the sections on tobacco smoking and physical activity. These analyses show that the association was strongest for drug dependence and nicotine dependence but was also significant for alcohol dependence, with the most deprived individuals being nearly three times more likely to receive a diagnosis of alcohol dependence (see Figure 3).

Figure 3: Deprivation score and risk of dependence

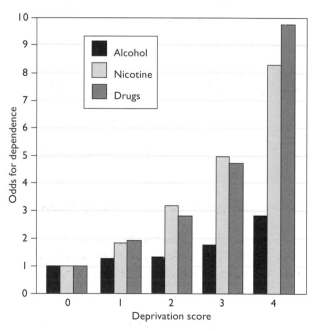

Source: OPCS Psychiatric Morbidity Survey

Alcohol use in youth

Among youth, heavy drinking is strongly associated with both delinquency and criminality, but the direction of the effect is not clear and this association may indeed simply reflect a constellation of behaviours which is more often associated with lower class status (Jessor and Jessor, 1977). What seems clear from the literature is that young and disadvantaged people, particularly males, are more

likely to engage in drinking patterns which sometimes have serious consequences for themselves and for society as a whole. The degree to which these drinking patterns remain chronic (and in the long run are highly associated with severe dependence) is a question that a cross-sectional study cannot answer. It is complex, in part, because deprivation may contribute to the probability of continuing to drink in a hazardous fashion and, as has been suggested for tobacco consumption, deprivation may inhibit opportunities for positive changes in such behaviours.

There is a need for some better longitudinal studies that could examine the social, environmental and peer influences on drinking behaviour especially within the young group among whom the greatest reported rates of problems occur.

Policy implications

The data presented above suggest a complex relationship between socio-economic deprivation and alcohol consumption. Average consumption varies little across social class groups, but there are indications of differences in the impact of alcohol. More deprived groups have higher levels of all alcohol-related problems ranging from self-reported difficulties or drunkenness, to dependence and alcohol-related deaths. These differences may relate to the patterning of consumption, which in turn could be a feature of the social context of consumption. Excessive alcohol use may well be a cause of downward social mobility, which appears likely to be the case among some of the homeless population. These considerations mean that policy implications are unlikely to be straightforward.

Price as an instrument of alcohol policy

The taxation of alcohol has been advocated specifically to modulate overall population consumption (Edwards et al, 1994). The impact of income on consumption is complex and not well studied among population sub-groups, although there are indications of differential response by income group, with heavy drinking more responsive at lower income levels (Sutton and Godfrey, 1995). Some recent US work suggests that pricing may influence poor heavy drinkers to drink cheaper and poorer quality alcohol (Kerr, 1997), but extrapolation to the UK situation is difficult.

Targeting heavy drinking among young adults

One of the questions for future policy initiatives is the potential to modify heavy drinking, especially among young drinkers. Education-based programmes which focused on teaching about 'sensible drinking' might target the aspect of drinking behaviour which is most closely linked to deprivation.

Controls on access to drink for young people might also have a part to play. For example the 'designer drinks' have been shown to be attractive to the younger age groups, but they have also been found to be associated with drinking in less-controlled environments, heavier drinking and greater drunkenness (Hughes et al, 1997). Regulation of advertising of drink to the youth market, or control of access to youth-oriented drinks may be one route.

PART 3: INEQUALITIES IN PHYSICAL ACTIVITY

Physical activity and health

Increased physical activity is associated with lower mortality rates, and decreased risks of cardiovascular mortality, colon cancer and non-insulin dependent diabetes. Regular physical activity prevents or delays the development of high blood pressure, reduces blood pressure in those with hypertension and relieves the symptoms of depression and anxiety. Weight bearing physical activity has a role in the development of bone mass during childhood and adolescence which may be important in reducing the likelihood of developing osteoporosis (USDHHS, 1996). A meta-analysis of observational studies has concluded that more physically active and physically fit individuals are at a lower risk for coronary heart disease; the relative risk of developing coronary heart disease in the least active compared to the most active was found to be 1.9 [(95%CI 1.6 -2.2) (Berlin and Colditz, 1990)]. Physical activity also has an important role in the prevention of weight gain and obesity (Haapanen et al, 1997).

Data from a review of epidemiological evidence supports the view that there is a dose–response relationship between physical activity and mortality (Blair and Connelly, 1996). The review found that greater amounts of activity or fitness provide greater benefits, although an optimal dose and intensity of exercise cannot be defined and concluded that "some activity is better than none and low to moderate intensity is better than remaining sedentary".

Although there is no disease as directly linked to lowered levels of physical activity as lung cancer is with smoking or liver cirrhosis with alcohol, obesity is likely to be a marker for lowered levels of energy output. As shown in Table 8, there is a higher level of obesity in more deprived people, with a sharper gradient in women than in men.

Table 8: Body mass index by deprivation score

	Deprivation score			
	0	**1**	**2**	**3+**
Men				
% BMI < 20	3.5	3.8	6.1	8.3
% BMI > 30	13.3	13.4	13.8	17.0
Women				
% BMI < 20	6.6	7.1	8.6	10.1
% BMI > 30	14.9	16.0	21.0	25.2

Source: HSE (1994)

Recommended levels of physical activity

Based on the existing epidemiological data, the Department of Health published a *Strategy statement on physical activity* in 1996 (DoH, 1996a) with three key objectives:

* to promote the value of moderate activity on a regular basis for sedentary people;
* to inform people of the value of maintaining 30 minutes of moderate activity on at least five days a week for those who already take some moderate activity;
* advocate, for those already taking some vigorous activity, the maintenance of a total of three periods of vigorous activity of 20 minutes a week.

Until 1995, the amount of exercise recommended in order to benefit health had been 3-5 days a week at 60-90% of maximum heart rate (that is, vigorous exercise) for 20-60 minutes on each occasion. The type of activity to be encouraged was defined as "any activity that uses large muscle groups, is rhythmical in nature, can be maintained continuously and is aerobic in nature". This recommendation was primarily concerned with improving functional capacity rather than reducing the risk of chronic disease (USDHHS, 1996). In 1995, the Centers for Disease Control in the US together with the American College of Sports Medicine (1995) published new recommendations which had a more public health focus, recommending that all adults should exercise on at least five days of the week at a moderate intensity for 30 minutes or more on each occasion (Pate et al, 1995). Brisk walking is the most commonly cited moderate intensity exercise. The new recommendation is not meant to replace the old one, but rather complement it.

Levels of physical activity and socio-economic status

Three sources of data have been used for this report: the Health Survey for England 1994 (HSE) (Joint Health Surveys Unit, 1996), the General Household Survey 1993 (GHS) (OPCS, 1993) and the National Fitness Survey 1992 (NFS) (Sports Council and Health Education Authority, 1992). Although the three surveys used varied in the method of assessing and reporting physical activity, similar trends can be seen in them.

Moderate to vigorous activity

GHS data show that rates of participation in physical activity (including sports and walking) are higher in men than women in all social classes, and higher in non-manual than manual groups for both sexes (Table 9). The results from the HSE and the NFS, in which respondents are classified by overall level of activity, confirm the gender difference (albeit somewhat attenuated), but show levels of moderate to vigorous activity (levels 3, 4 and 5) to be higher in manual than non-manual groups (Table 9). The difference is likely to be accounted for by differences in the occupational physical activity, which is higher in manual groups and is included in figures for overall physical activity (see Table 13). To complicate the situation further, results from the HSE based on deprivation rather than social class to characterise disadvantage, show that fewer men from the most deprived group are reporting moderate or vigorous physical activity (Table 10).

Table 9: Participation in physical activities in the four weeks before interview by socio-economic group and sex: age-standardised

	Professional	Employers and managers	Intermediate and junior non-manual	Skilled manual and own account non-professional	Semi-skilled manual and personal services	Unskilled manual
Men						
Observed%	84	74	78	66	65	62
Expected %	72	69	73	70	71	73
Standardised ratio	117*	108*	107*	94*	92*	86*
Base = 100%	561	1,509	1,322	2,764	1,052	318
Women						
Observed%	73	66	61	49	48	42
Expected%	60	57	58	54	55	51
Standardised ratio	123*	116*	106*	90*	86*	84*
Base = 100%	147	853	4,286	722	1,926	846

* Ratio significantly different from 100 (p<0.05).

Source: GHS (1993)

smoking, drinking, physical activity and screening uptake

Table 10: Age-standardised proportions of physical activity level by own social class

	Total	I and II	IIINM	IIIM	IV and V
		Social class groups			
Activity levels 3,4 and 5					
Men	51	46	45	54	55
Women	38	40	34	41	42
Activity levels 1 and 2					
Men	33	40	40	29	26
Women	43	42	47	38	38
Activity level 0					
Men	16	14	14	18	19
Women	19	17	19	21	20

Source: HSE (1994)

Sedentary behaviour

As an alternative to focusing on activity, it may be important to look at inactivity. Results from both the HSE and the NFS indicate that a higher proportion of the manual groups report being entirely sedentary (not having undertaken any episode of exercise in the last four weeks). In both the HSE and the NFS, the proportion of men classified as sedentary (activity level 0) is significantly higher in classes IIIM to V (Tables 11 and 12). A similar, non-significant, difference is seen for women.

Analysis of HSE data by deprivation level shows that the most deprived people are twice as likely to be sedentary as the most affluent (28.9% versus 14.3% among men and 31.5% versus 14.5% among women – see Table 10). The NFS also provides data on activity levels in relation to educational level and housing tenure. The proportion of people classified as inactive is lower for those with professional/technical qualifications at all age groups and in both sexes, and lower for those who own their homes.

Table 11: Proportion of those active at levels 0-5 by Deprivation Score

	0	1	2	3+
		Deprivation Index		
Male				
Activity level				
Level 0	14.3	14.5	21.0	28.9
Level 1,2	41.6	30.3	27.8	29.4
Level 3,4,5	44.0	55.1	51.1	41.7
Female				
Activity level				
Level 0	14.5	17.3	24.6	31.5
Level 1,2	47.1	41.0	40.6	35.9
Level 3,4,5	38.3	41.7	34.8	32.7

Source: HSE (1994)

Table 12: Activity averages for social class

		Men	Women
		No reported activity (Level 0)	
Age group 16-34		%	%
Social class	I and II	6	6
	IIINM	7	7
	IIIM	9	10
	IV & V	6	14
Age group 35-54			
Social class	I and II	9	9
	IIINM	8	13
	IIIM	13	10
	IV & V	14	16
Age group 55-74			
Social class	I and II	31	28
	IIINM	40	33
	IIIM	38	31
	IV & V	36	32

Source: NFS (1992)

Trends by type of activity

The trends observed for overall physical activity are not the same when types of physical activity are considered separately. Unsurprisingly, the manual social class groups have higher levels of moderate or vigorous occupational activity. Only 9% of men are active in their occupations at this level in social classes I and II, compared with 32% in social classes IV and V (Table 13). By contrast, there is a clear inverse relationship between social class and participation in sport activity, while home activity (heavy housework, gardening) varies little by social class.

Table 13: Age-standardised proportions of those active at a moderate or vigorous level for each activity type by sex and own social class

Type of activity	Total	I &II	IIINM	IIIM	IV and V
		Social class of informant			
% active at moderate or vigorous level (3, 4 or 5)					
Occupation					
Men	20	9	13	31	32
Women	11	13	5	16	18
Home					
Men	64	66	64	65	62
Women	70	69	71	69	72
Walking					
Men	32	39	34	25	27
Women	22	26	21	19	17
Sports (of 20 mins)					
Men	42	47	46	37	36
Women	42	42	35	31	26

Source: HSE (1994)

The pattern for participation in walking is complex. Table 13 shows that the frequency of reporting brisk walking shows an inverse relationship with social class in both men and women. Most of this difference is accounted for by how respondents assessed their usual walking pace. Although data are not provided, the HSE reports that people in social classes IIIM to V walked more than those in other social classes but were less likely to define their walking pace as brisk or fast.

Popularity of types of activity

Walking is the most common form of activity across all socio-economic groups, although the National Travel Survey shows that over the last 10 years the number of journeys made on foot has fallen by 13% (DETR, 1997). Walking is followed by swimming, keep-fit/yoga and cycling, although swimming is much more popular in professional groups (Table 14). Snooker/pool/billiards are particularly popular with younger men, but increased participation in this

sport is unlikely to lead to noticeable health benefits. Keep-fit/yoga ranks high mainly due to its popularity with women across all age groups.

Policy implications

Experimental evaluations of interventions aimed at changing levels of physical activity have generally been directed towards white, middle-aged, well-educated men and women (Hillsdon and Thorogood, 1996). Interventions targeted at individuals achieve modest increases in activity which can be sustained for up to two years (King et al, 1995). Interventions where the mode of exercise being encouraged is walking appear to be more effective than those that depend on attending a facility to practice games and sports (Hillsdon and Thorogood, 1996). Little is known about the effectiveness of interventions in other socio-economic groups, and evidence about the effectiveness of different types of interventions is scarce.

Table 14: Sports, games and physical activities: participating rates in the four weeks before interview by socio-economic group

Persons aged 16 and over
Active sports, games
Socio-economic group and
physical activities*

	Professional	Employers and managers	Intermediate and junior non-manual	Skilled manual and own account non-professional	Semi-skilled manual and personal service	Unskilled manual	Total+
Walking	57	46	42	39	36	31	41
Any swimming	27	19	18	10	11	8	15
Snooker/pool/billiards	11	12	8	17	10	9	12
Keep fit/yoga	13	12	18	6	9	8	12
Cycling	14	9	9	10	8	9	10
Darts	6	5	4	8	6	6	6
Weightlifting/training	7	5	5	6	4	3	5
Golf	9	10	5	6	2	2	5
Running (jogging etc)	11	6	4	3	2	2	5
Any soccer	6	3	3	6	3	3	4
Tenpin bowl skittles	5	5	4	4	3	2	4
Badminton	5	3	3	1	1	1	3
Tennis	5	2	2	1	1	1	2
Fishing	3	3	1	3	2	1	2
Any bowls	1	2	2	2	2	2	2
Squash	4	3	2	1	1	0	2
Table tennis	3	2	1	1	1	1	2
Horse riding	1	1	1	0	1	1	1
Cricket	2	1	1	1	0	1	1

Notes:
* Includes activities in which more than 1% of adults participated in the four weeks before interview.
+ Total includes full-time students, members of the Armed Forces, those who have never worked, and those whose job was inadequately desrcibed.
Source: GHS (1993)

Building more leisure centres, even if they are built in relatively deprived areas, is unlikely to reduce inequalities in participation in games and sports. Indeed, such leisure centres are more likely to increase inequalities, because this form of exercise is most popular with the least deprived, and is also relatively expensive and therefore out of the reach of those on low incomes. Provision of low-cost, keep-fit classes, in existing local facilities such as community centres or schools, may increase participation among women, since this form of exercise is popular.

It would seem to be logical to put more emphasis on encouraging walking, since it requires no expensive equipment or training for the individuals concerned and can be easily incorporated into everyday routines. More deprived sectors of the community need improved access to pleasant areas to increase opportunities for leisure time walking, while more affluent sectors of the community need changes in transport policy to get them out of their cars more often.

PART 4: INEQUALITIES IN BREAST AND CERVICAL SCREENING UPTAKE

Contrasting patterns of mortality by socio-economic position are seen for cervical cancer and breast cancer (Table 15). Whereas there is a sharp gradient toward higher mortality from cervical cancer in poorer women, there is currently no significant variation in breast cancer deaths by social class, reversing a previous trend to higher death rates in non-manual groups. National data on inequalities in breast and cervical screening uptake are available from two sources: Department of Health returns and occasional national surveys.

Department of Health returns

Information on coverage and uptake of screening by regional health authority and health district is published annually (for example, DoH, 1996b, 1997). An unpublished analysis conducted by the Department's Statistics Division shows a relationship between the Townsend deprivation score and coverage for both breast and cervical screening. For

Table 15: Breast and cervical mortality by social class

Cervical cancer mortality by social class

		SMR*
I	Professional	29
II	Employers and managers	60
III	Skilled non-manual	73
III	Skilled manual	112
IV	Semi-skilled	124
V	Unskilled	186

* Standardised Mortality Ratio, Great Britain = 100

Source: Occupational Mortality Decennial Supplement No 6

Breast cancer mortality by social class
Mortality Rate Ratios for breast cancer by social class:
Longitudinal study cohort, England and Wales 1976-92
Women aged 35-64

	1976-81	1981-85	1986-92
I/II	0.85	1.30	1.14
IIINM	1.23	1.24	1.06
IIIM	1.00	1.00	1.00
IV/V	0.78	0.88	1.17
Manual v non-manual	0.87	0.72	1.00

Source: Harding et al (1997); Crown Copyright

example, dividing health districts into quintiles on the basis of deprivation score, coverage of breast screening in 1995/96 was 68.5% in the least deprived districts and 58.0% in the most deprived districts. The corresponding figures for cervical screening coverage were 87.5% and 77.9% (see Figure 4). In principle, this analysis could be extended to take account of other district level variables derived from Census data and other sources (eg percentage of population in non-white ethnic groups; percentage of GP practices with practice nurses). Coverage rates for cervical screening have increased dramatically since the introduction of the computerised call-recall system and target payments to GPs. Department of Health data could be analysed to examine whether the gap in coverage rates between the more and less deprived districts has decreased in recent years, as might be expected.

National surveys

Questions on breast and cervical screening are not included in regular national surveys such as the General Household Survey and the Health Survey for England. However, several surveys conducted by the Health Education Authority have included relevant questions. The 1992 Health and Lifestyles Survey (Health Education Authority, 1995) showed a social class gradient in cervical smear uptake: 92% of women in social classes I-II said they had had a cervical smear compared with 82% among those in social classes IV-V and 78% among those not working (see Figure 5). There was a similar gradient for breast screening but the question was asked only indirectly. Similar questions were used in the Black and Minority Ethnic Groups Health and Lifestyles Survey conducted in 1992 (Health Education Authority, 1994). The percentage of African-Caribbean women who reported having had a smear test in the last five years was 81% (similar to the UK average) but the figures for the South Asian women were considerably lower: 63% for Indian women, 45% for Pakistani women and only 33% for Bangladeshi women. Breast screening showed similar differences by ethnic group (see Figure 6).

Figure 4: Breast and cervical screening coverage by deprivation index (1995/96)

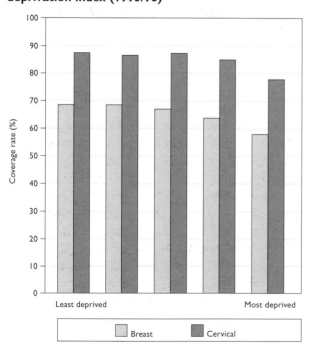

Source: Based on data provided by Peter Steele, Department of Health, Statistics Division

Figure 5: Breast and cervical screening coverage by deprivation index (1995/96)

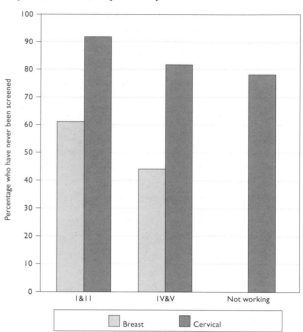

Figures are based on women aged 55-64 (breast) and 16-74 (cervical).
The HEA report does not give a figure for breast screening in the not working group.

Source: HEA (1995)

Figure 6: Breast and cervical screening uptake by ethnic group

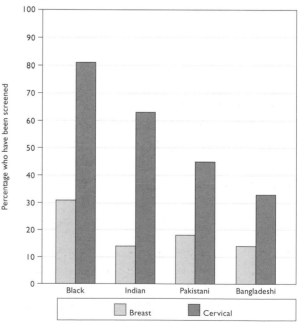

Figures are based on women aged 50-74 (breast) and 16-74 (cervical) and show the % who have been screened 'ever' (breast) and 'in the last five years' (cervical).
Source: HEA (1994)

Policy initiatives

A number of strategies have been suggested for reducing inequalities in screening uptake (and increasing overall uptake). There is little evidence currently available for judging their likely effectiveness and cost-effectiveness. They include:

- Introducing a system of target payments to GPs for breast screening similar to that for cervical screening. This is a controversial proposal. GPs have less involvement in the breast screening programme than they have in the cervical screening programme and therefore have less potential for influencing screening uptake. An ongoing Medical Research Council-funded trial should yield valuable information on the efficacy, and cost, of encouraging and helping primary care teams to become more involved in the breast screening programme. The establishment of a system of target payments to GPs also makes it more difficult to introduce changes in the screening programme in the future.
- Improving the accuracy of registers. Inaccuracy of registers is a major problem in inner cities. Initiatives to increase the accuracy of GP and health authority lists could help to reduce inequalities in screening uptake.
- Employing outreach workers to contact women in ethnic minority groups.
- Education campaigns targeted at women living in deprived areas.

Appendix A: Gender differences in cigarette smoking and smoking cessation in the UK

Introduction

Historically, smoking rates among men in the UK have been far higher than in women. Men started smoking in large numbers some 20 or 30 years earlier than women, and their cigarette smoking prevalence peaked at close to 80% in the years following the Second World War, compared to a peak of about 45% in women in the early 1970s. In recent years smoking rates in men and women have moved much closer, as a cohort of older women for whom never smoking was the norm has been replaced by younger women with smoking habits more similar to those among men.

Much recent comment, particularly in the media, has drawn attention to an emerging problem of smoking in young women. It is frequently suggested that smoking in young women is on the increase and is now outstripping that in young men, and there is a suggestion that policy initiatives should target smoking in young women. In the recently released figures from the 1996 General Household Survey (L. Jarvis, 1997a), it was noted that cigarette smoking prevalence increased from 26% to 28% in women compared with 1994, while in men the increase over the same period from 28% to 29% was not statistically significant. Women aged 25-34 were the only age group for whom the increase in prevalence was statistically significant.

The purpose of this brief note is to critically examine the evidence that there is an emerging problem of smoking specifically in young women.

OPCS/ONS surveys of schoolchildren's smoking

Regular national surveys of schoolchildren's smoking have been conducted since 1982. Over the whole of this period girls have tended to be more likely to smoke than boys. The 1996 survey (L. Jarvis, 1997b) reported that 15% of girls aged 11-15 in England were regular smokers of one or more cigarettes per week compared to 11% of boys. Girls were also more likely to report occasional smoking of less than one cigarette per week (10% versus 8%). At age 15, 33% of girls compared with 28% of boys were regular smokers. Figure 7 shows that girls have consistently been more likely to smoke than boys at age 15 over the whole period since 1982, although there has been no clear pattern of increasing prevalence in either sex over this period.

If these gender differences are carried forward into adult life, there should now be evidence of higher rates of smoking in women than in men among the age group 16-24, and to a lesser extent in those aged 25-34.

Figure 7: Smoking prevalence among 15-year-olds (OPCS/ONS 1982-96)

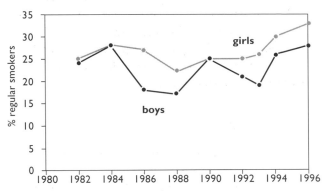

Source: ONS National Survey of smoking in secondary schoolchildren

Table 16: Cigarette smoking prevalence in men and old women aged 16-34, Great Britain (1982-96)

	Men			Women		
	16-24	25-34	All 16-34	16-24	25-34	All 16-34
1982	35.9	40.3	38.1	35.1	36.9	36.0
1984	35.0	40.3	37.7	34.4	35.8	35.2
1986	36.1	36.9	36.5	34.6	35.3	35.0
1988	33.2	36.9	35.2	33.3	34.6	34.0
1990	33.3	36.3	35.0	35.8	34.1	34.8
1992	34.9	34.3	34.6	32.3	33.7	33.1
1994	34.8	34.0	34.3	33.7	30.2	31.5
1996	35.1	38.4	37.1	34.1	34.2	34.2

	Men			Women		
Bases	16-24	25-34	All 16-34	16-24	25-34	All 16-34
1982	1,617	1,646	3,263	1,677	1,812	3,489
1984	1,462	1,576	3,038	1,528	1,748	3,276
1986	1,493	1,651	3,144	1,554	1,852	3,406
1988	1,352	1,543	2,895	1,524	1,796	3,320
1990	1,165	1,577	2,742	1,280	1,845	3,125
1992	1,149	1,571	2,720	1,359	1,695	3,054
1994	951	1,389	2,340	1,069	1,823	2,892
1996	877	1,322	2,199	970	1,615	2,585

Source: General Household Survey

Cigarette smoking in adults aged 16-34

Table 16 presents cigarette smoking prevalence among young adults aged less than 35 for the period 1982 to 1996 using data from the General Household Survey. There was a significant overall decline between 1982 and 1994 which was reversed in 1996 when prevalence did not differ significantly from that in 1982. Across the whole of this period women aged under 35 were significantly less likely to smoke cigarettes than men ($p<.0001$). The interaction term for gender by year of survey did not reach significance ($p=0.80$), indicating that trends in men and women over this period were similar. In the age group 16-24, there was no significant variation in prevalence between 1982 and 1996 ($p=0.61$) and no gender difference ($p=0.36$). Among those aged 25-34 women were less likely to smoke than men ($p<0.0001$), and prevalence declined initially but then returned close to 1982 levels in 1996, with no significant interaction by sex ($p=0.74$).

Since the cohort of 15-year-old girls with higher smoking rates than boys would have passed through the 16-24 year old group as surveyed by the General Household Survey during this period, these figures strongly suggest that the gender difference observed at age 15 is a transient phenomenon which is no longer in evidence in young adults aged 16-24. In this age group there would currently appear to be complete equality between the sexes in rates of cigarette smoking, and no trend to either increasing or decreasing prevalence. In slightly older adults aged 25-34, men are significantly more likely to

smoke than are women. There is no evidence from successive surveys since 1982 for the emergence of any different pattern of gender differences. The most disturbing aspect of the data is the significant increase in prevalence in 1996, an effect which was of similar magnitude in men and women, and which returned prevalence in young adults close to the level of 14 years previously.

Gender differences in rates of smoking cessation

Rates of smoking cessation can be estimated by calculating ex-smokers as a proportion of ever-regular smokers. This is sometimes known as the quit ratio, and it has been shown to be a reasonably robust indicator of trends in the population. Analyses comparing the quit ratio in men and women for the years 1988, 1990 and 1992 have been published based on data from the General Household Survey (M.J. Jarvis, 1994). Table 17 gives the observed rates of cessation in men and women in various age groups up to 35 (top) and odds ratios for cessation in women relative to men (bottom). Women had higher rates of cessation at all ages up to 35. This difference did not reach significance in adults aged 16-25, but was significant in those aged 25-34. It would therefore seem that women's lower rates of smoking in this age group may largely be attributable to their higher probability of giving up.

Table 17: Rates of smoking cessation in young adults

	1988		1990		1992	
	Men	Women	Men	Women	Men	Women
16-19	11	14	12	16	14	16
20-24	18	18	14	17	16	20
25-29	21	29	22	26	23	29
30-34	28	34	28	32	33	32

Odds of smoking cessation in women relating to men

	1988		1990		1992	
	OR	95%CI	OR	95%CI	OR	95%CI
16-25	1.00	(0.75-1.34)	1.26	(0.92-1.72)	1.23	(0.90-1.66)
26-35	1.30	(1.06-1.60)	1.32	(1.07-1.64)	1.19	(0.97-1.47)

Source: General Household Survey

Table 18: Predictors of current cigarette smoking

		Men		Women	
		OR	95%CI	OR	95%CI
Age	<35	1.00		1.00	
	35+	0.75	(0.71-0.79)	0.78	(0.74-0.82)
Deprivation score	0	1.00		1.00	
	1	1.56	(1.47-1.65)	1.44	(1.37-1.53)
	2	2.30	(2.15-2.46)	2.03	(1.91-2.15)
	3	3.27	(3.02-3.53)	2.54	(2.37-2.72)
	4	5.62	(4.91-6.45)	3.55	(3.04-4.15)
	5	8.28	(5.65-12.14)	5.81	(2.57-13.11)
Marital status and spouse smoking:					
Spouse never smoker		0.57	(0.54-0.60)	0.47	(0.44-0.50)
Spouse ex-smoker		0.58	(0.54-0.62)	0.65	(0.61-0.68)
Spouse current smoker		2.71	(2.57-2.85)	2.57	(2.46-2.69)
Single		0.93	(0.87-0.98)	0.99	(0.94-1.04)
Widowed		0.75	(0.68-0.82)	0.60	(0.56-0.64)
Divorced/separated		1.77	(1.62-1.92)	1.87	(1.76-1.99)
Year of survey					
	1988	1.00		1.00	
	1990	0.97	(0.91-1.05)	1.01	(0.95-1.08)
	1992	0.92	(0.85-0.95)	0.96	(0.90-1.02)
	1994	0.88	(0.82-0.95)	0.83	(0.77-.88)
	1996	0.91	(0.84-0.98)	0.94	(.88-1.00)

Note: reference group for marital status and spouse smoking is population average.
Source: General Household Survey (1988-96)

Predictors of current cigarette smoking in men and women in the UK

Table 18 shows some of the main predictors of cigarette smoking in men and women in Great Britain over the period 1988-96. What is striking is the lack of difference between the sexes, with odds ratios being very similar in almost every instance. The major predictors of smoking in both men and women are: age; marital status and spouse's smoking habits; socio-economic circumstances; and year of survey. Lower smoking prevalence is predicted by older age; having a non-smoking partner; being less deprived; and declined in successive surveys. The strength and similarity of these predictors in both men and women contrasts markedly with the weakness of gender as a predictor.

Conclusions

The supposed emergence of smoking in young women as a special problem is more myth than reality. Despite a transiently higher prevalence in girls in the mid-teen years, smoking rates in young adults, and their trends over time, show little difference by gender. By contrast, deprivation and family circumstances are major predictors of smoking, with similar associations to current cigarette smoking in men and in women. The reality of the current situation would appear to be that cigarette smoking is indeed a huge societal problem, but one that is not differentiated to any great extent by gender. Focusing on smoking in young women risks downplaying the extent of smoking in young men, and diverting attention from the factors that predict smoking in both young men and young women.

Appendix B: Inequalities in birth weight: are they mediated by smoking, or is smoking a proxy for socio-economic factors?

Cigarette smoking is consistently associated with lowered birth weight. On average, babies of women who smoke weigh about 200g less than those of non-smokers. Some have suggested that this association is not causal but explained by other factors, such as diet, personal characteristics, socio-economic status, or psychosocial stress, which may relate both to foetal growth and to smoking behaviour (Yerushalmy, 1971). Most, however, have concluded that the association is causal (USDHHS, 1980). In support of this interpretation is the dose response to number of cigarettes smoked, the existence of plausible biological pathways through which the effect might be mediated, and the fact that smoking cessation in pregnancy reduces or eliminates the birth weight difference (Li et al, 1993).

The St George's Birth Weight Study (Brooke et al, 1989) was set up to examine the role of personal, psychosocial and socio-economic factors, in addition to effects of smoking, drinking and caffeine consumption, on determining birth weight. A very wide range of variables was measured. Socio-economic status was represented by social class, housing tenure, educational level, income and receipt of benefits; social support by contact with neighbours, friends and relatives and by the presence of a confidant; psychological well-being by GHQ score, psychiatric history, feelings about the pregnancy, and life events. Of the total of over 40 indicators of socio-economic status and psychosocial stress only four were significantly associated with lowered birth weight, and these factors became non-significant when smoking was controlled for. The effect of smoking, by contrast, was robust to adjustment for socio-economic and psychosocial factors.

The findings of the St George's study have recently been extended by analysis of stored blood specimens for cotinine to provide a quantitative measure of inhaled smoke dose (Peacock et al, 1998). Birth weight adjusted for gestational age showed a graded decline with increasing cotinine concentration. This relationship was stronger than that with cigarette consumption, and remained significant after adjusting for cigarette consumption, strongly suggesting a biological effect of inhaled smoke dose. This was further suggested by the finding that a reduction in cotinine between booking and 28 weeks was associated with increased birth weight.

In summary, the evidence points strongly to a causal effect of cigarette smoking on lowering birth weight, but provides little support for any substantial effects of socio-economic or psychosocial factors.

Appendix C: Physical activity: details of population surveys consulted

Sources of data

Three main sources of data have been used for this report:

- Health Survey for England 1994 (HSE) (Colhoun and Prescott Clarke, 1996)
- General Household Survey 1993 (GHS) (OPCS, 1993);
- National Fitness Survey 1992 (NFS) (Sports Council and Health Education Authority, 1992).

All three surveys involved national samples and used face-to-face interviews to collect the data. The HSE interviewed 15,809 subjects aged 16 and over, the GHS 18,492 and the NFS 4,316. Unfortunately, methods for measuring and classifying physical activity differed between surveys.

Physical activity can be assessed in terms of *type*, *frequency*, *duration* and *intensity*.

Types of activity

The types of activity assessed in the three surveys included work activity, housework, gardening, walking, Do-It-Yourself (DIY) and sports and physical exercise. Both the HSE and NFS asked about occupational activity, housework, DIY/ building, walking and sports and exercise. The NFS also asked about stair climbing. The GHS asked about walking and sports/physical exercise, but Gardening and DIY were asked about separately and not used in summary measures of physical activity.

Frequency of activity

All three surveys assessed the frequency of activity by recording the number of occasions an activity was performed in the four weeks prior to the interview. Occupational activity was assumed to have been performed at least three times per week.

Duration of activity

No measure of duration was included in the GHS. In the other two surveys duration of activity was recorded in minutes and was usually determined by asking people about how long they 'usually' spent doing an activity or how long they spent on the most recent occasion. In the HSE only the duration of sports and exercise were assessed. The duration of walking was not assessed directly in any of surveys but 'occasions' of walking were only counted if they were one mile or longer in the HSE and two miles or longer in the NFS and GHS.

Intensity of activity

In the GHS no measure of intensity was included. The HSE and NFS both assigned scores to activities placing them in rank order on a scale which reflected the effort required for an average man to carry them out. Scores were expressed in terms of kilocalories per min (kcals/min). Variations in the intensity of activity at the individual level was taken into account by considering individual assessments of the amount of effort required to perform an activity. In the case of walking this depended on the 'usual' pace of walking, while for home activities respondents were given examples of what was meant by 'heavy' housework, DIY and gardening. Intensity classifications of sports and exercise were dependent on whether the person said the activity made them 'out of breath or sweaty'. The intensity of occupational activity was based on self-assessment of level of activity at work and lists of specific occupations that were known to involve greater levels of physical activity. Intensity measures in the HSE and HFS were summarised as follows:

Vigorous: some activity with an energy cost of 7.5 kcals/min or more;

Moderate: some activity with an energy cost of five kcals/min but less than 7.5 kcals/min;

Light: some activity with an energy cost of two kcals/min but less than five kcals/min.

Only sports, exercise and occupational activities could be classified as vigorous.

Summary measures

The HSE and NFS use a summary measure incorporating elements of frequency, intensity and duration. The reference period was the four weeks prior to interview.

Level 5:   twelve or more occasions of vigorous activity;

Level 4:   twelve or more occasions of a mix of moderate and vigorous activity;

Level 3:   twelve or more occasions of moderate activity;

Level 2:   five to eleven occasions of at least moderate activity;

Level 1   one to four occasions of at least moderate activity;

Level 0:   no occasions of moderate activity.

In the HSE sports and exercise occasions were only counted if they lasted for at least 20 minutes whereas in the NFS these plus home activities were only counted if they lasted 20 minutes.

The GHS did not consider duration or intensity, and therefore only reports the frequency of sports, exercise and walking occasions of any duration and intensity. Moreover, in the GHS the definition of 'sports' included snooker and darts which do not require sufficient intensity of physical activity to derive any health benefit.

References

American College of Sports Medicine (1995) *Guidelines for exercise testing and prescription*, 5th edn, Baltimore, MD: Williams and Wilkins.

Bennett, N., Jarvis, L., Rowlands, D., Singleton, N. and Haselden, L. (1996) *Living in Britain: Results from the 1994 General Household Survey*, London: HMSO.

Berlin, J.A. and Colditz, G.A. (1990) 'A meta-analysis of physical activity in the prevention of coronary heart disease', *American Journal of Epidemiology*, no 132, pp 639-46.

Blair, S.N. and Connelly, J.C. (1996) 'How much physical activity should we do: the case for moderate amounts and intensities of physical activity', *Research Quarterly for Exercise and Sport*, no 67, 193-205.

Bolinder, G. (1997) 'Smokeless tobacco a less harmful alternative?', in C.T. Bolliger and K.O. Fagerstrom (eds) *The tobacco epidemic*, Progress in Respiratory Research No 28, Basel: Karger, pp 199-212.

Bridgwood, A. and Malbon, G. (1995) *Survey of the physical health of prisoners*, London: HMSO.

Brooke, O.G., Anderson, H.R., Bland, J.M., Peacock, J.L. and Stewart, C.M. (1989) 'Effects on birth weight of smoking, alcohol, caffeine, socio-economic factors, and psychosocial stress', *British Medical Journal*, vol 298 (6676), pp 795-801.

Carroll, D., Bennett, P. and Davey Smith, G. (1993) 'Socio-economic health inequalities: their origins and implications', *Psychology and Health*, vol 8, pp 295-316.

Carstairs, V. and Morris, R. (1989) 'Deprivation and mortality: an alternative to social class?', *Community Medicine*, vol 11, pp 210-19.

Catalano, R. (1991) 'The health effects of economic insecurity', *American Journal of Public Health*, vol 81, no 9, pp 1148-52.

Clark, W.B. and Hilton, M.E. (eds) (1991) *Alcohol in America: Drinking practices and problems*, Albany, NY: State University of New York Press.

Cohen, S. and Lichtenstein, E. (1990) 'Perceived stress, quitting smoking, and smoking relapse', *Health Psychology*, no 9, pp 466-78.

Colhoun, H. and Prescott-Clarke, P. (eds) (1996) *Health Survey for England 1994*, London: HMSO.

Cox, B.D., Huppert, F. and Whichelow, M.J. (eds) (1993) *The Health and Lifestyle Survey: Seven years on*, Aldershot: Dartmouth.

Davey Smith, G. and Morris, J. (1994) 'Increasing inequalities in the health of the nation', *British Medical Journal*, vol 309, pp 1453-4.

DETR (Department of the Environment, Transport and the Regions) (1997) *National Travel Survey 1994/96*, London: The Stationery Office.

DoH (Department of Health) (1996a) *Strategy statement on physical activity*, London: DoH.

DoH (1996b) *Cervical screening programme, England: 1995-96*, Statistical Bulletin 1996/26, London.

DoH (1997) *Breast screening programme, England: 1995-96*, Statistical Bulletin 1997/3, London.

Doll, R., Peto, R., Wheatley, K., Gray, R. and Sutherland, I. (1994) 'Mortality in relation to smoking: 40 years' observations on male British doctors', *British Medical Journal*, no 309, pp 901-11.

Drever, F. and Bunting, J. (1997) 'Patterns and trends in male mortality', in F. Drever and M. Whitehead (eds) *Health inequalities*, London: HMSO, pp 95-107.

Drever, F. and Whitehead, M. (eds) (1997) *Health inequalities: Decennial supplement*, London: The Stationery Office.

Edwards, G., Anderson, P., Babor, T.F. et al (1994) *Alcohol policy and the public good*, New York, NY: Oxford University Press.

Ferri, E. (1993) *Life at 33: The fifth follow-up of the National Child Development Study*, London: National Children's Bureau.

Fiore, M.C., Smith, S.S., Jorenby, D.E. and Baker, T.B. (1994) 'The effectiveness of the nicotine patch for smoking cessation: a meta-analysis', *Journal of the American Medical Association*, no 271, pp 1940-7.

Fiore, M.C., Bailey, W.C., Cohen, S.J. et al (1996) *Smoking cessation*, Clinical Practice Guideline No 18, Rockville, MD: US Department of Health and Human Services, Agency for Health Care Policy and Research.

Forcier, M.W. (1988) 'Unemployment and alcohol abuse: a review', *Journal of Occupational Medicine*, vol 30, no 3, pp 246-51.

Fowler, G. (1997) 'Nicotine replacement should be prescribable on the NHS', *British Medical Journal*, vol 314, p 1827.

Gill, B., Meltzer, H., Hinds, K. and Pettigrew, M. (1996) *Psychiatric morbidity among homeless people*, OPCS Surveys of Psychiatric Morbidity in Great Britain Report 7, London: HMSO.

Glendinning, A., Shucksmith, J. and Hendry, L. (1994) 'Social class and adolescent smoking behaviour', *Social Science and Medicine*, vol 38, pp 1449-60.

Goldblatt, P. (ed) (1990) *Longitudinal study: Mortality and social organization*, London: HMSO.

Graham, H. (1987) 'Women's smoking and family health', *Social Science and Medicine*, vol 25, pp 47-56.

Graham, H. (1994) 'Gender and class as dimensions of smoking behaviour in Britain – insights from a survey of mothers', *Social Science and Medicine*, vol 38, pp 691-98.

Haapanen, N., Miilunpalo, S., Pasanen, M., Oja, P. and Vuori, I. (1997) 'Association between leisure time physical activity and 10-year body mass change among working-aged men and women', *International Journal of Obesity*, vol 21, pp 288-96.

Hall, W. and Farrell, M. (1997) 'Comorbidity of mental disorders with substance misuse', *British Journal of Psychiatry*, no 171, pp 4-5.

Hammarstroem, A. (1994) 'Health consequences of youth unemployment – review from a gender perspective', *Social Science and Medicine*, vol 38, no 5, pp 699-709.

Harding, S., Bethune, A., Maxwell, R. and Brown, J. (1997) 'Mortality trends using the Longitudinal Study', in F. Drever and M. Whitehead (eds) *Health inequalities*, London: HMSO, pp 143-55.

Health Education Authority (1994) *Black and minority ethnic groups in England*, London: Health Education Authority.

Health Education Authority (1995) *A Survey of the UK Population, Part 1*, London: Health Education Authority.

Hillsdon, M. and Thorogood, M. (1996) 'A systematic review of exercise promotion strategies', *British Journal of Sports Medicine*, no 30, pp 84-9.

Hilton, M. (1991) 'A note on measuring drinking problems in the 1984 National Alcohol Survey', in W.B. Clark and M.E. Hilton (eds) *Alcohol in America: Drinking practices and problems*, Albany, NY: State University of New York Press.

Hughes, J.R., Wadland, W.C., Fenwick, J.W., Lewis, J. and Bickel, W.K. (1991) 'Effect of cost on the self-administration and efficacy of nicotine gum: a preliminary study', *Preventive Medicine*, vol 20, pp 486-96.

Hughes, K., MacKintosh, A.M. and Hastings, G., Wheeler, C., Watson, J. and Inglis, J. (1997) 'Young people, alcohol, and designer drinks: quantitative and qualitative study', *British Medical Journal*, vol 314, pp 414-18.

Jarvis, L. (1997a) *Living in Britain: Preliminary results from the 1996 General Household Survey*, London: The Stationery Office.

Jarvis, L. (1997b) *Smoking among secondary school children in 1996: England*, London: The Stationery Office.

Jarvis, M.J. (1994) 'Gender differences in smoking cessation: real or myth?', *Tobacco Control*, vol 3, pp 324-8.

Jarvis, M.J. (1997) 'Patterns and predictors of unaided smoking cessation in the general population', in C.T. Bolliger and K.O. Fagerstrom (eds) *The tobacco epidemic*, Progress in Respiratory Research No 28, Basel: Karger, pp 151-64.

Jarvis, M.J. (1998) 'Supermarket cigarettes: the brands that dare not speak their name', *British Medical Journal*, vol 316, pp 929-31

Jessor, R. and Jessor, S.L. (1977) *Problem behaviour and psychosocial development: A longitudinal study of youth*, New York, NY: Academy Press.

Joint Health Surveys Unit (1996) *Health Survey for England 1994*, London: HMSO.

Kauhanen, J., Kaplan, G.A., Goldberg, D.E. and Salonen, J.T. (1997) 'Beer binging and mortality: results from the Kuopio ischaemic heart disease risk factor study, a prospective population based study', *British Medical Journal*, vol 315, pp 846-51.

Kerr, W.C. (1997) 'Addiction, quality, choice and demand for alcohol', PhD dissertion, University of California.

King, A.C., Haskell, W.L., Young, D.R., Oka, R.K. and Stefanick, M.L. (1995) 'Long term effects of varying intensities and formats of physical activity on participation rates, fitness and lipoproteins in men and women aged 50-65 years', *Circulation*, no 91, pp 2596-604.

Li, C.Q., Windsor, R.A., Perkins, L. et al (1993) 'The impact on infant birth weight and gestational age of cotinine-validated smoking reduction during pregnancy', *Journal of the American Medical Association*, vol 269, no 12, pp 1519-24.

Makela, P., Valkonen, T. and Martelin, T. (1997) 'Contribution of deaths related to alcohol use of socio-economic variation in mortality: register based follow up study', *British Medical Journal*, vol 315, pp 211-16.

Marsh, A. and McKay, S. (1994) *Poor smokers*, London: Policy Studies Institute.

Meltzer, H., Gill, B., Pettigrew, M. and Hinds, K. (1995) *The prevalence of psychiatric morbidity among adults living in private households*, OPCS Surveys of Psychiatric Morbidity in Great Britain No 1, London: HMSO.

Meltzer, H., Gill, B., Pettigrew, M. and Hinds, K. (1996) *Economic activity and social functioning of adults with psychiatric disorders*, OPCS Surveys of Psychiatric Morbidity in Great Britain No 3, London: HMSO.

Morris, R. and Carstairs, V. (1991) 'Which deprivation? A comparison of selected deprivation indexes', *Journal of Public Health Medicine*, vol 13, pp 318-26.

Moser, K.A., Pugh, H.S. and Goldblatt, P. (1988) 'Inequalities in women's health: looking at mortality differentials using an alternative approach', *British Medical Journal*, vol 296, pp 1221-4.

OPCS (Office of Population Censuses and Surveys) (1993) *General Household Survey 1993*, London: HMSO.

Parrott, A.C. (1995) 'Stress modulation over the day in cigarette smokers', *Addiction*, no 90, pp 233-44.

Pate, R.R., Pratt, M., Blair, S.N., Haskell, W.L., Macera, C.A., Bouchard, C. et al (1995) 'Physical activity and public health: a recommendation from the Centers for Disease Control and Prevention and the American College of Sports Medicine', *Journal of the American Medical Association*, no 273, pp 402-7.

Peacock, J.L., Cook, D.G., Carey, I.M., Jarvis, M.J., Bryant, A.E., Anderson, H.R. and Bland, J.M. (1998) 'Maternal cotinine level during pregnancy and birthweight for gestational age', *International Journal of Epidemiology*, vol 27, pp 647-56.

Peto, R., Lopez, A.D., Boreham, J., Thun, M. and Heath, C. Jr (1992) 'Mortality from tobacco in developed countries: indirect estimation from national vital statistics', *Lancet*, no 339, pp 1268-78.

Peto, R., Lopez, A.D., Boreham, J., Thun, M. and Heath, C. (1994) *Mortality form smoking in developed countries 1950-2000: Indirect estimates from national vital statistics*, Oxford: Oxford University Press.

Pierce, J.P., Gilpin, E. and Farkas, A.J. (1995) 'Nicotine patch use in the general population: results from the 1993 California Tobacco Survey', *Journal of the National Cancer Institute*, no 87, pp 87-93.

Pugh, H., Power, C., Goldblatt, P. and Arber, S. (1991) 'Women's lung cancer mortality, socio-economic status and changing smoking patterns', *Social Science and Medicine*, vol 32, pp 1105-10.

Schoenborn, C.A. and Horm, J. (1993) *Negative moods as correlates of smoking and heavier drinking: Implications for health promotion*, Advance Data from Vital and Health Statistics, Hyattsville, MD: National Center for Health Statistics.

Silagy, C., Mant, D., Fowler, G. and Lodge, M. (1994) 'Meta-analysis on efficacy of nicotine replacement therapies in smoking cessation', *Lancet*, no 43, pp 139-42.

Smith, J. and Harding, S. (1997) 'Mortality of women and men using alternative social classifications', in F. Drever and M. Whitehead (eds) *Health inequalities: Decennial supplement*, London: The Stationery Office, pp 168-83.

Sonderskov, J., Olsen, J., Sabroe, S., Meillier, L. and Overvad, K. (1997) 'Nicotine patches in smoking cessation: a randomized trial among over-the-counter customers in Denmark', *American Journal of Epidemiology*, no 145, pp 309-18.

Sports Council and Health Education Authority (1992) *Allied Dunbar National Fitness Survey: Main findings*, London: HEA.

Sutherland, G., Russell, M.A.H., Stapleton, J.A. and Feyerabend, C. (1993) 'Glycerol particle cigarettes: a less harmful option for chronic smokers', *Thorax*, no 48, pp 385-7.

Sutton, M. and Godfrey, C. (1995) 'A grouped data regression approach to estimating economic and social influences on individual drinking behaviour', *Health Economics*, vol 4, pp 237-47.

Tang, J.L., Law, M. and Wald, N. (1994) 'How effective is nicotine replacement therapy in helping people to stop smoking?', *British Medical Journal*, vol 308, pp 21-6.

Thomas, M., Walker, A., Wilmot, A. and Bennett, N. (1998) *Living in Britain: Results from the 1996 General Household Survey*, London: The Stationery Office.

Townsend, P., Phillimore, P. and Beattie, A. (1998) *Health and deprivation: Inequality and the North*, London: Croom Helm.

Townsend, J., Roderick, P. and Cooper, J. (1994) 'Cigarette smoking by socio-economic group, sex, and age: effects of price, income, and health publicity', *British Medical Journal*, vol 309, pp 923-7.

USDHHS (US Department of Health and Human Services) (1980) *The health consequences of smoking for women: A report of the Surgeon General*, Rockville, MD: USDHHS, Office on Smoking and Health.

USDHHS (1996) *Physical activity and health: A report of the Surgeon General*, Atlanta, GA: USDHHS, Centers for Disease Control and Prevention, National Center for Chronic Disease Prevention and Health Promotion.

Warner, K.E., Slade, J. and Sweanor, D.T. (1997) 'The emerging market for long-term nicotine maintenance', *Journal of the American Medical Association*, no 278, pp 1087-92.

Westman, E.C., Behm, F.M., Simel, D.L. and Rose, J.E. (1997) 'Smoking behavior on the first day of a quit attempt predicts long-term abstinence', *Archives of Internal Medicine*, no 157, pp 335-40.

Yerushalmy, J. (1971) 'The relationship of parents' cigarette smoking to outcome of pregnancy – implications as to the problem of inferring causation from observed associations', *American Journal of Epidemiology*, no 93, pp 443-56.

17

Inequalities in oral health

Aubrey Sheiham and Richard G. Watt

Executive summary

General

- Dramatic improvements in dental health in children and young adults have taken place in the past 20 years. The levels of caries in permanent teeth of children is low.
- Inequalities in oral health exist between social classes, regions of England, and among ethnic groups in preschool children.
- Main social class and ethnic differences in dental caries is in preschool children.
- Wide district and regional differences exist in prevalence of caries in young children.
- The area differences relate very strongly to deprivation.
- In adults the differences in decay experience is less unequal than in children but there are marked social class inequalities in toothlessness of adults.
- Dental caries decreased in all social classes in the United Kingdom between 1983 and 1993.
- The main causes of the inequalities are differences in patterns of consumption of non-milk extrinsic sugars (NMES) and fluoridated toothpaste.
- Improvements in oral health that have occurred over the last 30 years have been largely a result of fluoride toothpaste and social, economic and environmental factors.
- Oral health inequalities will only be reduced through the implementation of effective and appropriate oral health promotion policy. Treatment services will never successfully tackle the underlying cause of oral diseases.

Policy 1 **Amendment of the 1985 Water Fluoridation Act is urgently required to facilitate the extension of this proven public health measure.**

Benefits
- Fluoridation of public water supplies is a proven public health measure that has been demonstrated to reduce caries experience, especially among socially deprived communities.
- An overall 44% reduction in caries in five-year-old children has been achieved by water fluoridation.
- The greatest benefit are achieved in the most deprived areas. Water fluoridation therefore reduces oral health inequalities.

Evidence Water fluoridation is supported as a safe and effective means of preventing caries by a wide range of leading medical, dental and scientific organisations in the UK and throughout the world.

Policy 2 **The Treasury should reduce the VAT levied on fluoride toothpaste to reduce the cost of this preventive agent.**

Benefits
- Flouride toothpaste is the single most important reason for the dramatic decline in caries in the past 20 years.
- Patterns of consumption of toothpaste vary by social class.

Evidence Fluoride in toothpastes have made a marked contribution to the reduction in caries in most industrialised countries.

Policy 3 **The Departments of Education and Health should expand the Health Promoting Schools Programme to include all schools in socially deprived locations.**

Benefits • The creation of safe and health enhancing social and physical environments.

• The development of school nutrition, smoking and accident prevention policies.

Evidence The World Health Organisation health promoting schools network has already achieved impressive results in many schools across the UK. These benefits need to be extended to schools with the greatest health and social needs.

Policy 4 **The Minister of Public Health should create an interdepartmental forum to integrate government policy to improve diet and nutrition.**

Benefits • Development of policies which coordinate the diverse perspectives of government, industry and consumers.

• Creation of wide range of complementary policies to increase the availability of affordable, safe and healthy foods and drinks.

• An ultimate reduction in the prevalence of diet-related health problems including caries.

Evidence A reduction in the frequency and total consumption of NMES will only be achieved through a national food policy, supported by regional and local initiatives.

Policy 5 **The Minister of Public Health should review and extend government action on preventing and reducing smoking, especially among young people. Stricter controls on the advertising and marketing activities of the cigarette industry would be an essential element of such a policy.**

Benefits • A reduction in smoking would improve periodontal health and reduce oral cancer rates.

• Stricter controls on tobacco advertising and marketing would reduce the numbers of young people experimenting with cigarettes.

Evidence Reducing smoking rates especially among young people requires a coordinated strategic policy that addressees the underlying reasons behind smoking and deals with the social, economic and political determinants of teenage smoking.

Policy 6 **Regulations on the importation, labelling and sale of paan and associated products (betel nut) should be enacted and enforced alongside the regulations on the sale and promotion of tobacco.**

Benefits • The development and effective enforcement of regulations controlling the sale of paan and associated products would enable consumers to select healthier and safer options.

• Oral cancer rates among South Asian communities would ultimately be reduced.

Evidence Effective prevention of oral cancer is dependent upon developing culturally sensitive interventions that address the social and structural basis of paan and tobacco use among high-risk populations. Regulatory policies would be a core component of this preventive strategy.

Policy 7 **The health education components of the National Curriculum should be strengthened and incorporated across appropriate aspects of schools curriculum.**

Benefits • Integrated health education would facilitate the development of the necessary skills and knowledge required to make informed health choices.

• Reintroduction of cooking and budgeting skills is essential to enable young people to prepare and cook healthier food options.

Evidence Integrated oral health education input into the national curriculum is essential to foster the development of the necessary knowledge, attitudes and skills to promote oral health.

Policy 8 **All health authorities should develop and implement an oral health strategy which specifies preventive and health promotion measures relevant to local needs and designed to reduce inequalities.**

Benefits • Coordinate action within and beyond the NHS to address local oral health priorities.

• To set equity-based goals and establish monitoring systems to assess changes in oral health status, especially among populations with high treatment needs.

Evidence The NHS has a key role to play in promoting and developing policies to tackle oral health inequalities. Commissioning authorities have a responsibility to target resources where oral health needs are greatest. Effective actions could include population based preventive programmes and schemes to increase prescription of sugar-free medications.

Evidence on inequalities in oral health

General

• Moderate inequalities in oral health exist by social classes, regions of England, and among ethnic groups in pre-school children.
• There are wide regional and area differences in caries.
• Much of the inequalities relate to how dental caries is treated.
• The policy implications of those findings may appear clear cut but there is no good evidence that increasing dental care would reduce inequalities in oral health.

Social class and deprivation

Inequalities in caries in children

There are inequalities in caries by social class and deprivation in the primary dentition.

• Among toddlers of 1½ to 4½ years, 40% from manual social classes had decay experience compared to 16% in those from non-manual classes (Hinds and Gregory, 1995).
• In children aged 5 to 15 years, the only variable strongly and independently associated with the number of decayed and/or filled primary teeth was the pattern of the child's dental attendance. For both 12- and 15-year-olds there was an association between social class and decay (O'Brien, 1994).
• In 12-year-olds there was a strong independent association with dental attendance and decay. For both 12- and 15-year-olds there was an independent association between social class and the number of Decayed, Missing and Filled (DMF) permanent teeth.
• For 12-year-olds, the children of skilled manual workers had a mean DMF a little lower than the overall mean and there were significant differences between children from manual and non-manual households. The DMF for children of non-manual parents was 1.1, skilled manual 1.4, and children of semi-skilled and unskilled workers, 2.0.

- At 15 years the DMF children from non-manual classes was 2.0 compared to 2.7 among children of SC III manual, and 3.4 among those from SC IV and V (O'Brien, 1994).
- Despite the social class inequalities O'Brien found that:

   ... these social and background variables together explained very little of the variation between children in the mean numbers of decayed primary teeth. For five- and eight-year-olds, the combination of these variables explain only 8% of the variation in the level of known decay in the primary dentition, and for 12- and 15-year-olds they explain 7% and 8% respectively of the variation in the decay experience of the permanent dentition. (O'Brien, 1994, p 48)

- Dental caries decreases in all social classes in the UK between 1983 and 1993. The greatest improvements were among 12- and 15-year-old children from skilled manual households and the least was among children from semi-skilled and unskilled households, so the gap between the classes has widened from 0.9 teeth in 1983 to 1.4 in 1993 among 15-year-olds (O'Brien, 1994).
- Two other dental conditions, periodontal disease and dental trauma vary by social class and ethnicity. People in the lower social classes have more severe periodontal disease than those in the higher classes. Asians and Afro-Caribbeans have more severe periodontal diseases than whites.
- Trauma to teeth, a condition which affects 17% of 8- to 15-year-olds (O'Brien, 1994), is more common in lower than upper classes, although the trend appears to be changing.

Inequalities in caries in the permanent dentition in adults

- In adults the differences in decay experience is less unequal than in children but there are marked social class inequalities in toothlessness of adults.
- In the latest national adult survey, whereas 14% of social classes I, II, III NM had no teeth, 24% of IIIM and 32% of IV and V had no teeth. The differences increased between 1978 and 1988; it was 16% in 1978 (22 versus 38) and 18% in 1988 (14 versus 32) (Todd and Lader, 1991).

- The large social class differences in edentulousness did not exist in the dentate. More lower social classes had 18 or more sound and untreated teeth; 41% in social classes IV and V compared to 33% in I, II, IIINM. And, despite the higher percentage of social class I-IIINM (39%) with filled teeth than those in social class IV and V (18%), the difference in missing teeth by social class was only 1.4 – the mean numbers of missing teeth in social class IV and V was 8.6 compared to 7.2 in social class I, II, III NM. Higher percentages of social class IV and V had decayed/unsound teeth (59%) than in social class III NM but the mean numbers of teeth was not great: 1.8 compared to 1.4 (Todd and Lader, 1991).
- An encouraging trend is that the mean numbers of decayed/unsound teeth decreased more in social class IV and V between 1978 and 1988 than in the highest classes – from 2.7 to 1.8 compared to 1.5 to 0.8 in the upper socio-economic groups (Todd and Lader, 1991).

Inequalities in oral health of ethnic minorities

- Being a minority in the UK does not necessarily correspond to having poorer dental health.
- Caries experienced in the primary dentition is higher in Asian than in white children but when matched for social class and mothers' ability to speak English there were no differences (Bedi and Uppal, 1996).
- In the permanent dentition, Asian children had less caries than whites (Beal, 1990; Bedi and Uppal, 1996). Asians and Afro-Caribbean children had similar permanent teeth decayed scores as whites (Perkins, 1981; Bradnock et al, 1988; Booth and Ashley, 1989; Prendegast et al, 1989).
- There are no differences in oral health among ethnic groups of the same socio-economic status.
- The inclusion of ethnicity as a variable for dental caries may no longer be relevant as it could divert attention from more important variables such as income and social class (Plamping et al, 1985).

National and regional and district inequalities

Area-based indicators are better predictors of oral health status than measures of socio-economic status. Moreover they add additional explanatory power to models of health inequalities (Locker, 1993).

- Wide regional differences exist in prevalence of caries. Children in the North East Region had more decay than those in other parts of England. 43% of the 3½- to 4½-year-olds in the North East had decay compared to a quarter in the rest of England (Hinds and Gregory, 1995).
- The regional and national inequalities persisted in older children. In the UK, there is nearly a threefold difference in the dental health of five-year-old children from the relatively prosperous region in the South West Region and the relatively deprived regions of the North West. At six years old the DMF levels were 1.8 and 2.6 respectively (O'Brien, 1994). In 1992/93 the mean DMFT scores of the 12-year-olds in the two North West regions were 1.9 and 1.5 compared with 0.8 in South West Thames. The regional and district differences in caries are related to deprivation. Jones et al (1997a, 1997b) showed correlations of from r = 0.88 and r = 0.46 between caries levels in five-year-olds and Jarman scores.
- In adults there are marked regional inequalities in dental status, mainly in relation to toothlessness. For example, in the Southern Region of England 19% of females were edentulous compared to 33% in the Northern Region (Todd and Lader, 1991).

Inequalities by gender

- No differences by gender exists in the proportions of dentate males and females with 21 or more teeth – the percentages are identical at 80%.
- Unsurprisingly, the mean numbers of missing teeth in males and females is similar – 7.6 compared to 7.9.
- There is a consistent trend at all ages for a higher percentage of females to have fillings. For example at ages 35-44, 43% of males compared to 56% of females had 12 or more fillings. Females

generally had less periodontal disease than males (Todd and Lader, 1991).
- More females than males are edentulous. 25% of females in the UK were edentulous compared to 16% of males (Todd and Lader, 1991).

The causes for inequalities

The main reasons for the dramatic decrease in dental caries are the wide-scale use of fluoridated toothpastes, change in diet and infant feeding patterns, and lastly reduction in smoking and an improvement in oral cleanliness and socio-economic factors – the McKeown theory (McKeown, 1979). There is little evidence that better treatment or preventive care or increased availability of dental manpower dentists has contributed significantly to the improvement in dental caries. Dental services explained 3% of the variation in changes in 12-year-olds in 18 industrialised countries caries levels in the 1970s whereas broad socio-economic factors including fluoridated toothpastes explained 65% (Nadanovsky and Sheiham, 1994, 1995). So it appears that the increase in allocation of the budget spent on traditional dental care has only a marginal effect on the population's oral health status.

There is overwhelming evidence to support the link between sugars consumption and dental caries. It has now reached the status of an unequivocal axiom (DoH, 1989a). Sugars consumption varies by social class. National food surveys reveal a higher consumption of sugar and sugar containing foods and drinks among low income groups (Department of Health, 1989b; Gregory et al, 1990, 1995). Explanations for this pattern are complex but economic and structural factors play a significant role (Leather, 1996).

The causes of dental caries, periodontal diseases and dental trauma vary by social class, sugars ingestion, cleanliness and cigarette smoking and accidents respectively. Nevertheless the main social class differences in oral status are from the treatment for caries in the permanent dentition. In the upper social classes more teeth are filled and less extracted than in the lower classes.

In most countries the socio-economic gradient in utilisation of dental services is well documented, not only in terms of relatively lower frequency of dental visits for low-income and less-educated children and adult groups, but also in relation to lower consumption of preventive services (Petersen and Holst, 1995).

Policy options

Oral health inequalities will only be reduced through the implementation of effective and appropriate oral health promotion policies (Watt et al, 1996). Treatment services will never successfully tackle the underlying cause of oral diseases (Royal Commission on the National Health Services, 1979). Improvements in oral health that have occurred over the last 30 years have been largely a result of social, economic and environmental factors (Nadanovsky and Sheiham, 1994, 1995). To extend these improvements further and thereby reduce widening oral health inequalities therefore requires a strategic oral health promotion approach.

Recent systematic effectiveness reviews of dental health education have highlighted the limitations of existing dental health education interventions (Sprod et al, 1996; Kay and Locker, 1996, 1997). Interventions were shown to be ineffective at producing long-term sustainable changes in oral health behaviours and failed to address inequalities. Indeed the narrow individualist approach adopted actually increased oral health inequalities (Schou and Wight, 1994). A more progressive health promotion approach which recognises the importance of tackling the underlying social, political and environmental determinants of oral health is therefore needed. For this approach to be successful in achieving sustainable changes in oral health, multi-sectoral working is an essential requirement.

The Ottawa Charter provides a useful framework outlining the five strategic aims of health promotion:

- creating supportive environments;
- building healthy public policy;
- strengthening community action;
- developing personal skills;
- reorienting health services (WHO, 1986).

This framework will now be used to review the available options to reduce oral health inequalities.

Creating supportive environments

Policy 1   Fluoridating the mouth: amendment of the 1985 Water (Fluoridation) Act is urgently required to facilitate the extension of this proven public health measure.

Action by government is needed to amend the 1985 Water (Fluoridation) Act so that it works in the way that Parliament intended; or, to use the words of Robin Cook's 1992 Health Manifesto, action is needed to ensure that: "water undertakers implement water fluoridation schemes promptly and at reasonable cost when asked to do so by health authorities". In drafting an amendment to the Act, government should make clear that in the event of a dispute between a health authority and a water undertaker over the technical feasibility of water fluoridation, the final arbiter shall be the Secretary of State for the Environment.

The 1985 Water (Fluoridation) Act, and the associated guidance from the Department of Health, clearly places the responsibility for decisions about water fluoridation with health authorities who, under the terms of the Act, are required to consult widely – including with local authorities – and to debate and make their decision in a public, rather than a closed, meeting of the health authority. Health authorities must allow a period of at least three months for this consultation process before making a final decision; then, following a request from a health authority, water undertakers may fluoridate the appropriate supply. The Department of Health's Circular (HC(87)18) indicates that, in arriving at their decision, the "chief concern" of water undertakers "will be the technical feasibility of water fluoridation". However, the water undertakers have interpreted the word 'may' in the Act as giving them very wide discretion. This is the crux of the disagreement between health authorities and the water undertakers, and is currently the subject of judicial review. Indeed, since the 1985 Water (Fluoridation) Act received the Royal Assent on 30 October 1985, no new fluoridation scheme has been introduced – other than those in the West Midlands for which legally binding agreements existed prior to the Act. To date, over 60 health authorities have completed the publicity and consultation required by the Act, but implementation of their fluoridation policies is being frustrated by the water undertakers.

Fluoridation of public water supplies is a proven public health measure that has been demonstrated to reduce caries experience, especially among socially deprived communities. Water fluoridation led to a 44% overall reduction in caries in five-year-old children. The greatest benefit was in the most deprived areas. Water fluoridation reduced oral health inequalities among the child population (Jones et al, 1997a). This finding is supported by studies in the UK and Australia (Carmicheal et al, 1989; Slade et al, 1996). Water fluoridation provided benefits for all social classes but the effects were more pronounced in lower social class children, particularly in the primary dentition (Slade et al, 1996).

Policy 2   Fluoridating the mouth: the Treasury should reduce the VAT levied on fluoride toothpastes to reduce the cost of this proven preventive agent.

Fluoride toothpaste is the single most important reason for the dramatic decline in caries in the past 20 years. Patterns of consumption of toothpaste vary by social class. Fluoride in toothpastes made a marked contribution to caries in most industrialised countries. The decline in caries in England is 55% in the deciduous teeth of five-year-old children, 75% in the permanent teeth of the 12-year-old population and 74% in 14-year-old adolescents. The DMF in 15-year-olds decreased from 5.9 in 1983 to 2.5 in 1993 (O'Brien, 1994). The percentages with no caries experience increased from 28 to 55% in five-year-olds; from 7 to 50% in 12-year-olds. The decreases in caries have increased the inequalities in caries by social class.

Policy 3   Health Promoting Schools: the Departments of Education and Health should expand the Health Promoting Schools Programme to include all schools in socially deprived locations.

This World Health Organisation initiative aims at:

... achieving healthy lifestyles for the total school population by developing supportive environments

conducive to the promotion of health. It offers opportunities for, and requires commitments to, the provision of safe and health enhancing social and physical environment. (WHO, Council for Europe and European Commission, 1993)

Of particular relevance to oral health promotion would be nutrition, smoking and accident prevention policies. In addition, efforts such as the Schools Meals Campaign and School Nutrition Action Groups (SNAG) are initiatives which aim to provide students with a range of food choices within schools including nutritional options (Caroline Walker Trust, 1992; Harvey and Passmore, 1994). Such initiatives recognise the importance of increasing the availability of cheap and appealing nutritious foods and drinks within school canteens, tuck shops and vending machines.

Building healthy public policy

Policy 4   National food policy: the Minister of Public Health should create an inter-departmental forum to integrate government policy to improve diet and nutrition.

A reduction in the frequency and total consumption of NMES will only be achieved through a national food policy, supported by regional and local initiatives. Such a policy requires government support to facilitate legislative, fiscal, educational and organisational policies. Elements of this policy could include nutritional guidelines on the content of nursery school meals, school meals, and guidelines for food in residential homes (Caroline Walker Trust, 1992, 1995, 1998). Consultation with major supermarkets to provide a wider range of low- and no-sugar confectionery, drinks, biscuits, cereals, and to introduce clear shelf, as well as product, labelling of NMES content of all products would also be needed. Developments in welfare and social policies which focus upon the impact of food poverty which is affecting an increasing proportion of the population, are urgently required (Leather, 1996).

Policy 5   Smoking policy: the Minister of Public Health should review and extend government action on preventing and reducing smoking,

especially among young people. Stricter controls on the advertising and marketing activities of the cigarette industry would be an essential element of such a policy.

Smoking is an aetiological factor associated with periodontal diseases and oral cancer. Currently the dental profession is not actively involved in the prevention of smoking. Reducing smoking rates especially among young people requires a coordinated strategic policy that addressees the underlying reasons behind teenage smoking and deals with the social, economic and political determinants of this behaviour (Stead et al, 1996).

Policy 6   Paan policy: regulations on the importation, labelling and sale of paan and associated products should be enacted and enforced alongside the regulations on sale and promotion of tobacco

Oral cancer rates among South Asian communities in the UK are higher than in the indigenous community. Effective prevention is dependent upon developing culturally sensitive interventions that address the social and structural basis of tobacco use among high-risk populations. Sale of tobacco containing paan (betel nut) is largely unregulated and many teenagers use these products (Islam et al, 1996).

Developing personal skills

Policy 7   Oral health education: the health education components of the National Curriculum should be strengthened and incorporated across appropriate aspects of the curriculum.

Health promotion supports personal and professional development through providing information, education for health, and helping people to develop the skills needed to make healthy choices. Integrated oral health education input into the national curriculum is essential to foster the development of the necessary knowledge, attitudes and skills to promote oral health. In particular skills training such as decision making, assertiveness training and cooking can be included in personal and social development courses.

Reorienting health services

Policy 8   Oral health strategies: all health authorities should develop and implement an oral health strategy which specifies preventive and health promotion measures relevant to local needs and designed to reduce inequalities.

Population preventive programmes

Fissure sealant population programmes targeted at schools with high caries levels is an effective preventive measure to reduce occlusal caries in high-risk child populations.

Prescription of sugar-free medications

Frequent use of sugar-based paediatric medicines is associated with increased risk of caries in vulnerable chronically sick children. Caries can be prevented by using sugar-free medicines (Bentley et al, 1994). Greater use of sugar-free medicines is dependent upon action by medical and pharmaceutical professions together with the pharmaceutical industry. For example, the computerised labelling of sugar-free options on GPs IT prescribing systems will encourage GPs to select these healthier choices.

Commissioning services

The NHS has a key role to play in promoting and developing purposive policies to tackle oral health inequalities. In particular commissioners of services have a major contribution to offer (Benzeval et al, 1995). Strategic developments which include equity-based goals, targeting of resources and the formation of healthy alliances with agencies and organisations outside of the NHS are all important commissioning functions.

References

Beal, J.F. (1990) 'The dental health of ethnic minority groups', in F. Esten (ed) *Good practices in health care of black and minority ethnic groups*, Public Health Report, Occasional Papers No 2, Yorkshire Health Authority, pp 15-18.

Bedi, R. and Uppal, R. (1996) 'The oral health of minority ethnic communities in the United Kingdom', in R. Bedi, V. Bahl and R.R. Rayan (eds) *Dentists, patients and ethnic minorities*, London: Royal College of Surgeons of England, pp 23-33.

Bentley, E., Mackie, I. and Fuller, S. (1994) 'Smile for sugar free medicines: a dental health education campaign', *Journal of the Institute of Health Education*, no 32, pp 36-8.

Benzeval, M., Judge, K. and Whitehead, M. (eds) (1995) *Tackling inequalities in health: An agenda for action*, London: King's Fund.

Booth, V. and Ashley, F. (1989) 'The oral health of 15-17 year old British school children of different ethnic origin', *Community Dental Health*, vol 6, pp 195-205.

Bradnock, G., Jadoua, S.I. and Hamburger, R. (1988) 'Dental health of indigenous and non-indigenous infant school children in West Birmingham', *Community Dental Health*, vol 1, pp 139-50.

Carmichael, C., French, A., Rugg-Gunn, A. and Ferrell, R. (1989) 'The relationship between fluoridation, social class and caries experience in 5 year old children in Newcastle and Northumberland in 1987', *British Dental Journal*, no 167, pp 57-61.

Caroline Walker Trust (1992) *Nutritional guidelines for school meals: Report of an expert working group*, London: Caroline Walker Trust.

Caroline Walker Trust (1995) *Eating well for older people: Practical and nutritional guidelines for food in residential and nursing homes and for community meals*, Report of an Expert Working Group, London: Caroline Walker Trust.

Caroline Walker Trust (1998) *Nutritional guidelines for under 5's in child care*, Report of an Expert Working Group, London: Caroline Walker Trust.

DoH (Department of Health) (1989a) *Dietary sugars and human disease*, Report of the Panel on Dietary Sugars of the Committee on Medical Aspects of Food Policy Report No 37, London: HMSO.

DoH (1989b) *The diets of British school children*, Report on Health and Social Subjects No 36, London: HMSO.

Gregory, J., Collins, D., Davies, P., Hughes, J. and Clarke, P. (1995) *National diet and nutrition survey: children aged 1½ to 4½ years*, Report of the Diet and Nutrition Survey, London: HMSO.

Gregory, J., Foster, K., Tyler, H. and Wiseman, M. (1990) *The dietary and nutritional survey of British adults*, MAFF and the DoH, London: HMSO.

Harvey, J. and Passmore, S. (1994) *School nutrition action groups: A new policy for managing food and nutrition in schools*, Birmingham: Health Education Unit.

Hinds, K. and Gregory, J.R. (1995) *National diet and nutrition survey: children aged 1½ to 4½ years*, Volume 2: Report of the Dental Survey, London: HMSO.

Islam, S., Croucher, R. and O'Farrell, M. (1996) *Paan chewing in Tower Hamlets, London: A summary report of an investigation*, London: St Bartholomews and The Royal London School of Medicine.

Jones, C.M., Taylor, G.O., Whittle, J.G., Evans, D. and Trotter, D.P. (1997a) 'Water fluoridation, tooth decay in 5 year olds, and social deprivation measured by the Jarman score: analysis of data from British dental surveys', *British Medical Journal*, vol 315, pp 514-7.

Jones, C.M., Taylor, G.O., Woods, K., Whittle, G., Evans, D. and Young, P. (1997b) 'Jarman underprivileged area scores, tooth decay and the effect of water fluoridation', *Community Dental Health*, vol 14, pp 156-60.

Kay, L. and Locker, D. (1996) 'Is dental health education effective? A systematic review of current evidence', *Community Dentistry and Oral Epidemiology*, vol 24, pp 231-5.

Kay, L. and Locker, D. (1997) *Effectiveness of oral health promotion: A review*, London: Health Education Authority.

Leather, S. (1996) *The making of modern malnutrition: An overview of food poverty in the UK*, London: Caroline Walker Trust.

Locker, D. (1993) 'Measuring social inequality in dental health services research: individual, household and area-based measures', *Community Dental Health*, vol 10, pp 139-50.

McKeown, T. (1979) *The role of medicine*, Oxford: Basil Blackwell.

Nadanovsky, P. and Sheiham, A. (1994) 'The relative contribution of dental services to the changes and geographical variations in caries status of 5 and 12 year-old children in England and Wales in the 1980s', *Community Dental Health*, vol 11, pp 215-23.

Nadanovsky, P. and Sheiham, A. (1995) 'The relative contribution of dental services to the changes in caries levels of 12 year-old children in 18 industrialized countries in the 1970s and early 1980s', *Community Dentistry Oral Epidemiology*, vol 23, pp 231-9.

O'Brien, M. (1994) *Children's dental health in the United Kingdom 1993*, London: HMSO.

Perkins, P.C. (1981) 'Dental caries in children of 9 and 14 years in three ethnic groups in north-west London', *British Dental Journal*, no 150, pp 194-5.

Petersen, P.E. and Holst, D. (1995) 'Utilization of dental health services', in L.K. Cohen and H.C. Gift (eds) *Disease prevention and oral health promotion*, Copenhagen: Munksgaard, pp 341-86.

Plamping, D., Bewley, R.N. and Gelbier, S. (1985) 'Dental health and ethnicity', *British Dental Journal*, no 158, pp 261-3.

Prendegast, M.J., Williams, S.A. and Curzon, M.E.J. (1989) 'An assessment of dental caries prevalence among Gujurati, Pakistani and white Caucasian five-year-old children resident in Dewsbury, West Yorkshire', *Community Dental Health*, vol 6, pp 223-32.

Royal Commission on the National Health Service (1979) *Report*, Cmnd 7615 (Chairman, Sir Alex Merrison), London: HMSO.

Schou, L. and Wight, C. (1994) 'Does dental health education affect inequalities in dental health?', *Community Dental Health*, vol 11, pp 97-100.

Slade, G.D., Spencer, A.J., Davies, M.J. and Stewart, J.F. (1996) 'Influence of exposure to fluoridated water on socio-economic inequalities in children's caries exposure', *Community Dentenistry Oral Epidemiology*, vol 24, pp 89-100.

Sprod, A., Anderson, R. and Treasure, E. (1996) *Effective oral health promotion: Literature review*, Health Promotion Wales.

Stead, M., Hastings, G. and Tudor-Smith, C. (1996) 'Preventing adolescent smoking: a review of options', *Health Education Journal*, vol 55, pp 31-54.

Todd, J.E. and Lader, D. (1991) *Adult dental health 1988 United Kingdom*, London: HMSO.

Watt, R.G., Daly, B. and Fuller, S. (1996) *Strengthening oral health promotion in the commissioning process*, Manchester: Eden Bianchi Press.

WHO (World Health Organisation) (1986) *The Ottawa Charter for Health Promotion*, Health Promotion 1. iii-v, Geneva: WHO.

WHO, Council for Europe and European Commission (1993) *The European network of health promoting schools*, Copenhagen: WHO.

Index

and health inequalities 197–205
  policy recommendations 197–8
and health promotion needs of older people 198,
  204–5
and life expectancy 37, 81–2
and mental health 208, 209–10
and morbidity rates 201
and mortality rates 148, 197, 199–201
and obesity 126–7
and oral health 244
and osteoporosis 136
and primary care access 105–6
sensitivity to in health provision 197, 198–9
and smoking 210, 213, 231–3
and transport 175–6, 188, 202
women neglected in mainstream healthcare and
  research 197, 199
General Medical Services (GMS) 89–90, 92, 93
general practitioners
  access to female practitioners 105–6, 163–4
  and ethnic minority groups 163–4, 166
  in rural areas 187
  uneven distribution 89–90, 92, 93, 102-3, 105,
    107–8
  see also primary care
geographical location and inequalities in health
  148–52
    effect on ethnic minorities 165–6
    inverse care law 151
    oral health inequalities 244
    and policy 150–2
Gillies, P. 139–40
Gilligan, J. 73
Ginn, J. 205
Gordon, D. 79
Green Commuter Plans 179
greengrocers in deprived areas 24, 30, 131
Gregory, J. 123
Grundy, E. 42

H

Hawtin, M. 52, 53
Headstart project 7, 140–1
Health Action Zones 64, 102, 112, 114, 143, 166
health behaviours
  and geographical location 148–52
  and inequalities in health 213–35
    policy implications 214–15
  older people 39

youth 17-18
  see also drinking; health screening; physical
    activity; smoking
health education *see* health promotion
Health Education Authority (HEA) 205, 230
Health Education Council 104
  report (1987) xiv
Health Education and Monitoring Survey (HEMS)
  205
Health Impact Assessment 114
Health Improvement Programmes 102, 104, 112, 113
Health and Lifestyle Survey 217, 230
Health of the Nation (White Paper and Working
  Group) 81, 88, 89, 91, 107, 205
health promotion
  and drinking 214, 225
  drug use and children 208, 209, 210–11
  and ethnic minority groups 155, 166
  and NHS 104–8, 112, 113
  and older people 204–5
  and oral health 242, 247
  in schools 143
    Health Promoting Schools 19, 141–2, 241, 246
  on smoking cessation 220
  and social capital 139–40
  and social class 210
Health and Safety Commission 23, 29
health screening uptake 214, 215, 229–31
health status inequalities 100–2
Health Survey for England 120, 217, 222, 226, 229–30,
  234, 235
Healthy Cities initiative 101, 142
healthy life expectancy 37, 38
Healthy Living Centres 167
Henwood, M. 205
Hertzman, C. 3-4, 138–9, 140
high cholesterol levels 121
Highscope project (Perry Project) 7, 140–1
Hillfields project, Coventry 142
hip replacement 109, 110
homelessness 3, 15, 45, 46
  among families 47–8, 52
  among single people 47, 52
  and drinking 222
  and drug use 18
  and health 52, 91
  youth 52
homicide and income distribution 73–4
Hospital and Community Health Services (HCHS)
  90, 103-4, 113
House, J.S. 73

decentralisation of services 177–8
and diet (access to food supply) 128, 151, 152, 174–5, 186-7, 188
and gender 175–6, 188, 202
high traffic volumes
    and access to healthcare 173–4, 177
    road modification to reduce 1
    in rural areas 174, 175, 190
Local Safety Scheme 178
and older people 34, 41, 42–3, 175, 177, 188, 202
policy recommendations 177–80, 191–4
    costs benefits 193–4
    effect on children 1, 7–8, 84, 176, 178
    to decrease car dependency 191, 192
pollution from *see* pollution and road transport
road pricing schemes 180
in rural areas 174–5, 186–7, 190
speed controls 178–9, 191, 192
traffic restraint measures 171, 178, 188, 191–2
in urban areas 173–4, 187–8
Transport Research Laboratory 178, 179, 194
triglycerides levels and diet 121
Tyler, H. 123

U

unemployment xiv, 14, 15
    and diet 129
    and drinking 222
    and drug use 18
    of ethnic minority groups 158, 160, 166
    and housing construction 60
    of long-term sick and disabled 81
    and mental health 17, 19, 209
    and smoking 216
    training for unemployed 23
United Nations (UN): Declaration and Programme of Action xix
United States: minimum income for pregnant women 4
University of York
    Budget Standards research 82–3
    homelessness survey 47

V

violence 28–9
    violent crime and income 73–4

W

Wadsworth, M.E.J. 139, 140, 142
walking
    access to healthcare 173–4
    decline in 170, 171, 175, 190
    and gender 175
    pedestrian infrastructure on roads 179, 192
    promotion to increase physical activity 214–15, 228, 229
    and social class 228
    see also pedestrian injuries
Water Fluoridation Act (1985) 240, 245–6
Welfare to Work programme 51, 60, 143, 207, 211
Wenlock, R.W. 123
West of Scotland Collaborative Study 25
White, A. 123
Whitehall Study 28, 134
Whitty, G. 140
WHO *see* World Health Organisation
Wiens, M. 3–4
Wilkinson, R.G. 140
Williams, D.R.R. 39
Willms, J.D. 139
Wing, J.K. 208
winter mortality rates 42, 52
WISE group 60
women
    body mass index 3, 4
    and diet 118, 119, 129
    housing and health 54
    as poor 79–80
    and primary care access 105–6
    use of public transport 175, 176, 188
    work and health 28
    see also gender; mothers; pregnancy
Women, Infants and Children (WIC) scheme 119, 130
Woodstock, Canada: interagency working 142
Working Families Tax Credit xv, xviii, xx
World Health Organisation (WHO) viii, 12
    Health Promoting Schools 241, 246
    Healthy Cities initiative 101, 142
World Summit on Social Development xix

Y

York: road user hierarchy in 171, 179
youth 12–19
    anaemia in 126